D1394369

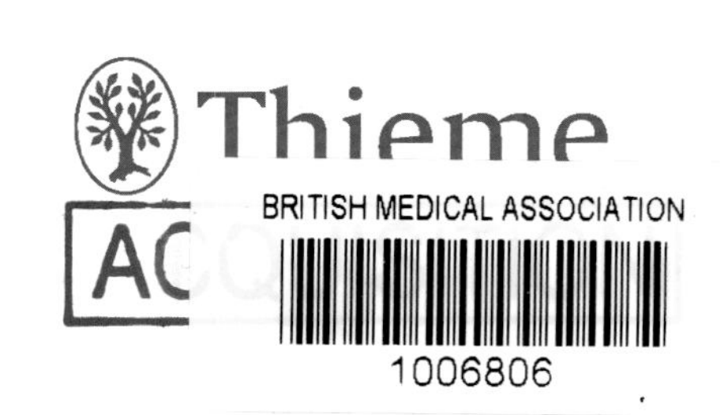
Thieme
BRITISH MEDICAL ASSOCIATION
1006806

The Audiogram Workbook

Kristi Oeding, AuD
Clinical Audiologist
Washington University in St. Louis - School of Medicine
St. Louis, Missouri, USA

Jennifer Listenberger, AuD
Clinical Audiologist
Washington University in St. Louis - School of Medicine
St. Louis, Missouri, USA

Steven Smith, AuD
Clinical Audiologist
Washington University in St. Louis - School of Medicine
St. Louis, Missouri, USA

126 illustrations

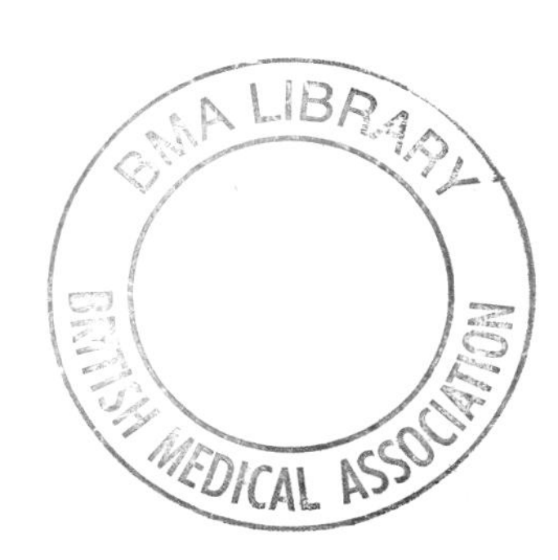

Thieme
New York • Stuttgart • Delhi • Rio de Janeiro

Executive Editor: Anne M. Sydor
Managing Editor: Elizabeth Palumbo
Director, Editorial Services: Mary Jo Casey
Production Editor: Torsten Scheihagen
International Production Director: Andreas Schabert
Vice President, Editorial and E-Product Development: Vera Spillner
International Marketing Director: Fiona Henderson
International Sales Director: Louisa Turrell
Director of Sales, North America: Mike Roseman
Senior Vice President and Chief Operating Officer: Sarah Vanderbilt
President: Brian D. Scanlan

Library of Congress Cataloging-in-Publication Data

Names: Oeding, Kristi, author. | Listenberger, Jennifer, author. | Smith, Steven (Clinical audiologist) author.
Title: The audiogram workbook / Kristi Oeding, Jennifer Listenberger, Steven Smith.
Description: First edition. | New York : Thieme, [2016] | Includes bibliographical references.
Identifiers: LCCN 2015047894| ISBN 9781626231757 (hardcover) | ISBN 9781626231955 (e-book)
Subjects: | MESH: Hearing Tests–methods | Hearing Loss–diagnosis | Problems and Exercises
Classification: LCC RF294 | NLM WV 18.2 | DDC 617.8/075–dc23 LC record available at http://lccn.loc.gov/2015047894

Important note: Medicine is an ever-changing science undergoing continual development. Research and clinical experience are continually expanding our knowledge, in particular our knowledge of proper treatment and drug therapy. Insofar as this book mentions any dosage or application, readers may rest assured that the authors, editors, and publishers have made every effort to ensure that such references are in accordance with **the state of knowledge at the time of production of the book.**

Nevertheless, this does not involve, imply, or express any guarantee or responsibility on the part of the publishers in respect to any dosage instructions and forms of applications stated in the book. **Every user is requested to examine carefully** the manufacturers' leaflets accompanying each drug and to check, if necessary in consultation with a physician or specialist, whether the dosage schedules mentioned therein or the contraindications stated by the manufacturers differ from the statements made in the present book. Such examination is particularly important with drugs that are either rarely used or have been newly released on the market. Every dosage schedule or every form of application used is entirely at the user's own risk and responsibility. The authors and publishers request every user to report to the publishers any discrepancies or inaccuracies noticed. If errors in this work are found after publication, errata will be posted at www.thieme.com on the product description page.

Some of the product names, patents, and registered designs referred to in this book are in fact registered trademarks or proprietary names even though specific reference to this fact is not always made in the text. Therefore, the appearance of a name without designation as proprietary is not to be construed as a representation by the publisher that it is in the public domain.

Thieme Publishers New York
333 Seventh Avenue, New York, NY 10001 USA
+1 800 782 3488, customerservice@thieme.com

Thieme Publishers Stuttgart
Rüdigerstrasse 14, 70469 Stuttgart, Germany
+49 [0]711 8931 421, customerservice@thieme.de

Thieme Publishers Delhi
A-12, Second Floor, Sector-2, Noida-201301
Uttar Pradesh, India
+91 120 45 566 00, customerservice@thieme.in

Thieme Publishers Rio de Janeiro, Thieme Publicações Ltda.
Edifício Rodolpho de Paoli, 25º andar
Av. Nilo Peçanha, 50 – Sala 2508
Rio de Janeiro 20020-906 Brasil
+55 21 3172-2297 / +55 21 3172-1896

Cover design: Thieme Publishing Group
Typesetting by DiTech Process Solutions

Printed in China by Everbest Printing Co. 5 4 3 2 1

ISBN 978-1-62623-175-7

Also available as an e-book:
eISBN 978-1-62623-195-5

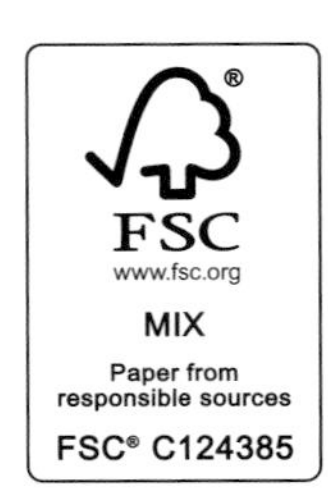

Contents

Acknowledgments

This book would not have been possible without the wonderful patients seen daily. Our patients are our true teachers; without them, we would not learn how to adapt our methods and individualize our care. We thank Mike Valente, PhD, for the opportunity for this experience. A special thank you goes to Katie Bergman for sharing her editing expertise. Our love and gratitude go to our families for their love, support, and patience—each new project means more time away from home.

1 Introduction

1.1 Interpreting an Audiogram

To interpret an audiogram, readers of this book must have a basic understanding of the graph, symbols, and tests. The following provides a basic overview of the graph and symbols and how to interpret their meaning. For purposes of consistency this book works with the interpretation criteria used in the authors' own clinic. Other clinics may use different standards—there are several available. Regardless of which criteria are chosen, it is important for everyone in a given clinic to use the same criteria for ease and consistency of interpretation.

1.1.1 Pure-Tone Air and Bone Conduction Thresholds

Pure-tone air and bone conduction thresholds are plotted on the audiogram graph. Pure-tone air and bone conduction thresholds are used to determine the degree and type of hearing loss.

Graph

The air and bone conduction symbols are plotted on the audiogram graph (▶ Fig. 1.1). The x-axis represents pitch or frequency. The x-axis goes from low to high frequencies from left to right. The y-axis represents the magnitude or degree of hearing loss. The y-axis goes from soft to loud sounds from top to bottom.

Symbols

There are specific symbols for the right and left ear (▶ Fig. 1.2). The air conduction symbol for the right ear consists of a circle (unmasked) or a triangle (masked), while the left ear symbol can be an X (unmasked) or a square (masked). For bone conduction, the right ear is represented by < (unmasked) or "[" (masked), whereas the left ear symbol is > (unmasked) or "]" (masked). When a response cannot be obtained at the limits of the audiometer (no response), the foregoing symbols have an arrow added to the bottom of the symbol. For unmasked air conduction, for example, the symbol for no response in the right ear is , whereas the symbol for the left ear is . The symbols are shown in red for the right ear and blue for the left ear. Sometimes an indication of whether masking could or could not be performed or whether a symbol was vibrotactile (felt) should be noted. A "c" or asterisk near the symbol can be used to indicate an air or bone conduction threshold that could not be masked. A "v" can be used to indicate a threshold that was vibrotactile. It is important that whatever indicator (letter, asterisk, etc.) you use that it is defined somewhere on the audiogram (ex. v = vibrotactile). Note, other symbols are used, such as an "S" for sound field testing. This book is going to focus on the most common symbols used for testing adults.

Configuration of Hearing Loss

Symmetric and Asymmetric Hearing Loss

Although this book provides a description of each ear, it is also possible to describe the two ears together or define whether the hearing loss is symmetric (equal hearing between ears) or asymmetric (different hearing between ears). Symmetric hearing loss is typically defined as hearing in which pure-tone air conduction thresholds in the right and left ear are separated by ≤ 10 dB HL across all frequencies. Although there is no consensus on defining asymmetric hearing loss, one interpretation of asymmetric hearing loss that may warrant a referral to an otologist is two pure-tone air conduction thresholds with a difference of ≥ 15 dB HL or one threshold with a difference of ≥ 20 dB HL.

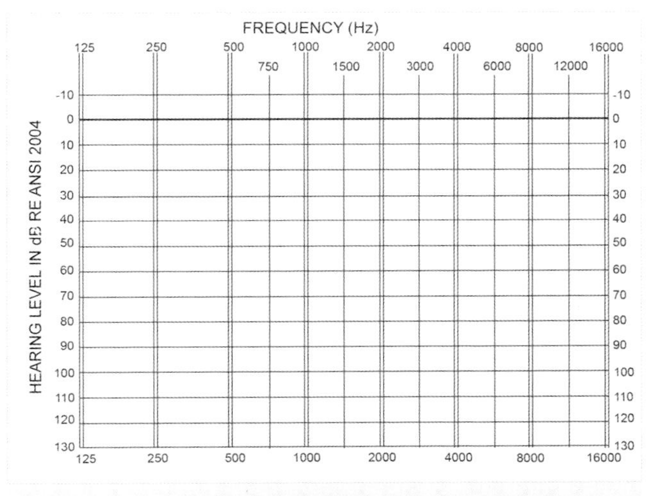

Fig. 1.1 Audiogram graph, with the x-axis, from left to right, representing low to high frequencies and the y-axis, from top to bottom, representing soft to loud sounds.

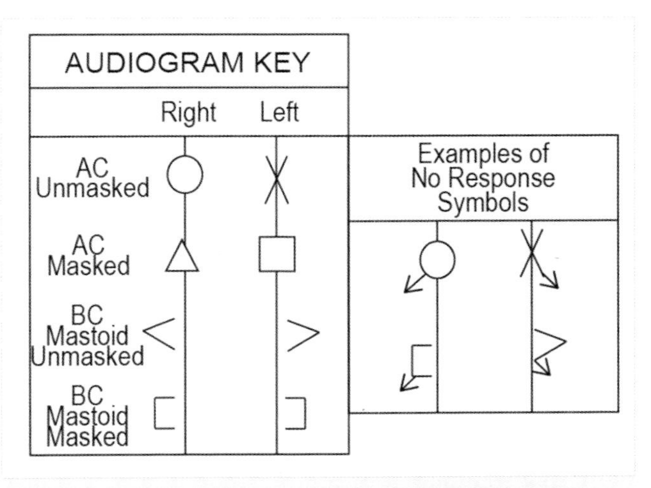

Fig. 1.2 A basic legend of symbols used to graph results on an audiogram.

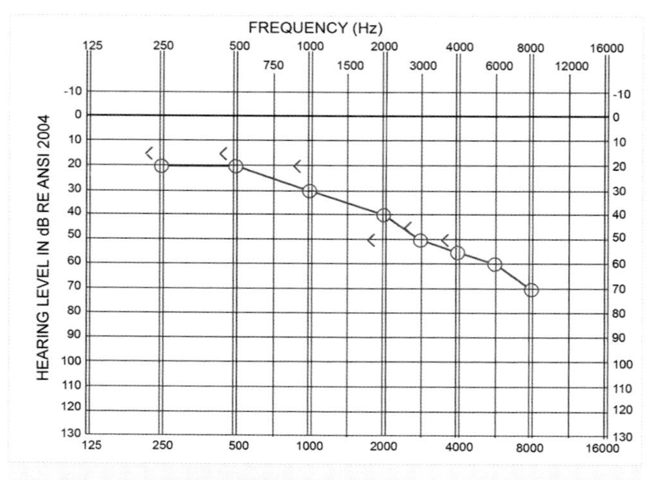

Fig. 1.3 Audiogram depicting a right ear with slight to moderately severe sensorineural hearing loss.

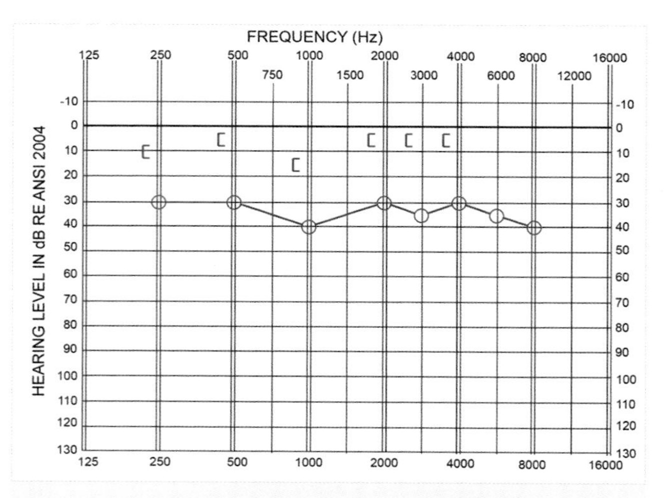

Fig. 1.4 Audiogram depicting a right ear with mild conductive hearing loss.

Degree of Hearing Loss

Degree of hearing loss is used to classify the magnitude or amount of hearing loss. Clark developed the following guidelines for determining the degree of hearing loss based on an air conduction PTA of 500, 1,000, and 2,000 Hz[1]:

Normal = –10 to 15 dB HL
Slight = 16 to 25 dB HL
Mild = 26 to 40 dB HL
Moderate = 41 to 55 dB HL
Moderately severe = 56 to 70 dB HL
Severe = 71 to 90 dB HL
Profound = ≥ 91 dB HL

For example, in ▶ Fig. 1.3, the hearing loss would be classified as a slight sloping to moderately severe hearing loss.

Types of Hearing Loss

Sensorineural Hearing Loss

This is the most common type of hearing loss that is seen clinically (▶ Fig. 1.3). A sensorineural hearing loss indicates hearing loss that involves the inner ear and/or the eighth (auditory) nerve. It can be caused by many factors, such as normal aging of the hearing system (presbycusis), genetics, or noise exposure. On the audiogram, this type of hearing loss is characterized by having an air–bone gap that is ≤ 10 dB HL (the bone conduction and air conduction thresholds are within 10 dB HL). ▶ Fig. 1.3 illustrates an example of sensorineural hearing loss. An example of an interpretation of this audiogram would be slight sensorineural hearing loss from 250 to 500 Hz, sloping from a mild to moderately severe hearing loss from 1,000 to 8,000 Hz. Note that there may sometimes be reverse air–bone gaps (the bone conduction threshold has greater hearing loss than the air conduction threshold, such as at 2,000 Hz). If the air–bone gap is reversed, even if it is > 15 dB, it is still considered a sensorineural hearing loss.

Conductive Hearing Loss

This type of hearing loss involves the outer and/or middle ear (▶ Fig. 1.4). It can be caused by many factors, such as a cerumen impaction, fluid in the middle ear, or disarticulation of the bones of the middle ear. On the audiogram, this type of hearing loss is characterized by having an air–bone gap that is > 10 dB HL and bone conduction thresholds that are within the normal range of hearing. ▶ Fig. 1.4 illustrates an example of conductive hearing loss. An example of an interpretation of this audiogram would be a mild conductive hearing loss from 250 to 8,000 Hz.

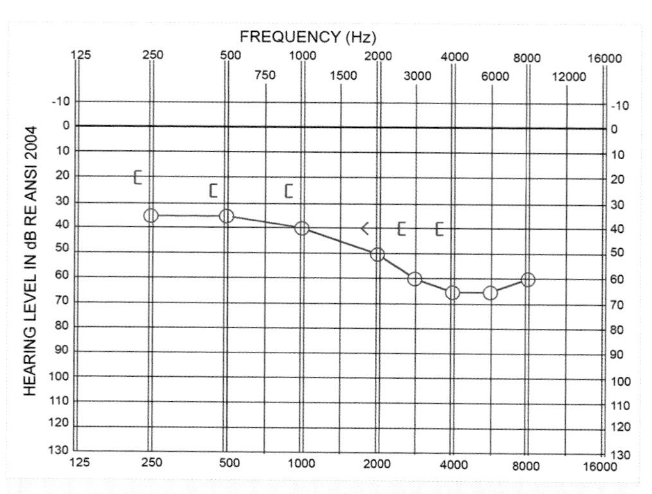

Fig. 1.5 Audiogram depicting a right ear with mild to moderately severe mixed hearing loss.

Mixed Hearing Loss

This type of hearing loss involves the outer and/or middle ear and the inner ear and/or eighth nerve (▶ Fig. 1.5). It can be caused by a combination of factors already mentioned. On the audiogram, this type of hearing loss can be characterized by having both the aforementioned characteristics and/or having an air–bone gap > 10 dB HL, but the bone conduction thresholds are not within the normal range of hearing. ▶ Fig. 1.5 illustrates an example of mixed hearing loss. An interpretation of this audiogram would be mild sloping to moderately severe mixed hearing loss.

1.1.2 Speech Awareness Thresholds and Speech Recognition Thresholds

A speech awareness threshold (SAT) is used to find the level at which the patient can detect spondee words 50% of the time. It is important to note the patient does not have to understand what was said, but rather needs only to detect the sound. An SAT can be used if the patient does not speak the language of the examiner or if the patient is unable to repeat the words due to the inability to talk or poor word recognition. A speech recognition threshold (SRT) is established by finding the level at which the patient can repeat or identify a spondee word 50% of the time. The SAT/SRT should be within ± 10 dB of the pure-tone average (PTA; average of 500, 1,000, and 2,000 Hz). A difference larger than this may indicate nonorganic (unreliable) hearing loss. It is also possible that a discrepancy will occur due to steeply sloping hearing loss or poor word recognition. SAT and SRT are interpreted the same way the degree of pure-tone air and bone conduction thresholds are interpreted. For example, an SRT of 15 dB HL would indicate a normal ability to receive speech, but an SRT of 50 dB HL would indicate a moderate loss in the ability to receive speech. An SAT of 50 dB HL would indicate a moderate loss in the ability to *detect* speech.

1.1.3 Word Recognition Scores

A word recognition score (WRS) provides information on the ability of the patient to understand or recognize speech. It reports how clear speech is to a patient when it is presented at a suprathreshold level (level that is audible and comfortable) and can be used to counsel the patient on realistic expectations for communication and possibly help predict benefit from hearing aids. The scale to interpret WRS is as follows:

Normal = 90 to 100%
Slight difficulty = 76 to 88%
Moderate difficulty = 60 to 74%
Poor recognition = 50 to 58%
Very poor recognition = < 50%

For example, a WRS of 64% would indicate a moderate difficulty in the ability to recognize speech.

1.1.4 Immittance Testing

Tympanometry

Tympanometry measures the integrity of the tympanic membrane and the middle ear. This book uses the following interpretation:

Ear canal volume normal range = 0.6 to 2 mL (a difference between ears of > 1 mL may indicate a perforation or patent pressure equalization (PE) tube)
Middle ear pressure normal range = ± 100 daPa
Static admittance normal range = 0.3 to 1.5 mL

A large ear canal volume, such as 4 mL in one ear, compared to 1.5 mL in the opposite ear may indicate a perforation in the tympanic membrane. The interpretation is stated as "large ear canal volume." Middle ear pressure of – 150 daPa indicates negative pressure behind the tympanic membrane and is interpreted as "excessive negative pressure." Static admittance of 0.1 mL is interpreted as hypocompliant, meaning the tympanic membrane is moving less than normal (fluid, etc.), and static admittance of 1.8 mL is interpreted as hypercompliant, meaning the tympanic membrane is moving more than normal (disarticulation of ossicles, etc.). Middle ear pressure and static admittance of no pressure or no peak (NP) is interpreted as flat (fluid, etc.).

1.1.5 Acoustic Reflex Thresholds

Acoustic reflex thresholds measure the acoustic reflex arc, which consists of the tympanic membrane, middle ear, inner ear, eighth nerve, auditory brain stem, seventh (facial) nerve, and stapedius muscle. The reflex occurs bilaterally; therefore, it is measured with ipsilateral and contralateral stimulation. Results from this test are used in conjunction with others to help determine conditions, such as a tumor on the eighth nerve. A reflex is considered present if a compliance change ≥ 0.02 mL is measured. Acoustic reflex thresholds are interpreted as follows:

Normal/present = ≤ 100 dB HL
Elevated = 105 to 110 dB HL
Absent = no response at 110 dB HL

Acoustic Reflex Decay

Acoustic reflex decay measures the ability of the acoustic reflex threshold to remain present for 10 seconds and not decay by 50% during this 10-second period. It has traditionally been used to aid in determining the presence of a tumor on the eighth nerve. When the reflex remains present and does not decay by 50% during the 10 seconds, the result is interpreted as negative (for retrocochlear pathology). If the reflex decays, for example, at 5 seconds, the result is interpreted as positive or abnormal, and the point at which it decays, 5 seconds in this example, is also stated.

1.2 Testing Considerations

1.2.1 Clinician–Patient Interaction

It is important to establish a rapport with the patient to make the patient feel comfortable for the hearing test. For some patients, having a hearing test can cause extreme anxiety. Obtaining a thorough case history, listening to the patient's concerns, and providing clear instructions as well as reassurance during testing will help make testing go smoothly.

1.2.2 Preparation for Testing

General maintenance of the equipment is important for obtaining accurate results. It is important to do daily listening checks of the equipment to ensure all transducers are functioning properly. Immittance probe tips should be examined and cleared of any debris. Annual calibration is required and quarterly calibration checks are recommended. The cords should be untangled to ensure ease of placement of the transducers on the patient. It is also important to disinfect the earphones, specula, and immittance probe tips to prevent the spread of infection. Otoscopy should be performed prior to testing to ensure clear ear canals. Also, if the patient reports a better ear, testing should start in the better ear.

1.2.3 Audiological Test Instructions and Masking

For tests involving pure-tone air and bone conduction, SAT/SRT, and WRS, it is recommended that patients face away from the examiner so they cannot anticipate when pure-tones or words are being presented and to prevent lip reading.

Pure-Tone Air Conduction

Supra-aural headphones or insert earphones are used for pure-tone air conduction testing. Patients are typically provided with a response button or asked to raise their hand when they hear a beep, even if it is very soft. Sometimes a patient will press the button too much and may have to be reinstructed to press the button only when the beep is heard.

Masking may be required if the patient has an asymmetric hearing loss. The purpose of masking is to prevent the better, nontest ear from hearing the test stimulus; otherwise, the thresholds reported on the hearing test may not reflect the true hearing loss in the ear being tested. A traditional rule is that masking is required if there is a difference of 40 dB HL between the air conduction threshold of the test ear and the bone conduction threshold of the nontest ear for headphones and 60 dB HL for insert earphones. When masking, the patient will be asked to ignore the new sound presented and continue to respond to the tone. The masking signal will be added to the opposite or nontest ear, and the tone will continue to be presented in the ear being tested. To mask, a typical rule is to add 10 dB HL to the threshold of the nontest ear and use a 15 dB plateau to obtain threshold. There are many methods for masking, and this topic is beyond the scope of this book, and the reader is referred to other sources.[2,3]

Pure-Tone Bone Conduction

A bone oscillator is used for pure-tone bone conduction testing. It is important to place the bone oscillator on the mastoid, and it should not touch the pinna. Bone conduction can help determine the type of hearing loss. As for pure-tone air conduction threshold testing, patients are typically provided with a button or asked to raise their hand when they hear a beep, even if it is very soft.

Masking will be required if there is an air–bone gap of ≥ 15 dB HL between the air conduction and bone conduction threshold of the test ear. If masking is needed, a headphone or insert earphone is placed on the nontest ear, and the bone oscillator remains on the mastoid of the test ear. Masking noise is then presented, and the method and response will be the same as for air conduction testing. The only difference between masking for bone and air conduction is additional masking may be needed to account for the occulsion effect at 250, 500, and 1,000 Hz.

SAT/SRT

SAT and SRT are typically completed using supra-aural headphones or insert earphones using a CD or monitored live voice (ensuring the examiner's voice peaks at 0 on the VU meter for the two syllables). The patient is instructed to press the button upon hearing two-syllable spondee words (SAT) or is asked to repeat the words (SRT). If the patient is unsure of a word, the patient is encouraged to guess.

Masking may be required if there is a difference of 40 dB between the unmasked SAT/SRT and the best bone conduction threshold of the nontest ear for headphones and 60 dB for insert earphones. Masking method and presentation are the same as for pure-tone testing.

WRS

WRS testing determines the speech recognition ability of a patient at a suprathreshold level using a CD recording because it is standardized and avoids the variability of a monitored live voice. There are different ways to determine the suprathreshold level of testing. One is to add + 30 to + 40 dB sensation level (SL) to the SRT. This may not be the best method for patients with a sloping hearing loss because an SRT of 10 dB with a + 40 dB SL for hearing loss that is moderately severe to severe at 2,000 Hz may not provide adequate high-frequency information. Another method, used in the authors' clinic, is the most intelligible level (MIL). This involves slowly increasing the volume of monitored live speech until a comfortable and intelligible level is determined. The patient is then instructed to repeat the last word of the sentence (which may vary depending on the test material used).

Masking may be required if there is a difference of 40 dB between the presentation level and the best bone conduction threshold of the nontest ear for headphones and 60 dB for insert earphones. One method for masking is to take the presentation level and subtract 20 dB to determine the masking presentation level for the nontest ear. This typically works for symmetric hearing. If there is an asymmetry, particularly for mixed or conductive hearing loss, the SRT should be examined as well as the pure-tone thresholds of the nontest ear to ensure effective masking is being used.

Tympanometry

A probe is placed in the patient's ear and positive and negative pressures are introduced. The patient is counseled that there will be a sensation of pressure and to be as quiet and still as possible. If a seal cannot be maintained, sometimes using a small amount of a water-based gel, such as that used for insertion of earmolds, on the tip of the probe may help maintain a seal for testing.

Acoustic Reflex Thresholds

The probe is placed in the test ear and the stimulus is presented ipsilaterally. Then a probe with a loudspeaker is placed in the contralateral ear and the stimulus is presented contralaterally. The patient is instructed to be as quiet and still as possible.

Acoustic Reflex Decay

The stimulus probe is placed in the contralateral ear and the measurement probe is placed in the test ear. The stimulus presentation level is determined by adding + 10 dB SL to the contralateral reflex threshold for 500 Hz and 1,000 Hz. The patient is instructed that a loud sound will be heard for 10 seconds and to remain as quiet and still as possible.

1.2.4 Patient Conditions and Circumstances Requiring Procedure Modifications

Atresia

Atresia of the ear is defined as the absence or closure of the ear canal. When a patient presents with atresia, air conduction thresholds can and should still be measured. Headphones must be used for this testing procedure because no ear canal is present for the use of insert earphones. The purpose of this is to measure the conductive component of the hearing loss. The ear without atresia should be masked in the conventional manner for this procedure. Bone conduction testing should also be performed to determine inner ear function and the magnitude of the air–bone gap. Immittance testing for the ear with atresia cannot be performed; however, tympanometry and ipsilateral acoustic reflexes should be obtained in the ear without atresia.

Collapsing Ear Canals

On occasion, a patient may have a collapsing ear canal when the headphones are placed. When performing otoscopy, it is important to note the size and shape of the ear canal. If an ear canal is narrow or the ear canal tissue and cartilage are more pliable, then there may be an increased probability of a collapsing ear canal. Even proper ear canal inspection may not reveal the presence of a collapsing ear canal. The weight and pressure of headphones placed on an ear canal that has the propensity to collapse will cause closure of the ear canal and thereby result in a false conductive/mixed hearing loss, particularly in the higher frequencies. To determine if the conductive component is caused by a collapsing ear canal, the clinician must integrate the patient's history with the testing results. If the patient's history does not indicate a conductive component but one is present, then a collapsed ear canal may be possible. Insert earphones can be used if a collapsing ear canal is suspected. This will avoid the false conductive/mixed hearing loss caused by the headphones. Also, if a collapsing canal is suspected, insert earphones can be used to determine if there are any threshold changes. If there is a threshold change with the use of inserts, then the patient likely has a collapsing ear canal. This should be noted in the patient's chart to prevent confusion of whether or not headphones or insert earphones would be more appropriate for future testing.

Headphone/Insert Earphone Placement

The placement of the headphones and insert earphones can affect the results of the hearing test. If the anatomy of the head and ear do not allow a tight seal of the headphones, a leak may occur and cause a false low-frequency hearing loss. This hearing loss will likely be conductive or mixed when one would not expect this result. Readjusting the headphones may alleviate this problem. For insert earphones, a deep and tight seal is needed; otherwise a loose seal may cause a leak and hearing loss in the low frequencies as well. Changing the size of the insert earphone or switching to headphones may alleviate this problem. When using traditional headphones, it is also important that the diaphragm of the headphone is over the ear canal, otherwise a null or hearing loss may appear, particularly at 6,000 Hz. This can be corrected by adjusting the headphones or using insert earphones.

Inability to Repeat Words

During clinical testing, there may be times when it is not possible to perform speech testing. This may occur when patients have other medical problems that prohibit speech, such as a tracheostomy or a breathing tube. Depending on the health conditions, these patients may be able to write out the words/responses. This may add a significant amount of time to the testing procedure, but can be useful for assessing word recognition. In addition to this, picture pointing tests, such as the Word Intelligibility by Picture Identification (WIPI)[4] and the Northwestern University–Children's Perception of Speech test (NU-CHIPS)[5] can also be used. Even though these are closed set tests, information obtained will be useful in determining word recognition.

A clinician may also test a patient that does not speak English. When a patient presents in the clinic that does not speak English, an interpreter is invaluable to determine the history and to provide testing instructions. The clinician should also remember that it is proper etiquette to speak directly to the patient instead of the interpreter. However, for these patients, speech testing may not be performed due to a lack of familiarity with the words and the unfamiliarity of the clinician to determine whether a word is repeated correctly and not due to dialect. If this is the case, speech testing may not be performed, and it should be noted on the test as to why this was not performed. Instead, an SAT should be obtained; knowledge of the words is not needed for this test, and it can be used to determine the accuracy of pure-tone thresholds.

Hyperacusis/Sensitivity to Sound

Some patients will present with sensitivity to sound. This may be through recruitment (abnormal growth of the loudness of sound) or through hyperacusis (sensitivity even to soft to moderate sounds). For these patients, counseling is a key factor in performing a comprehensive audiological evaluation. Patients should be advised of when louder sounds may be presented, such as masking, or any higher-intensity sound. A patient may feel more comfortable during testing because they have more control when they are warned that a sound may be uncomfortable. Also, an ascending approach (starting at a soft level and slowly increasing the volume) will prevent discomfort from the initial presentation of a suprathreshold pure-tone because the sensitivity level of the patient will likely be unknown. Special considerations should also be provided when acoustic reflex testing is performed. Some patients may prefer not to have acoustic reflex testing completed due to the aversion of specific tones or intensities. Once again, the patient must be made aware of the testing procedures. These patients also frequently have tinnitus. Using a pulsed pure-tone can make it easier for the patient to determine the pure-tone from the tinnitus.

Otorrhea

Otorrhea is liquid or mucus discharge from the ear that may or may not be infected. Otorrhea may also present as smelly discharge from the ear canal. When otorrhea is present in the ear canal, universal precautions should be followed. Medical gloves should be used to avoid contact with any discharge from the ear canal. Typically, this patient is referred to an ear, nose, and throat physician (ENT) for an evaluation prior to an audiological evaluation; however, there are times when the otorrhea cannot be cleared, and testing may be necessary to determine a path for medical care. If a hearing evaluation is performed, then protective covers should be used over headphones to avoid damage to and contamination of the equipment. It is not advised to perform immittance testing on an ear with otorrhea because the positive and negative pressure produced by the immittance unit may contaminate and/or damage the immittance unit. Equipment should be disinfected after testing.

Otosurgery

Ears that have had otosurgery (e.g., tympanoplasty, mastoidectomy, etc.) should be treated with extreme caution. Immittance is not recommended due to potential damage to the ear, unless it is recommended by the ENT. Otoscopy may reveal blood, or the patient may report tenderness of the ear if the surgery was recent, and care should be taken to prevent discomfort when headphones or inserts are used.

Stenger

Occasionally a patient will arrive in the clinic and provide unreliable results. Reinstructing the patient may help alleviate this problem. In addition, starting with SRT may help indicate if a patient is faking because this type of patient will often present with an SRT that is better than the pure-tone thresholds. If repeated reinstruction does not produce reliable results, the Stenger test may be performed. The Stenger test can be completed if there is a 20 dB difference between the better and poorer ear. The Stenger test is performed by interlocking the presentation of the right and left ears. The better ear is presented with a pure-tone that is 10 dB above threshold at one frequency (usually 1,000 Hz, but other frequencies can be used, and this can also be completed using SRT) and 10 dB below the threshold of the poorer ear. No instructions are provided to the patient if pure-tone thresholds are still being tested. If a different test was being completed, state that a few more beeps will be presented and to press the button when the beep is heard. If the patient does not respond to the beep, it means the patient heard the pure-tone in the poorer ear and did not respond because this is the ear he/she is trying to exaggerate hearing loss in. Therefore, the result is a positive Stenger test, indicating the patient is likely exaggerating hearing loss in this ear. If the patient responds to the beep, the hearing loss in the poorer ear is likely accurate.

1.3 Conclusion

When becoming a proficient clinician, an individual may find that there are many different methods to test a patient. Even though some of these methods may vary from clinician to clinician, the testing results will likely remain the same. A clinician may need to have experience in multiple testing methods in order to adapt to the needs and abilities of the patient. As experience is gained a clinician will become more comfortable when testing difficult patients or difficult audiological configurations. It was not noted in this book, but many different methods of testing may have been used by the authors to obtain the audiological testing results. The reader may notice that there are different methods of writing case histories as well as audiological reports. As long as the appropriate information is conveyed, readers should understand that there is more than one way to express the results of testing.

1.4 References

[1] Clark JG. Uses and abuses of hearing loss classification. ASHA 1981;23 (7):493–500
[2] Turner RG. Masking redux. I: An optimized masking method. J Am Acad Audiol 2004;15(1):17–28
[3] Yacullo W. Clinical Masking Procedures. Needham Heights, MA: Allyn and Bacon; 1996
[4] Ross M, Lerman J. A picture identification test for hearing-impaired children. J Speech Hear Res 1970;13(1):44–53
[5] Elliott L, Katz D. Northwestern University children's perception of speech (NU-CHIPS). St. Louis, MO: Auditec; 1980

2 Audiological Interpretation Cheat Sheet

2.1 Degree of Hearing Loss/SAT/ SRT (Air Conduction PTA of 500, 1,000, and 2,000 Hz)

Normal = – 10 to 15 dB HL
Slight = 16 to 25 dB HL
Mild = 26 to 40 dB HL
Moderate = 41 to 55 dB HL
Moderately severe = 56 to 70 dB HL
Severe = 71 to 90 dB HL
Profound = ≥ 91 dB HL

2.2 Type of Hearing Loss

Sensorineural hearing loss = hearing loss with an air–bone gap that is ≤ 10 dB HL (with the exception of reverse air–bone gaps where the bone conduction has a greater degree of hearing loss than the air conduction threshold; reverse air–bone gaps > 10 dB HL are still considered to be sensorineural)
Conductive hearing loss = hearing loss of an air conduction threshold with a normal bone conduction threshold with an air–bone gap that is > 10 dB HL
Mixed hearing loss = a combination of sensorineural and conductive hearing loss that may also include having an air–bone gap that is > 10 dB HL, but the bone conduction thresholds are not within the normal range of hearing

2.3 Speech Recognition/ Awareness Test

Agreement of ± 10 dB with PTA

2.4 Word Recognition Score

Normal = 90 to 100%
Slight difficulty = 76 to 88%
Moderate difficulty = 60 to 74%
Poor recognition = 50 to 58%
Very poor recognition = < 50%

2.5 Tympanometry

Ear canal volume normal range = 0.6 to 2 mL (a difference between ears of > 1 mL may indicate a perforation or patent pressure equalization tube)
Middle ear pressure normal range = ± 100 daPa
Static admittance normal range = 0.3 to 1.5 mL (< 0.3 = hypocompliant; > 1.5 = hypercompliant)

2.6 Acoustic Reflex Thresholds

Normal/present = ≤ 100 dB HL
Elevated = 105 to 110 dB HL
Absent = no response at 110 dB HL

2.7 Acoustic Reflex Decay

Negative = Reflex does not decay by 50% for 10 seconds.
Positive/abnormal = Reflex decays by 50% within 10 seconds.

2.8 The Stenger Test

Instructions: The better ear is presented with a pure-tone that is 10 dB above threshold at one frequency (usually 1,000 Hz, but other frequencies can be used, and this can also be completed using SRT) and 10 dB below the threshold of the poorer ear.
Negative = Patient responds to presentation—results are reliable.
Positive = Patient does not respond to presentation—results are not reliable.

3 Common Audiological Abbreviations

Absent (ABS)
Acoustic reflex decay (ARD)
Acoustic reflex threshold (ART)
Air conduction (AC)
Auditory brainstem response (ABR)
Auditory processing disorder (APD)
Behind-the-ear (BTE)
Benign paroxysmal positional vertigo (BPPV)
Bilateral contralateral routing of signals (BICROS)
Bone-anchored hearing aid (BAHA)
Bone conduction (BC)
Cochlear implant (CI)
Completely-in-the-canal (CIC)
Computerized axial tomography scan (CAT scan)
Computerized tomography (CT)
Contralateral routing of signals (CROS)
Could not mask (CNM)
Could not test (CNT)
Decibel (dB)
Did not test (DNT)
Distortion product otoacoustic emissions (DPOAE)
Ear, nose, and throat physician (ENT)
Electrocochleography (ECOG)
Electronystagmography (ENG)
Hearing aid (HA)
Hearing-assistive technology (HAT)
Hearing level (HL)
In-the-canal (ITC)
In-the-ear (ITE)
Magnetic resonance imagining (MRI)
Most intelligible loudness (MIL)
No peak/pressure (NP)
No response (NR)
Otoacoustic emissions (OAE)
Positron emission tomography scan (PET scan)
Pressure equalization (PE)
Pure-tone average (PTA)
Sensation level (SL)
Sound pressure level (SPL)
Speech awareness threshold (SAT)
Speech recognition threshold (SRT)
Transient evoked otoacoustic emissions (TEOAE)
Uncomfortable loudness (UCL)
Vestibular evoked myogenic potential (VEMP)
Volume unit (VU)
Word recognition score (WRS)

4 Normal Hearing Cases

4.1 Case 1

4.1.1 Case History

The patient was a 27-year-old woman who reported difficulty hearing in noise. She had noticed this for many years. She reported that she had meningitis when she was 16 and felt that this was when she started to notice difficulty with her hearing. Others had told her that she may have hearing loss, and she felt she needed to listen at a higher volume to understand the TV. She was a resident physician in the emergency room, and she reported difficulty hearing with the noise that was present in the emergency room. She noticed this more when she was performing tasks in the emergency room when others were speaking through face masks. She had trouble hearing in social settings and restaurants. She denied dizziness, tinnitus, or loud noise exposure. She denied pain, pressure, or fullness relating to her ears.

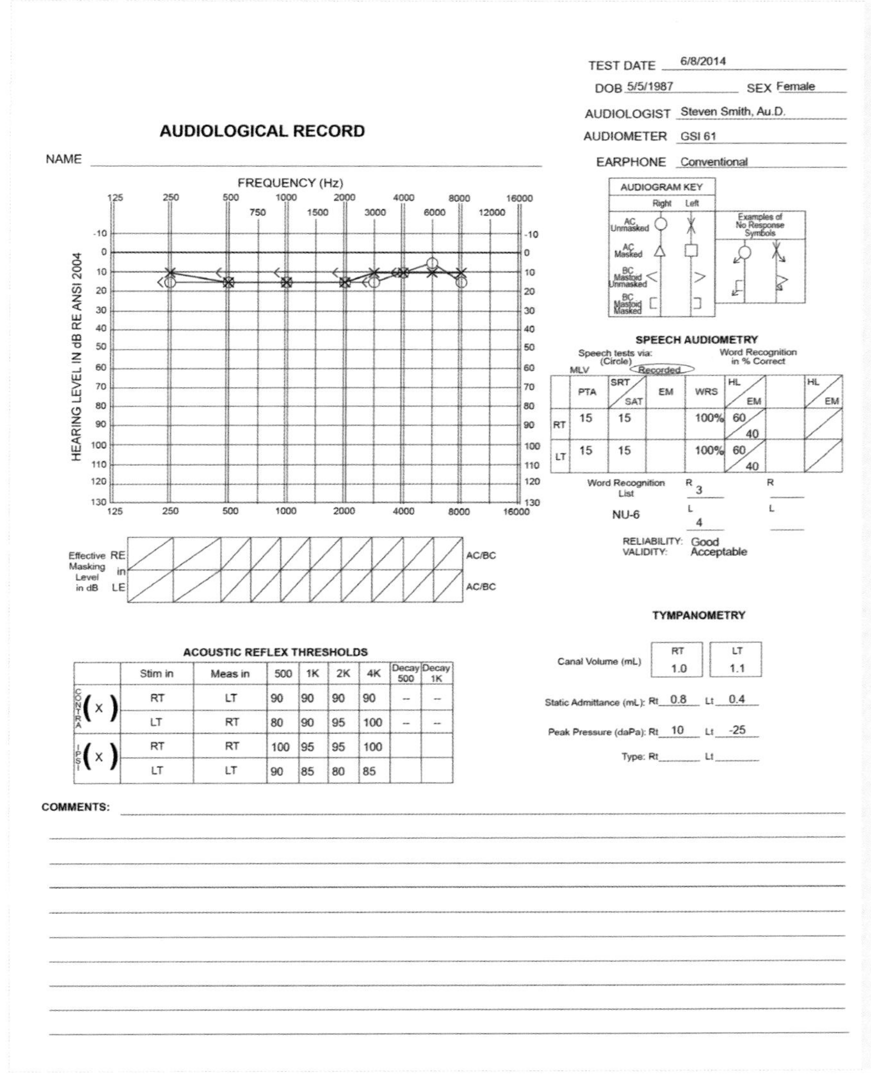

AUDIOLOGICAL RECORD

NAME ______

TEST DATE 6/8/2014
DOB 5/5/1987 SEX Female
AUDIOLOGIST Steven Smith, Au.D.
AUDIOMETER GSI 61
EARPHONE Conventional

SPEECH AUDIOMETRY

Speech tests via: (Circle) MLV (Recorded)

Word Recognition in % Correct

	PTA	SRT/SAT	EM	WRS	HL/EM		HL/EM
RT	15	15		100%	60/40		
LT	15	15		100%	60/40		

Word Recognition List: NU-6 R 3, L 4

RELIABILITY: Good
VALIDITY: Acceptable

TYMPANOMETRY

Canal Volume (mL)	RT	LT
	1.0	1.1

Static Admittance (mL): Rt 0.8 Lt 0.4

Peak Pressure (daPa): Rt 10 Lt -25

Type: Rt ______ Lt ______

ACOUSTIC REFLEX THRESHOLDS

	Stim in	Meas in	500	1K	2K	4K	Decay 500	Decay 1K
CONTRA (x)	RT	LT	90	90	90	90	--	--
	LT	RT	80	90	95	100	--	--
IPSI (x)	RT	RT	100	95	95	100		
	LT	LT	90	85	80	85		

COMMENTS: ______

Fig. 4.1 Audiogram of a patient with a possible central auditory processing disorder due to difficulty hearing in background noise. The patient also had a history of meningitis.

4.1.2 Interpretation

Right ear—Normal hearing. The SRT was normal and was in agreement with the PTA. The WRS was considered to be normal. Immittance testing revealed a normal tympanogram with normal ipsilateral and contralateral acoustic reflexes from 500 to 4,000 Hz. The contralateral acoustic reflex decay was negative.

Left ear—Normal hearing. The SRT was normal and was in agreement with the PTA. The WRS was considered to be normal. Immittance testing revealed a normal tympanogram with normal ipsilateral and contralateral acoustic reflexes from 500 to 4,000 Hz. The contralateral acoustic reflex decay was negative.

4.1.3 Intervention

The patient was counseled on her hearing evaluation results and that she had normal hearing. It was recommended that she pursue further testing for an evaluation for a central auditory processing disorder as well as a HAT evaluation.

4.2 Case 2

4.2.1 Case History

The patient reported that sounds such as people chewing, sniffling, coughing, and clicking an ink pen caused an instant feeling of anger. These symptoms started when she was around age 8, but she could not think of a specific event that caused her reaction. Her father and mother were the worst causes of the trigger sounds. She avoided situations where the trigger sounds could occur, or she left the situation where they were occurring. She instantly felt better and was able to relax when she was not around the trigger sounds. She did not report other otologic symptoms or history.

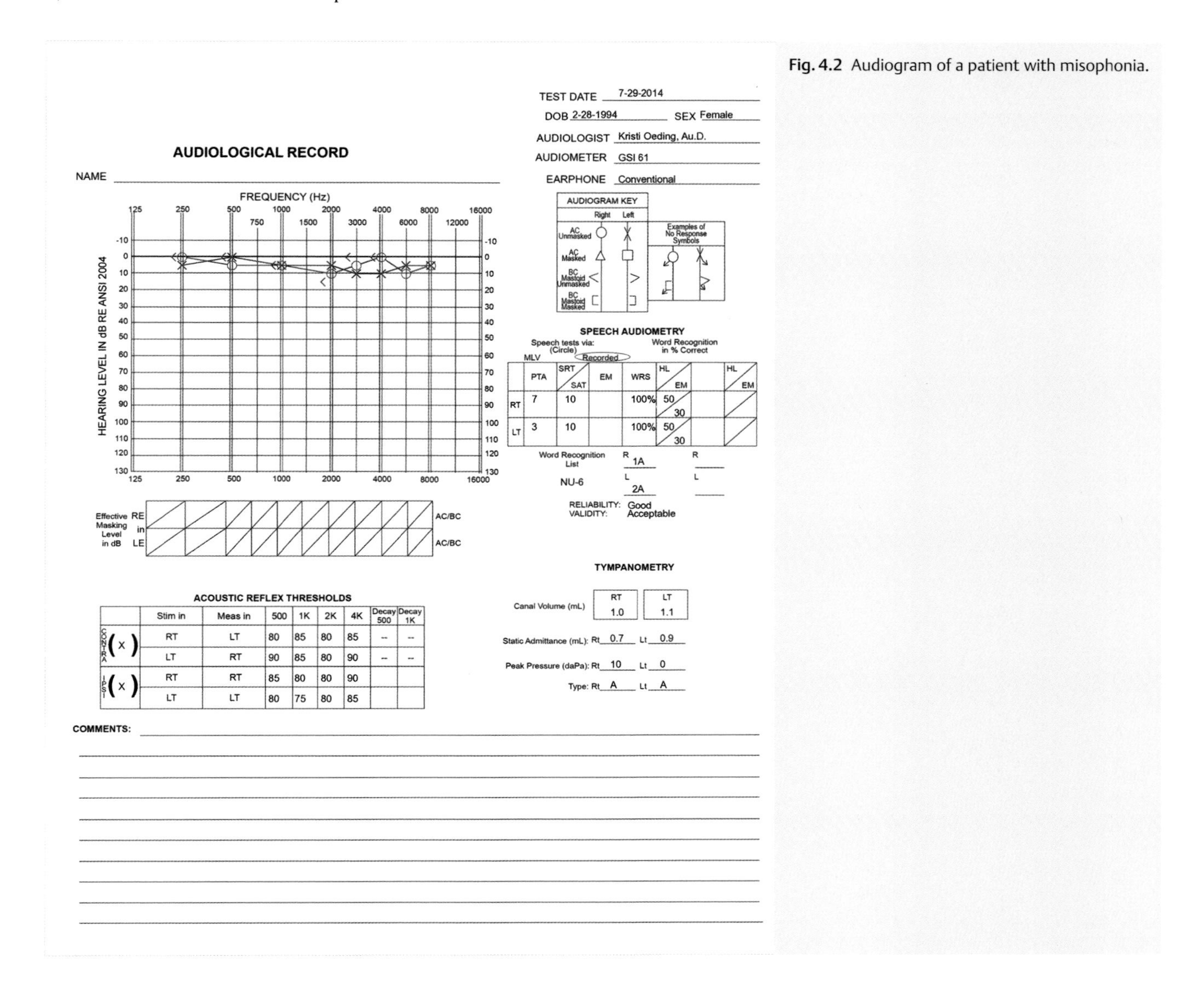

AUDIOLOGICAL RECORD

NAME

TEST DATE 7-29-2014
DOB 2-28-1994 SEX Female
AUDIOLOGIST Kristi Oeding, Au.D.
AUDIOMETER GSI 61
EARPHONE Conventional

SPEECH AUDIOMETRY

Speech tests via: (Circle) MLV Recorded

Word Recognition in % Correct

	PTA	SRT / SAT	EM	WRS	HL / EM		HL / EM
RT	7	10		100%	50 / 30		
LT	3	10		100%	50 / 30		

Word Recognition List NU-6: R 1A, L 2A; R ___, L ___

RELIABILITY: Good
VALIDITY: Acceptable

TYMPANOMETRY

	RT	LT
Canal Volume (mL)	1.0	1.1

Static Admittance (mL): Rt 0.7 Lt 0.9
Peak Pressure (daPa): Rt 10 Lt 0
Type: Rt A Lt A

ACOUSTIC REFLEX THRESHOLDS

	Stim in	Meas in	500	1K	2K	4K	Decay 500	Decay 1K
CONTRA (X)	RT	LT	80	85	80	85	--	--
	LT	RT	90	85	80	90	--	--
IPSI (X)	RT	RT	85	80	80	90		
	LT	LT	80	75	80	85		

COMMENTS:

Fig. 4.2 Audiogram of a patient with misophonia.

4.2.2 Interpretation

Right ear—Pure-tone thresholds were within normal limits from 250 to 8,000 Hz. The SRT revealed a normal ability to receive speech and was in agreement with the PTA. The WRS revealed a normal ability to recognize speech. Immittance testing revealed a normal tympanogram. The acoustic reflex thresholds were normal with ipsilateral and contralateral stimulation from 500 to 4,000 Hz. The acoustic reflex decay was negative at 500 and 1,000 Hz.

Left ear—Pure-tone thresholds were within normal limits from 250 to 8,000 Hz. The SRT revealed a normal ability to receive speech and was in agreement with the PTA. The WRS revealed a normal ability to recognize speech. Immittance testing revealed a normal tympanogram. The acoustic reflex thresholds were normal with ipsilateral and contralateral stimulation from 500 to 4,000 Hz. The acoustic reflex decay was negative at 500 and 1,000 Hz.

4.2.3 Intervention

The patient was referred to an ENT specialist and no medical complications were found. She was diagnosed with misophonia and decided to try sound therapy with BTE sound generators as well as counseling with a cognitive behavioral therapist. Other audiological recommendations included retesting her hearing as needed and hearing protection in noise.

4.3 Case 3

4.3.1 Case History

The patient reported a 2-month history of constant tinnitus in the right ear that presented suddenly. Reportedly, the tinnitus remained unchanged. It was described as a constant low-level ringing sound that was extremely distracting and interfered with the patient's ability to fall asleep. The tinnitus was reported to be loudest upon waking in the morning. The patient denied any hearing loss or dizziness. There was no reported history of ear pathology, familial hearing loss, or noise exposure. No significant health history was reported. The patient changed her diet to limit caffeine and sodium, and she reported that this did not seem to change the tinnitus.

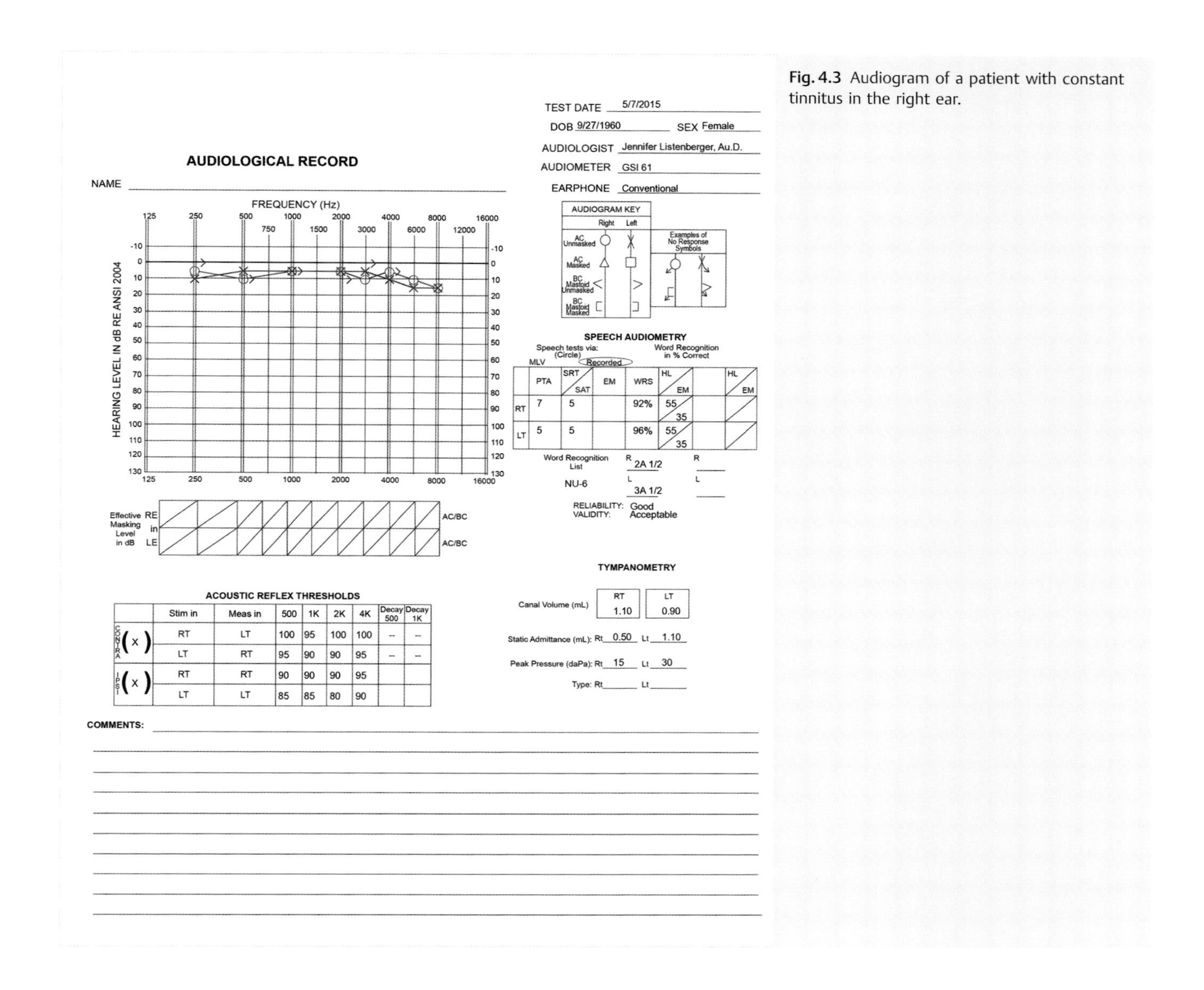

AUDIOLOGICAL RECORD

NAME

TEST DATE 5/7/2015
DOB 9/27/1960 SEX Female
AUDIOLOGIST Jennifer Listenberger, Au.D.
AUDIOMETER GSI 61
EARPHONE Conventional

SPEECH AUDIOMETRY

Speech tests via: (Circle) MLV Recorded — Word Recognition in % Correct

	PTA	SRT / SAT	EM	WRS	HL / EM		HL / EM
RT	7	5		92%	55 / 35		
LT	5	5		96%	55 / 35		

Word Recognition List: R 2A 1/2; L 3A 1/2 — NU-6

RELIABILITY: Good
VALIDITY: Acceptable

TYMPANOMETRY

	RT	LT
Canal Volume (mL)	1.10	0.90
Static Admittance (mL)	0.50	1.10
Peak Pressure (daPa)	15	30
Type		

ACOUSTIC REFLEX THRESHOLDS

	Stim in	Meas in	500	1K	2K	4K	Decay 500	Decay 1K
CONTRA (x)	RT	LT	100	95	100	100	--	--
	LT	RT	95	90	90	95	--	--
IPSI (x)	RT	RT	90	90	90	95		
	LT	LT	85	85	80	90		

COMMENTS:

Fig. 4.3 Audiogram of a patient with constant tinnitus in the right ear.

4.3.2 Interpretation

Right ear—Pure-tone air and bone conduction threshold testing revealed normal hearing sensitivity at 250 through 8,000 Hz. The SRT revealed a normal ability to receive speech and was in agreement with the PTA. The WRS revealed a normal ability to recognize speech. Immittance testing revealed a normal tympanogram. The acoustic reflex thresholds were within normal limits for ipsilateral and contralateral stimulation at 500 through 4,000 Hz. The contralateral acoustic reflex decay was negative at 500 and 1,000 Hz.

Left ear—Pure-tone air and bone conduction threshold testing revealed normal hearing sensitivity at 250 through 8,000 Hz. The SRT revealed a normal ability to receive speech and was in agreement with the PTA. The WRS revealed a normal ability to recognize speech. Immittance testing revealed a normal tympanogram. The acoustic reflex thresholds were within normal limits for ipsilateral and contralateral stimulation at 500 through 4,000 Hz. The contralateral acoustic reflex decay was negative at 500 and 1,000 Hz.

4.3.3 Intervention

The patient was encouraged to continue with the scheduled consultation with the otologist. Audiological recommendations included follow-up testing as needed, use of hearing protection in noise, and consultation for tinnitus management if the tinnitus did not improve.

4.4 Case 4

4.4.1 Case History

The patient was an 18-year-old man who was studying music education. He reported playing the piano and singing for most of his life. He began to use non-custom musician earplugs a few months ago when practicing. He wanted his hearing evaluated to establish a baseline. He denied hearing loss and tinnitus as well as dizziness.

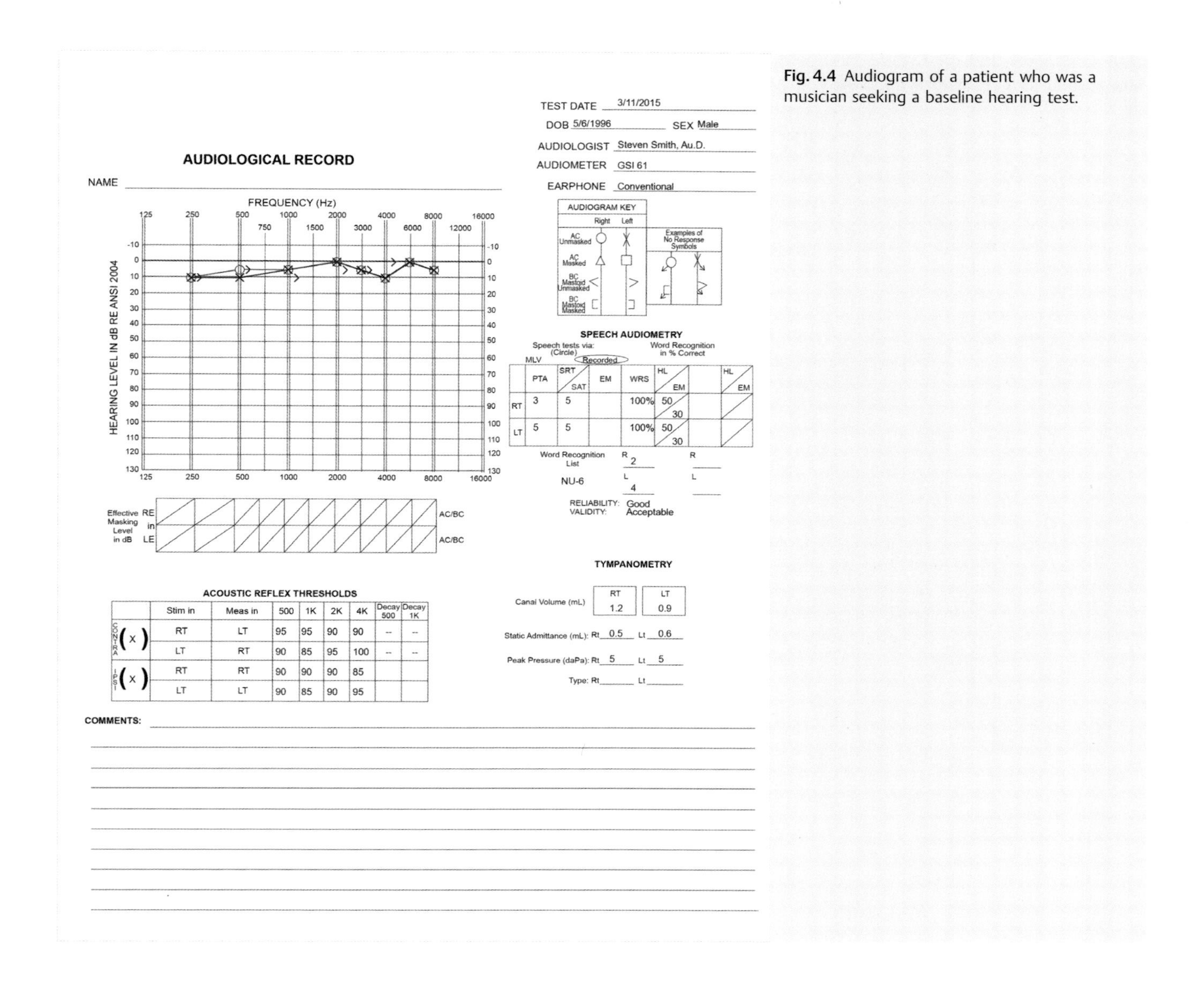

AUDIOLOGICAL RECORD

NAME

TEST DATE 3/11/2015

DOB 5/6/1996 SEX Male

AUDIOLOGIST Steven Smith, Au.D.

AUDIOMETER GSI 61

EARPHONE Conventional

SPEECH AUDIOMETRY

Speech tests via: (Circle) MLV Recorded

Word Recognition in % Correct

	PTA	SRT / SAT	EM	WRS	HL / EM	HL / EM
RT	3	5		100%	50 / 30	
LT	5	5		100%	50 / 30	

Word Recognition List: R 2, L 4; R ___, L ___

NU-6

RELIABILITY: Good

VALIDITY: Acceptable

TYMPANOMETRY

	RT	LT
Canal Volume (mL)	1.2	0.9

Static Admittance (mL): Rt 0.5 Lt 0.6

Peak Pressure (daPa): Rt 5 Lt 5

Type: Rt ___ Lt ___

ACOUSTIC REFLEX THRESHOLDS

	Stim in	Meas in	500	1K	2K	4K	Decay 500	Decay 1K
CONTRA (x)	RT	LT	95	95	90	90	--	--
	LT	RT	90	85	95	100	--	--
IPSI (x)	RT	RT	90	90	90	85		
	LT	LT	90	85	90	95		

COMMENTS:

Fig. 4.4 Audiogram of a patient who was a musician seeking a baseline hearing test.

4.4.2 Interpretation

Right ear—Normal hearing. The SRT revealed a normal ability to receive speech and was in agreement with the PTA. The WRS was normal. Immittance testing revealed a normal tympanogram. Acoustic reflexes with ipsilateral and contralateral stimulation were normal from 500 to 4,000 Hz. The contralateral acoustic reflex decay was negative at 500 and 1,000 Hz

Left ear—Normal hearing. The SRT revealed a normal ability to receive speech and was in agreement with the PTA. The WRS was normal. Immittance testing revealed a normal tympanogram. Acoustic reflexes with ipsilateral and contralateral stimulation were normal from 500 to 4,000 Hz. The contralateral acoustic reflex decay was negative at 500 and 1,000 Hz

4.4.3 Intervention

The patient was counseled to continue to monitor his hearing. He was encouraged to continue the use of the non-custom musician earplugs and was advised custom musician earplugs could be used if desired.

4.5 Case 5

4.5.1 Case History

The patient reported a sudden hearing loss in the right ear about 10 months ago. An audiogram from a previous clinic revealed a moderately severe mixed hearing loss rising to within normal limits in the right ear and normal hearing sensitivity in the left ear. She noted slight improvement after intratympanic steroid injections, but she still noticed difficulty hearing with multiple talkers and hearing speech from a distance. She also noted episodic dizziness with nausea that occurred twice per week and was undergoing vestibular rehabilitation, which had been helping. She experienced intermittent tinnitus, pressure, and otalgia in the right ear. She did not report other otologic symptoms or history.

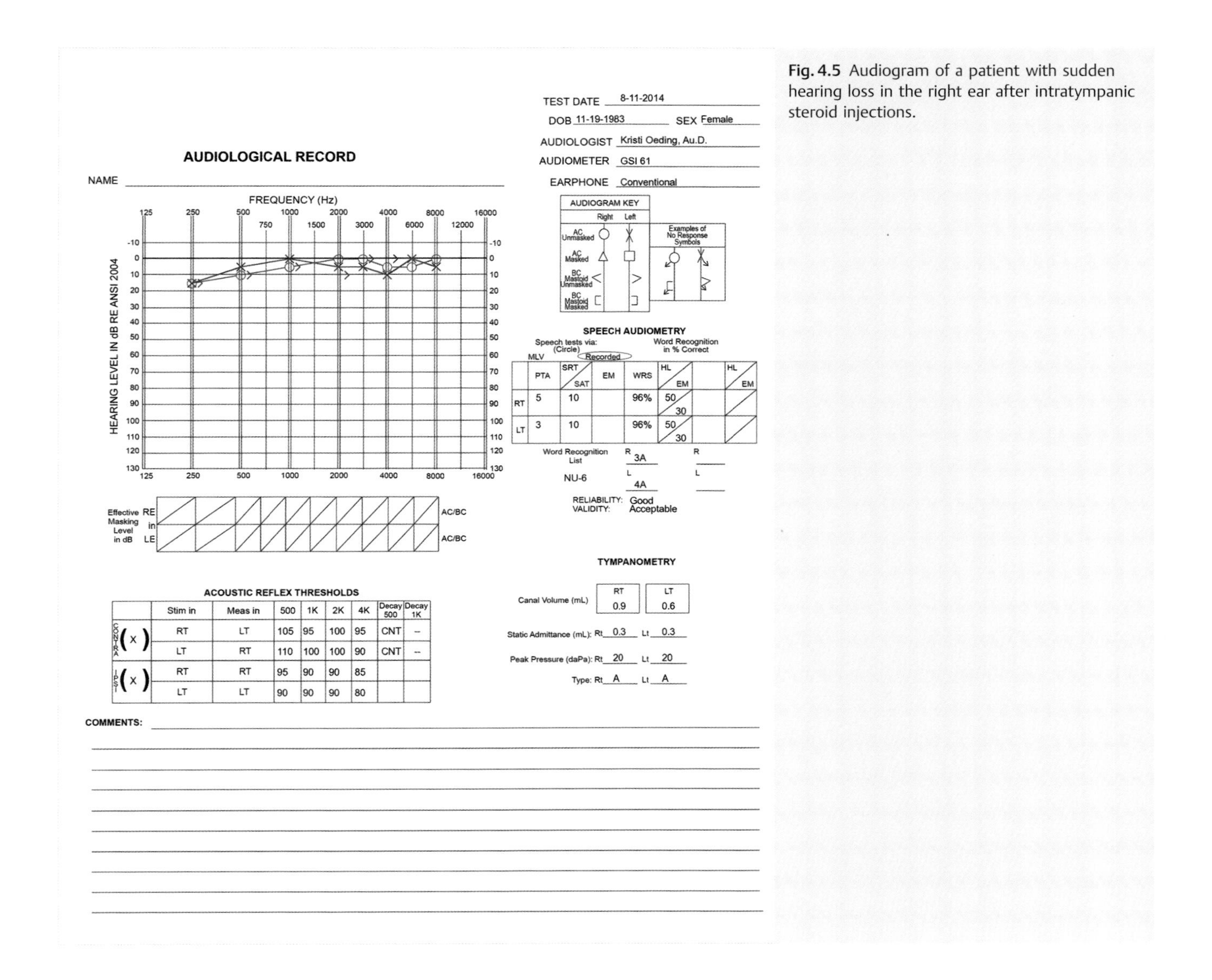

AUDIOLOGICAL RECORD

NAME

TEST DATE 8-11-2014
DOB 11-19-1983 SEX Female
AUDIOLOGIST Kristi Oeding, Au.D.
AUDIOMETER GSI 61
EARPHONE Conventional

SPEECH AUDIOMETRY

Speech tests via: (Circle) MLV Recorded

Word Recognition in % Correct

	PTA	SRT / SAT	EM	WRS	HL / EM		HL / EM
RT	5	10		96%	50 / 30		
LT	3	10		96%	50 / 30		

Word Recognition List: R 3A; L 4A (NU-6)

RELIABILITY: Good
VALIDITY: Acceptable

TYMPANOMETRY

	RT	LT
Canal Volume (mL)	0.9	0.6
Static Admittance (mL)	0.3	0.3
Peak Pressure (daPa)	20	20
Type	A	A

ACOUSTIC REFLEX THRESHOLDS

	Stim in	Meas in	500	1K	2K	4K	Decay 500	Decay 1K
CONTRA (x)	RT	LT	105	95	100	95	CNT	--
	LT	RT	110	100	100	90	CNT	--
IPSI (x)	RT	RT	95	90	90	85		
	LT	LT	90	90	90	80		

COMMENTS:

Fig. 4.5 Audiogram of a patient with sudden hearing loss in the right ear after intratympanic steroid injections.

4.5.2 Interpretation

Right ear—Pure-tone thresholds were within normal limits from 250 to 8,000 Hz. The SRT revealed a normal ability to receive speech and was in agreement with the PTA. The WRS revealed a normal ability to recognize speech. Immittance testing revealed a normal tympanogram. The acoustic reflex thresholds were normal with ipsilateral stimulation from 500 to 4,000 Hz and normal with contralateral stimulation from 1,000 to 4,000 Hz and elevated at 500 Hz. The acoustic reflex decay was negative at 1,000 Hz and could not be measured at 500 Hz due to an elevated contralateral acoustic reflex threshold.

Left ear—Pure-tone thresholds were within normal limits from 250 to 8,000 Hz. The SRT revealed a normal ability to receive speech and was in agreement with the PTA. The WRS revealed a normal ability to recognize speech. Immittance testing revealed a normal tympanogram. The acoustic reflex thresholds were normal with ipsilateral stimulation from 500 to 4,000 Hz and normal with contralateral stimulation from 1,000 to 4,000 Hz and elevated at 500 Hz. The acoustic reflex decay was negative at 1,000 Hz and could not be measured at 500 Hz due to an elevated contralateral acoustic reflex threshold.

4.5.3 Intervention

The patient was interested in assistive hearing devices and was counseled on HAT. Other audiological recommendations included retesting hearing as needed and hearing protection in noise.

4.6 Case 6

4.6.1 Case History

An 18-year-old woman was accompanied by her father. Her father reported that the family had concerns regarding her hearing loss due to how loud her voice was when she talked. The patient reported some need for repetition in noisy places, such as her dance studio. She denied any tinnitus, dizziness, or aural pressure.

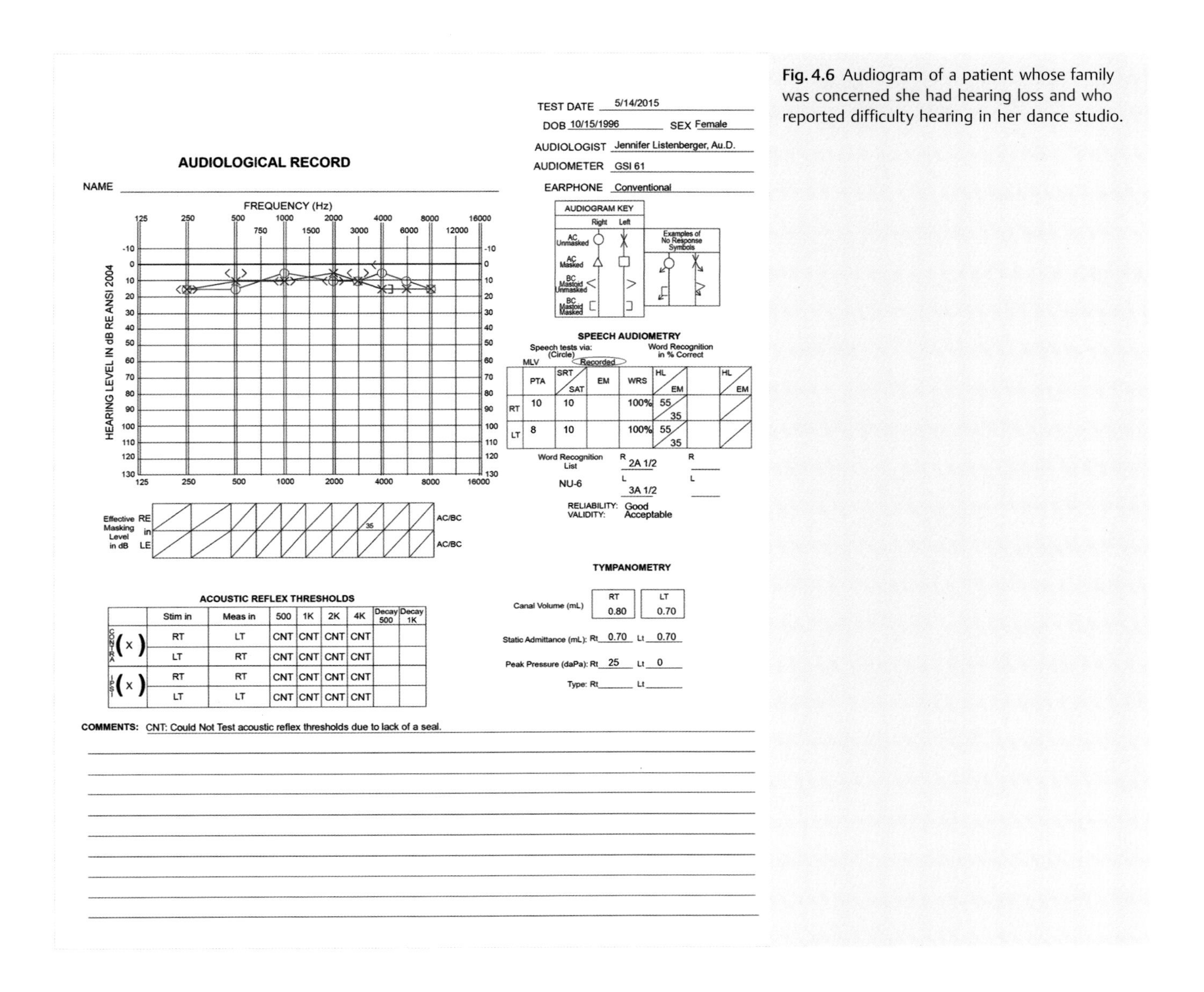

AUDIOLOGICAL RECORD

NAME

TEST DATE 5/14/2015

DOB 10/15/1996 SEX Female

AUDIOLOGIST Jennifer Listenberger, Au.D.

AUDIOMETER GSI 61

EARPHONE Conventional

SPEECH AUDIOMETRY

Speech tests via: (Circle) MLV Recorded

Word Recognition in % Correct

	PTA	SRT / SAT	EM	WRS	HL / EM	HL / EM
RT	10	10		100%	55 / 35	
LT	8	10		100%	55 / 35	

Word Recognition List NU-6: R 2A 1/2; L 3A 1/2

RELIABILITY: Good

VALIDITY: Acceptable

TYMPANOMETRY

	RT	LT
Canal Volume (mL)	0.80	0.70

Static Admittance (mL): Rt 0.70 Lt 0.70

Peak Pressure (daPa): Rt 25 Lt 0

Type: Rt ____ Lt ____

ACOUSTIC REFLEX THRESHOLDS

	Stim in	Meas in	500	1K	2K	4K	Decay 500	Decay 1K
CONTRA (x)	RT	LT	CNT	CNT	CNT	CNT		
	LT	RT	CNT	CNT	CNT	CNT		
IPSI (x)	RT	RT	CNT	CNT	CNT	CNT		
	LT	LT	CNT	CNT	CNT	CNT		

COMMENTS: CNT: Could Not Test acoustic reflex thresholds due to lack of a seal.

Fig. 4.6 Audiogram of a patient whose family was concerned she had hearing loss and who reported difficulty hearing in her dance studio.

4.6.2 Interpretation

Right ear—Pure tone air and bone conduction threshold testing revealed normal hearing sensitivity at 250 through 8,000 Hz. The SRT revealed a normal ability to receive speech and was in agreement with the PTA. The WRS revealed a normal ability to recognize speech. Immittance testing revealed a normal tympanogram. The acoustic reflex threshold and decay testing were not measured due to the inability to maintain a seal.

Left ear—Pure-tone air and bone conduction threshold testing revealed normal hearing sensitivity at 250 through 8,000 Hz. The SRT revealed a normal ability to receive speech and was in agreement with the PTA. The WRS revealed a normal ability to recognize speech. Immittance testing revealed a normal tympanogram. The acoustic reflex threshold and decay testing were not measured due to the inability to maintain a seal.

4.6.3 Intervention

The patient will follow up with the otologist as scheduled. The audiological recommendation was to return for a hearing test as needed.

4.7 Case 7

4.7.1 Case History

The patient reported that he started his car and the radio was on full volume. Ever since then, he had noted tinnitus and sensitivity to loud sounds. Everyday sounds were too loud, such as driving in a car and eating in a restaurant. High-frequency sounds were particularly bothersome. He also noted a sensation of aural pressure bilaterally. The patient wore earplugs or earmuffs when leaving his house in order to drive in a car or be in public. He did not report other otologic symptoms or history.

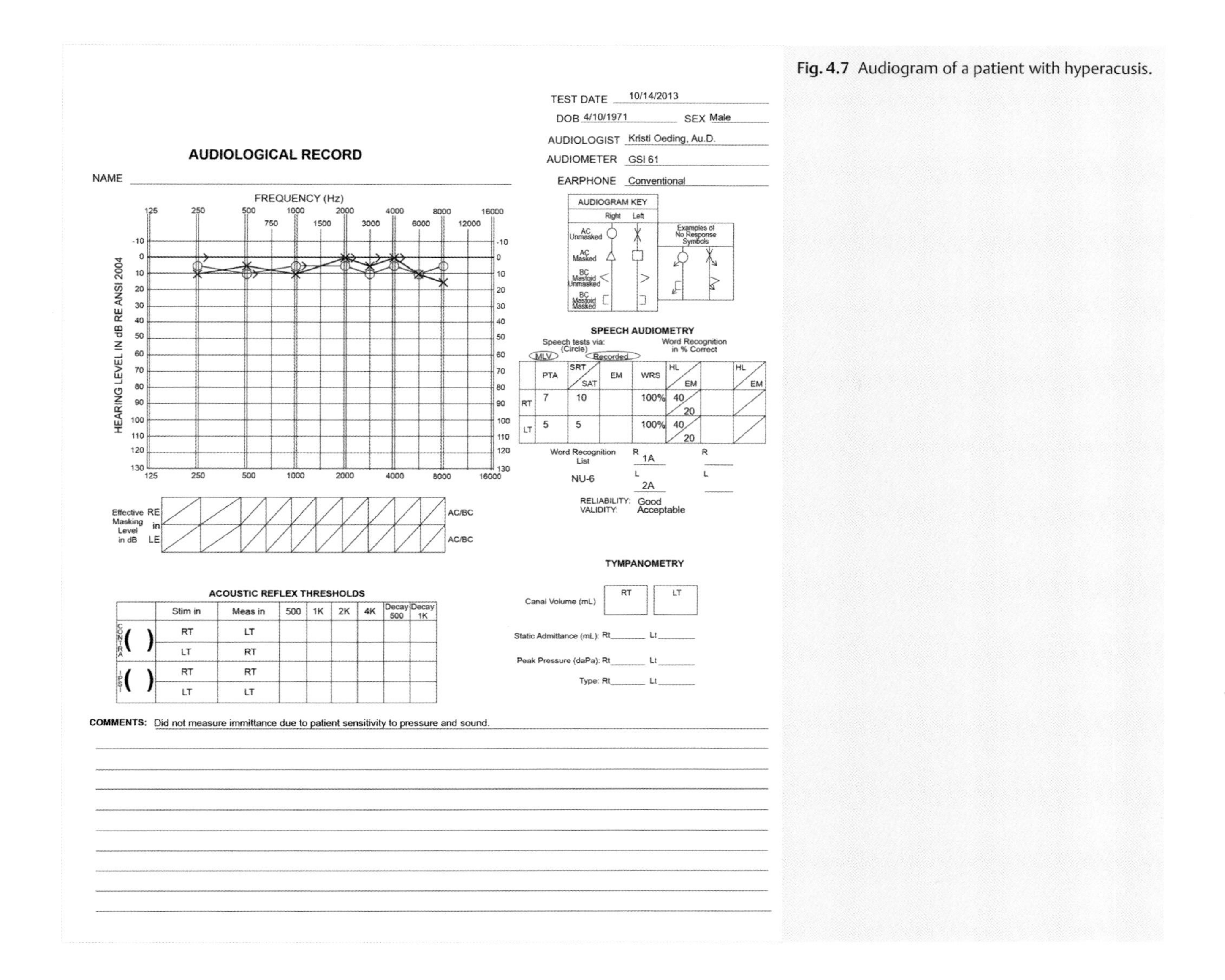

AUDIOLOGICAL RECORD

TEST DATE 10/14/2013
DOB 4/10/1971 SEX Male
AUDIOLOGIST Kristi Oeding, Au.D.
AUDIOMETER GSI 61
EARPHONE Conventional
NAME

SPEECH AUDIOMETRY

Speech tests via: (Circle) MLV Recorded

	PTA	SRT / SAT	EM	WRS	HL / EM	HL / EM
RT	7	10		100%	40 / 20	
LT	5	5		100%	40 / 20	

Word Recognition List: R 1A; L 2A
NU-6

RELIABILITY: Good
VALIDITY: Acceptable

TYMPANOMETRY

Canal Volume (mL): RT ___ LT ___
Static Admittance (mL): Rt ___ Lt ___
Peak Pressure (daPa): Rt ___ Lt ___
Type: Rt ___ Lt ___

ACOUSTIC REFLEX THRESHOLDS

	Stim in	Meas in	500	1K	2K	4K	Decay 500	Decay 1K
CONTRA	RT	LT						
	LT	RT						
IPSI	RT	RT						
	LT	LT						

COMMENTS: Did not measure immittance due to patient sensitivity to pressure and sound.

Fig. 4.7 Audiogram of a patient with hyperacusis.

4.7.2 Interpretation

Right ear—Pure-tone thresholds were within normal limits from 250 to 8,000 Hz. The SRT revealed a normal ability to receive speech and was in agreement with the PTA. The WRS revealed a normal ability to recognize speech. Immittance testing was not performed due to the patient's sensitivity to pressure and sound.

Left ear—Pure-tone thresholds were within normal limits from 250 to 8,000 Hz. The SRT revealed a normal ability to receive speech and was in agreement with the PTA. The WRS revealed a normal ability to recognize speech. Immittance testing was not performed due to the patient's sensitivity to pressure and sound.

4.7.3 Intervention

The patient was referred to an ENT specialist, and no medical complications were found. Loudness discomfort levels were performed and were approximately 50–60 dB HL, indicating hyperacusis. He was fitted with BTE sound generators to improve his tolerance for sound. He also saw a cognitive behavioral therapist due to his fear of sound hurting his ears. Other audiological recommendations included having his hearing retested as needed, wearing hearing protection in noise, and avoiding overprotecting his ears.

4.8 Case 8

4.8.1 Case History

The patient reported decreased hearing in the left ear for many years. She described the hearing in the left as being muffled and stated that it may fluctuate. She reported that a constant left aural fullness had existed for a few years, and the fullness may be worse with bad weather. She also reported a long-standing history of vertigo that appeared to increase in frequency over the past few months. She denied any tinnitus or fifth or seventh nerve symptoms. She reported some past difficulty with ear infections, but had had none for 8 years. She denied any otosurgery, noise exposure, or familial hearing loss. She reported having chronic pancreatitis, but had no other significant health history.

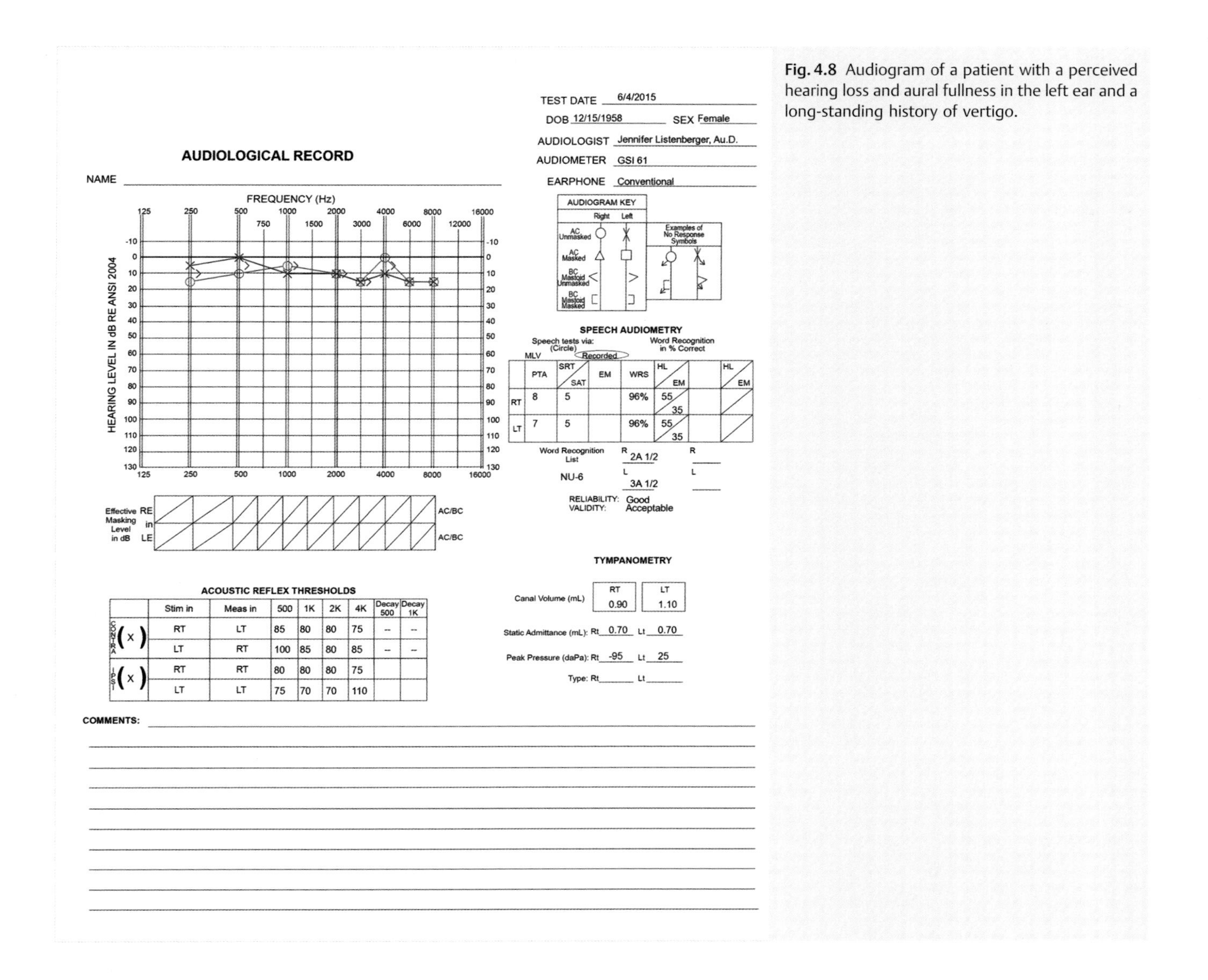

AUDIOLOGICAL RECORD

NAME

TEST DATE 6/4/2015
DOB 12/15/1958 SEX Female
AUDIOLOGIST Jennifer Listenberger, Au.D.
AUDIOMETER GSI 61
EARPHONE Conventional

SPEECH AUDIOMETRY

Speech tests via: (Circle) MLV Recorded

Word Recognition in % Correct

	PTA	SRT / SAT	EM	WRS	HL / EM		HL / EM
RT	8	5		96%	55 / 35		
LT	7	5		96%	55 / 35		

Word Recognition List: R 2A 1/2; L 3A 1/2 (NU-6)

RELIABILITY: Good
VALIDITY: Acceptable

ACOUSTIC REFLEX THRESHOLDS

	Stim in	Meas in	500	1K	2K	4K	Decay 500	Decay 1K
CONTRA (x)	RT	LT	85	80	80	75	--	--
	LT	RT	100	85	80	85	--	--
IPSI (x)	RT	RT	80	80	80	75		
	LT	LT	75	70	70	110		

TYMPANOMETRY

	RT	LT
Canal Volume (mL)	0.90	1.10

Static Admittance (mL): Rt 0.70 Lt 0.70
Peak Pressure (daPa): Rt -95 Lt 25
Type: Rt ____ Lt ____

COMMENTS:

Fig. 4.8 Audiogram of a patient with a perceived hearing loss and aural fullness in the left ear and a long-standing history of vertigo.

4.8.2 Interpretation

Right ear—Pure-tone air and bone conduction threshold testing revealed normal hearing sensitivity at 250 through 8,000 Hz. The SRT revealed a normal ability to receive speech and was in agreement with the PTA. The WRS revealed a normal ability to recognize speech. Immittance testing revealed a normal tympanogram. The acoustic reflex thresholds were present and normal for ipsilateral and contralateral stimulation at 500 to 4,000 Hz. The acoustic reflex decay with contralateral stimulation at 500 and 1,000 Hz was negative.

Left ear—Pure-tone air and bone conduction threshold testing revealed normal hearing sensitivity at 250 through 8,000 Hz. The SRT revealed a normal ability to receive speech and was in agreement with the PTA. The WRS revealed a normal ability to recognize speech. Immittance testing revealed a normal tympanogram. The acoustic reflex thresholds were present and normal for ipsilateral stimulation from 500 to 2,000 Hz and elevated at 4,000 Hz and present for contralateral stimulation at 500 to 4,000 Hz. The acoustic reflex decay with contralateral stimulation at 500 and 1,000 Hz was negative.

4.8.3 Intervention

The patient will follow up with the otologist as scheduled. The audiological recommendation was to return for a hearing test as needed.

4.9 Case 9

4.9.1 Case History

The patient was a 25-year-old woman who was diagnosed with ovarian cancer and was scheduled to be treated with cisplatin. She stated she was unsure of the number of treatments she would be receiving. She reported her hearing was good bilaterally. She denied tinnitus or dizziness. She did not report otalgia and/or fullness in her ears. She stated that she did work around louder noises in a cheese production factory.

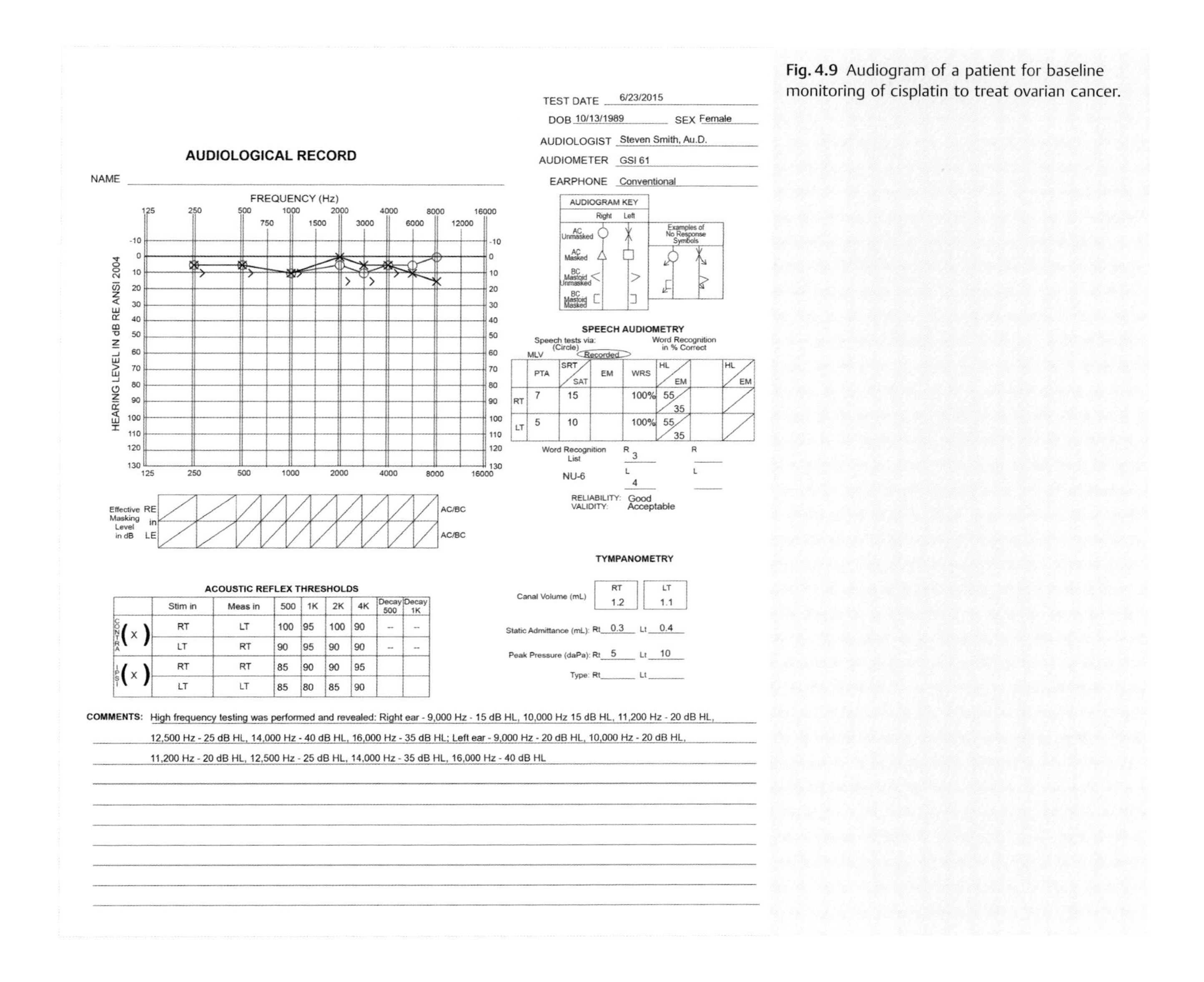

TEST DATE 6/23/2015
DOB 10/13/1989 SEX Female
AUDIOLOGIST Steven Smith, Au.D.
AUDIOMETER GSI 61
EARPHONE Conventional

AUDIOLOGICAL RECORD

NAME

Effective Masking Level in dB — RE in AC/BC; LE in AC/BC

SPEECH AUDIOMETRY

Speech tests via: (Circle) MLV Recorded (circled)

Word Recognition in % Correct

	PTA	SRT / SAT	EM	WRS	HL / EM		HL / EM
RT	7	15		100%	55 / 35		
LT	5	10		100%	55 / 35		

Word Recognition List: R 3, L 4 (NU-6); R ___, L ___

RELIABILITY: Good
VALIDITY: Acceptable

TYMPANOMETRY

	RT	LT
Canal Volume (mL)	1.2	1.1

Static Admittance (mL): Rt 0.3 Lt 0.4
Peak Pressure (daPa): Rt 5 Lt 10
Type: Rt ___ Lt ___

ACOUSTIC REFLEX THRESHOLDS

	Stim in	Meas in	500	1K	2K	4K	Decay 500	Decay 1K
CONTRA (x)	RT	LT	100	95	100	90	--	--
	LT	RT	90	95	90	90	--	--
IPSI (x)	RT	RT	85	90	90	95		
	LT	LT	85	80	85	90		

COMMENTS: High frequency testing was performed and revealed: Right ear - 9,000 Hz - 15 dB HL, 10,000 Hz 15 dB HL, 11,200 Hz - 20 dB HL, 12,500 Hz - 25 dB HL, 14,000 Hz - 40 dB HL, 16,000 Hz - 35 dB HL; Left ear - 9,000 Hz - 20 dB HL, 10,000 Hz - 20 dB HL, 11,200 Hz - 20 dB HL, 12,500 Hz - 25 dB HL, 14,000 Hz - 35 dB HL, 16,000 Hz - 40 dB HL

Fig. 4.9 Audiogram of a patient for baseline monitoring of cisplatin to treat ovarian cancer.

4.9.2 Interpretation

Right ear—Normal hearing. The SRT was normal and was in agreement with the PTA. The WRS was normal. Immittance testing revealed a normal tympanogram with normal ipsilateral and contralateral acoustic reflex thresholds from 500 to 4,000 Hz. The contralateral acoustic reflex decay was negative. High-frequency baseline testing was performed at 9,000 through 16,000 Hz to monitor for ototoxic effects.

Left ear—Normal hearing. The SRT was normal and was in agreement with the PTA. The WRS was normal. Immittance testing revealed a normal tympanogram with normal ipsilateral and contralateral acoustic reflex thresholds from 500 to 4,000 Hz. The contralateral acoustic reflex decay was negative. High-frequency baseline testing was performed at 9,000 through 16,000 Hz to monitor for ototoxic effects.

4.9.3 Intervention

The patient was counseled on her hearing evaluation results. She was provided with information regarding cisplatin and hearing loss. It was recommended to her that she have a hearing evaluation prior to her next dose of cisplatin to further monitor her hearing. She agreed to this and will follow up for subsequent testing. She was advised to use hearing protection at her job at the cheese production facility. She was made aware that ototoxic medication, in addition to noise, may cause more damage to her ears. She agreed that she will wear hearing protection at work.

4.10 Case 10

4.10.1 Case History

A 59-year-old woman reported a 2-month history of a plugged right ear. She was seen by an ENT specialist and referred for testing due to the continued sensation of her right ear being full of fluid even though, per the reviewed medical report, the fluid seemed to have resolved. There was no reported hearing loss prior to the ear infection.

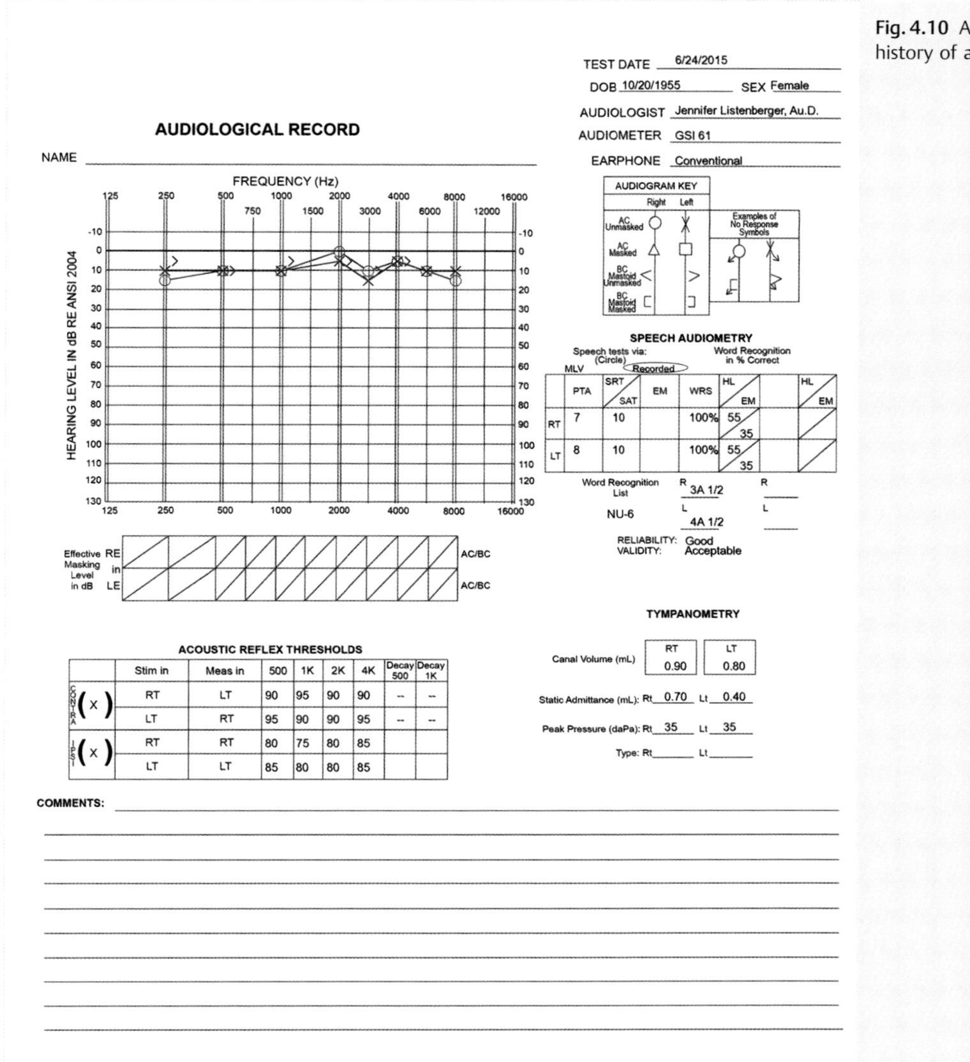

AUDIOLOGICAL RECORD

TEST DATE 6/24/2015
DOB 10/20/1955 SEX Female
AUDIOLOGIST Jennifer Listenberger, Au.D.
AUDIOMETER GSI 61
EARPHONE Conventional

NAME

SPEECH AUDIOMETRY

Speech tests via: (Circle) MLV Recorded

Word Recognition in % Correct

	PTA	SRT/SAT	EM	WRS	HL/EM		HL/EM
RT	7	10		100%	55/35		
LT	8	10		100%	55/35		

Word Recognition List NU-6: R 3A 1/2; L 4A 1/2

RELIABILITY: Good
VALIDITY: Acceptable

TYMPANOMETRY

	RT	LT
Canal Volume (mL)	0.90	0.80
Static Admittance (mL)	0.70	0.40
Peak Pressure (daPa)	35	35
Type		

ACOUSTIC REFLEX THRESHOLDS

	Stim in	Meas in	500	1K	2K	4K	Decay 500	Decay 1K
CONTRA	RT	LT	90	95	90	90	--	--
	LT	RT	95	90	90	95	--	--
IPSI	RT	RT	80	75	80	85		
	LT	LT	85	80	80	85		

COMMENTS:

Fig. 4.10 Audiogram of a patient with a 2-month history of a sensation of a plugged right ear.

4.10.2 Interpretation

Right ear—Pure-tone air and bone conduction threshold testing revealed normal hearing sensitivity at 250 through 8,000 Hz. The SRT revealed a normal ability to receive speech and was in agreement with the PTA. The WRS revealed a normal ability to recognize speech. Immittance testing revealed a normal tympanogram. The acoustic reflex thresholds were present and normal for ipsilateral and contralateral stimulation for 500 to 4,000 Hz. The acoustic reflex decay was negative for contralateral stimulation at 500 and 1,000 Hz.

Left ear—Pure-tone air and bone conduction threshold testing revealed normal hearing sensitivity at 250 through 8,000 Hz. The SRT revealed a normal ability to receive speech and was in agreement with the PTA. The WRS revealed a normal ability to recognize speech. Immittance testing revealed a normal tympanogram. The acoustic reflex thresholds were present and normal for ipsilateral and contralateral stimulation for 500 to 4,000 Hz. The acoustic reflex decay was negative for contralateral stimulation at 500 and 1,000 Hz.

4.10.3 Intervention

The patient was recommended to follow up with the otologist as scheduled. The audiologic recommendation was to return for a hearing test as needed.

5 Sensorineural Hearing Loss Cases

5.1 Case 1

5.1.1 Case History

The patient reported that his hearing began to decrease bilaterally over 20 years ago. He stated he began to use amplification approximately 12 years ago and now was on his second pair of hearing aids. He reported his hearing has continued to decline, and he was noting that he was struggling to hear in most situations. He also stated that if he did not look at the person who was speaking he could not understand what was said. He did not feel he could use the phone any longer because, although he could hear the caller talking, he was not able to understand what was being said.

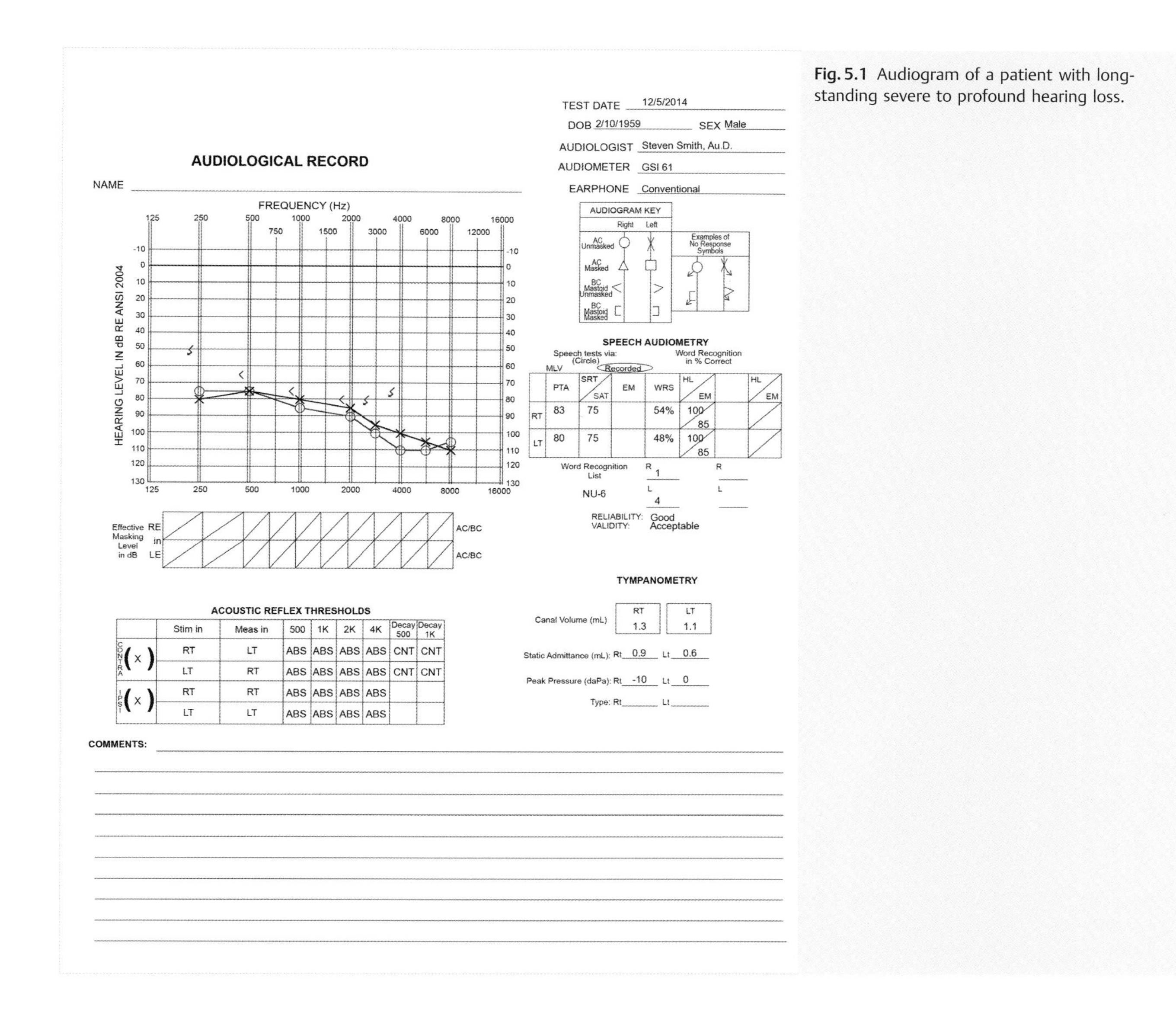

AUDIOLOGICAL RECORD

NAME

TEST DATE 12/5/2014
DOB 2/10/1959 SEX Male
AUDIOLOGIST Steven Smith, Au.D.
AUDIOMETER GSI 61
EARPHONE Conventional

SPEECH AUDIOMETRY

Speech tests via: (Circle) MLV Recorded

Word Recognition in % Correct

	PTA	SRT / SAT	EM	WRS	HL / EM		HL / EM
RT	83	75		54%	100 / 85		
LT	80	75		48%	100 / 85		

Word Recognition List: R 1, L 4 — NU-6

RELIABILITY: Good
VALIDITY: Acceptable

TYMPANOMETRY

	RT	LT
Canal Volume (mL)	1.3	1.1

Static Admittance (mL): Rt 0.9 Lt 0.6
Peak Pressure (daPa): Rt -10 Lt 0
Type: Rt ____ Lt ____

ACOUSTIC REFLEX THRESHOLDS

	Stim in	Meas in	500	1K	2K	4K	Decay 500	Decay 1K
CONTRA	RT	LT	ABS	ABS	ABS	ABS	CNT	CNT
	LT	RT	ABS	ABS	ABS	ABS	CNT	CNT
IPSI	RT	RT	ABS	ABS	ABS	ABS		
	LT	LT	ABS	ABS	ABS	ABS		

COMMENTS:

Fig. 5.1 Audiogram of a patient with long-standing severe to profound hearing loss.

5.1.2 Interpretation

Right ear—Severe sensorineural hearing loss at 250 through 2,000 Hz, sloping to profound at 3,000 through 8,000 Hz. The SRT revealed a severe loss in the ability to receive speech and was in agreement with the PTA. The WRS was poor. Immittance testing revealed a normal tympanogram with absent acoustic reflexes with ipsilateral and contralateral stimulation from 500 to 4,000 Hz. Reflex decay was not measured due to absent reflex thresholds.

Left ear—Severe sensorineural hearing loss at 250 through 2,000 Hz, sloping to profound at 3,000 through 8,000 Hz. The SRT revealed a severe loss in the ability to receive speech and was in agreement with the PTA. The WRS was very poor. Immittance testing revealed a normal tympanogram with absent acoustic reflex thresholds with ipsilateral and contralateral stimulation from 500 to 4,000 Hz. Reflex decay was not measured due to absent reflex thresholds.

5.1.3 Intervention

The patient was referred to an ENT specialist for consideration for cochlear implantation due to poor and very poor word recognition. He was found to be a surgical candidate for a cochlear implant and was referred for a formal cochlear implant evaluation.

5.2 Case 2

5.2.1 Case History

The patient reported decreased hearing bilaterally for 4 to 6 months due to air bag deployment from a car accident. He also noted constant and bothersome tinnitus. He thought the left ear was poorer than the right ear. A computerized tomography scan was performed, and the results were normal. He also noticed a sensation of ear pressure. He had a hearing test prior to the accident that was used for comparison to today's hearing test. He did not report other otologic symptoms or history.

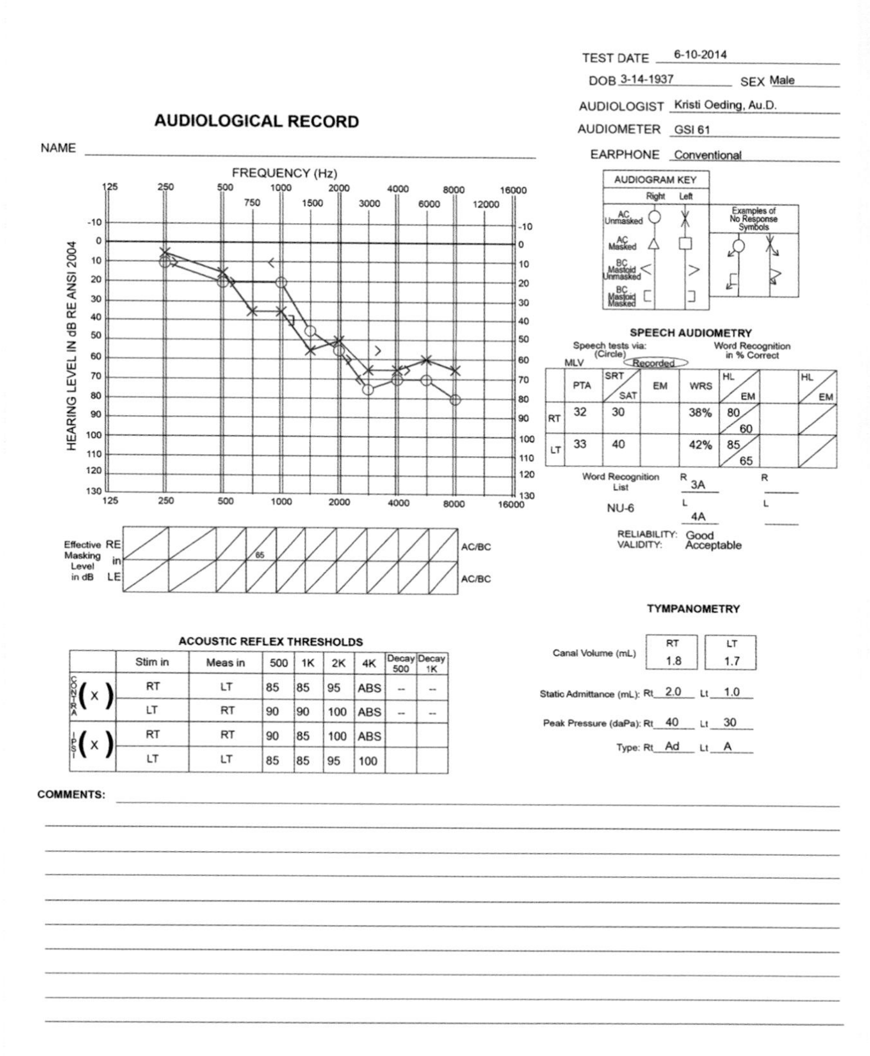

AUDIOLOGICAL RECORD

NAME

TEST DATE 6-10-2014
DOB 3-14-1937 SEX Male
AUDIOLOGIST Kristi Oeding, Au.D.
AUDIOMETER GSI 61
EARPHONE Conventional

FREQUENCY (Hz): 125, 250, 500, 750, 1000, 1500, 2000, 3000, 4000, 6000, 8000, 12000, 16000

HEARING LEVEL IN dB RE ANSI 2004: -10 to 130

AUDIOGRAM KEY (Right / Left): AC Unmasked; AC Masked; BC Mastoid Unmasked; BC Mastoid Masked. Examples of No Response Symbols

Effective Masking Level in dB: RE in LE — AC/BC; 85

SPEECH AUDIOMETRY

Speech tests via: (Circle) MLV Recorded (circled)

Word Recognition in % Correct

	PTA	SRT / SAT	EM	WRS	HL / EM		HL / EM
RT	32	30		38%	80 / 60		
LT	33	40		42%	85 / 65		

Word Recognition List NU-6: R 3A; L 4A

RELIABILITY: Good
VALIDITY: Acceptable

TYMPANOMETRY

Canal Volume (mL): RT 1.8; LT 1.7
Static Admittance (mL): Rt 2.0 Lt 1.0
Peak Pressure (daPa): Rt 40 Lt 30
Type: Rt Ad Lt A

ACOUSTIC REFLEX THRESHOLDS

	Stim in	Meas in	500	1K	2K	4K	Decay 500	Decay 1K
CONTRA (X)	RT	LT	85	85	95	ABS	--	--
	LT	RT	90	90	100	ABS	--	--
IPSI (X)	RT	RT	90	85	100	ABS		
	LT	LT	85	85	95	100		

COMMENTS:

Fig. 5.2 Audiogram of a patient who had a decrease in hearing after a car accident with airbag deployment.

5.2.2 Interpretation

Right ear—Pure-tone thresholds were within normal limits to a slight sensorineural hearing loss from 250 to 1,000 Hz, then sloping to a moderate to severe sensorineural hearing loss from 1,500 to 8,000 Hz. The SRT revealed a mild loss in the ability to receive speech and was in agreement with the PTA. The WRS revealed a very poor ability to recognize speech. Immittance testing revealed a hypercompliant tympanic membrane with normal acoustic reflex thresholds to ipsilateral and contralateral stimulation from 500 to 2,000 Hz and absent acoustic reflex thresholds at 4,000 Hz for ipsilateral and contralateral stimulation. Acoustic reflex decay was negative at 500 Hz and 1,000 Hz.

Left ear—Pure-tone thresholds were within normal limits from 250 to 500 Hz and sloping from a mild to moderately severe sensorineural hearing loss from 750 to 8,000 Hz. The SRT revealed a mild loss in the ability to receive speech and was in agreement with the PTA. The WRS revealed a very poor ability to recognize speech. Immittance testing revealed a normal tympanogram with normal acoustic reflex thresholds to ipsilateral and contralateral stimulation from 500 to 4,000 Hz, except for an absent acoustic reflex threshold at 4,000 Hz for contralateral stimulation. Acoustic reflex decay was negative at 500 and 1,000 Hz.

5.2.3 Intervention

A significant decrease was noted in pure-tone thresholds and the WRS decreased by approximately 50% and 70% in the left and right ears, respectively. The patient was referred for a cochlear implant evaluation, but preferred the cosmetics of hearing aids and was fit with hearing aids and HAT for the TV, phone, and computer. Other audiological recommendations included an annual hearing test and hearing protection in noise.

5.3 Case 3

5.3.1 Case History

The patient was a 40-year-old man with Alport's syndrome and reported a diagnosis of some hearing loss during grade school with stable hearing until college. He reported a rapid decline in hearing over the past 2 years with a noticeable increase in the need for repetition in quiet settings at home and work, as well as increased difficulty understanding speech in noisy situations. He denied any tinnitus, dizziness, or aural pressure or fullness at that time. There was no significant history of ear pathology, ear surgery, or noise exposure. The patient's mother has Alport's syndrome and a significant hearing loss. He reported having a kidney transplant approximately 20 years ago that failed within 5 years of completion of the procedure. He was currently on kidney dialysis. There were no hearing tests available for comparison. The patient had not used hearing aids, but did use HAT for the television and theater.

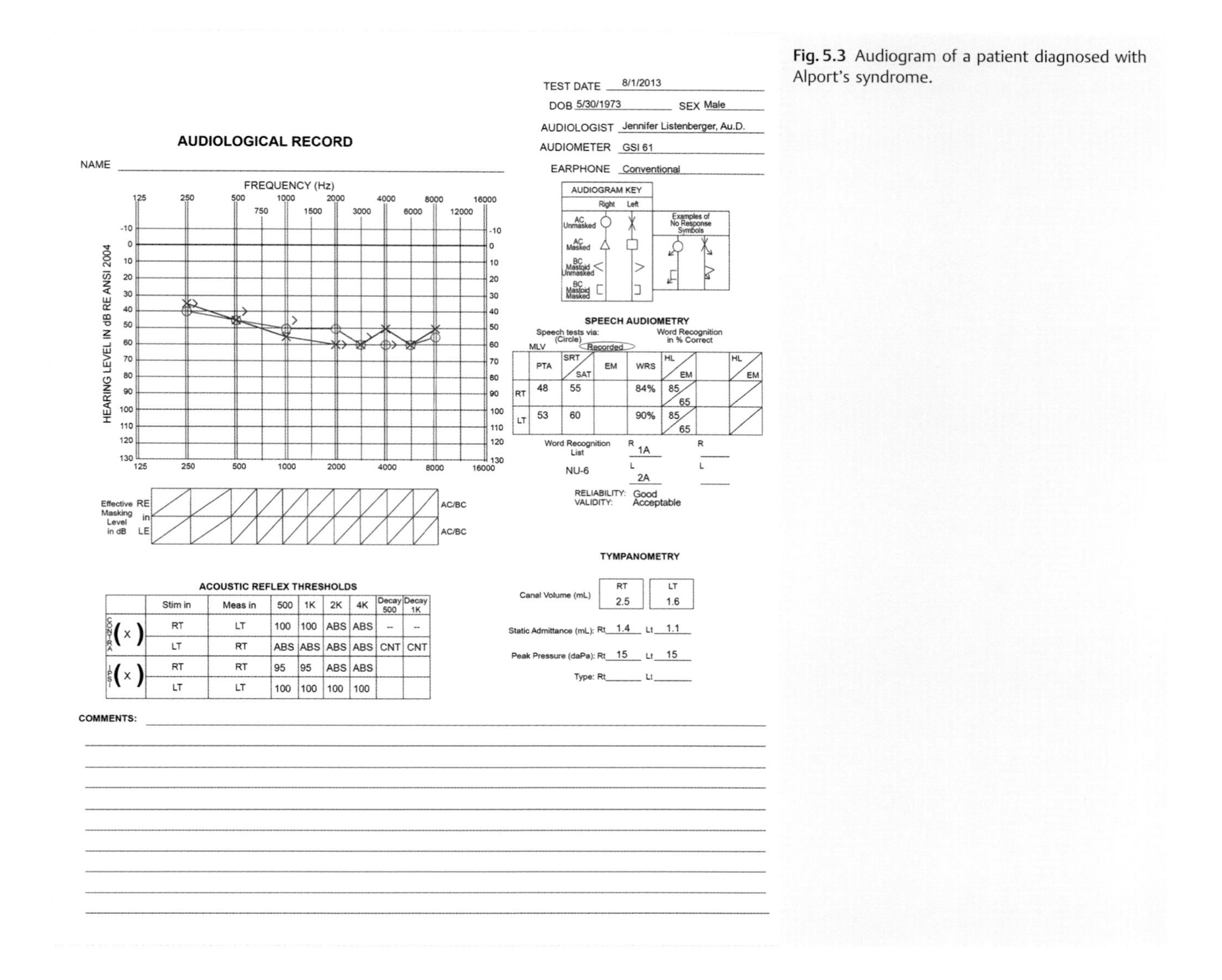

AUDIOLOGICAL RECORD

NAME

TEST DATE 8/1/2013
DOB 5/30/1973 SEX Male
AUDIOLOGIST Jennifer Listenberger, Au.D.
AUDIOMETER GSI 61
EARPHONE Conventional

SPEECH AUDIOMETRY

Speech tests via: (Circle) MLV Recorded

Word Recognition in % Correct

	PTA	SRT/SAT	EM	WRS	HL/EM		HL/EM
RT	48	55		84%	85/65		
LT	53	60		90%	85/65		

Word Recognition List NU-6: R 1A, L 2A; R ___, L ___

RELIABILITY: Good
VALIDITY: Acceptable

Effective Masking Level in dB: RE in AC/BC; LE in AC/BC

TYMPANOMETRY

	RT	LT
Canal Volume (mL)	2.5	1.6

Static Admittance (mL): Rt 1.4 Lt 1.1
Peak Pressure (daPa): Rt 15 Lt 15
Type: Rt ___ Lt ___

ACOUSTIC REFLEX THRESHOLDS

	Stim in	Meas in	500	1K	2K	4K	Decay 500	Decay 1K
CONTRA (X)	RT	LT	100	100	ABS	ABS	--	--
	LT	RT	ABS	ABS	ABS	ABS	CNT	CNT
IPSI (X)	RT	RT	95	95	ABS	ABS		
	LT	LT	100	100	100	100		

COMMENTS:

Fig. 5.3 Audiogram of a patient diagnosed with Alport's syndrome.

5.3.2 Interpretation

Right Ear—Mild sensorineural hearing loss at 250 Hz, sloping to moderate at 500 to 2,000 Hz, sloping to moderately severe at 3,000 to 6,000 Hz, and rising to moderate at 8,000 Hz. The SRT revealed a moderate loss in the ability to receive speech and was in agreement with the PTA. The WRS revealed slight difficulty in the ability to recognize speech. Immittance testing revealed a normal tympanogram and normal acoustic reflex thresholds from 500 to 1,000 Hz and absent from 2,000 to 4,000 Hz to ipsilateral stimulation and absent thresholds from 500 to 4,000 Hz to contralateral stimulation. Acoustic reflex decay could not be measured.

Left Ear—Mild sensorineural hearing loss at 250 Hz, sloping to moderate to moderately severe at 500 to 3,000 Hz, and rising and sloping to moderate and moderately severe at 4,000 to 6,000 Hz, and rising to moderate at 8,000 Hz. The SRT revealed a moderately severe loss in the ability to receive speech and was in agreement with the PTA. The WRS revealed a normal ability to recognize speech. Immittance testing revealed a normal tympanogram, normal acoustic reflex thresholds from 500 to 4,000 Hz to ipsilateral stimulation, and normal acoustic reflex thresholds from 500 to 1,000 Hz and absent from 2,000 to 4,000 Hz to contralateral stimulation, and negative contralateral reflex decay at 500 and 1,000 Hz.

5.3.3 Intervention

An ENT specialist medically cleared the patient for amplification. Audiological recommendations included annual hearing testing to monitor progression of hearing loss, evaluation for amplification and HAT options, and hearing protection in noise.

5.4 Case 4

5.4.1 Case History

The patient, a professor, started to notice difficulty hearing students in class a few years prior. He reported that students sounded like they were mumbling, and he asked them to repeat. He also stated he had difficulty hearing speech in noise.

The patient reported a long-standing history of tinnitus bilaterally. Seemingly, the intensity of the tinnitus had increased in the last 2 months. He denied dizziness, otalgia, or aural pressure.

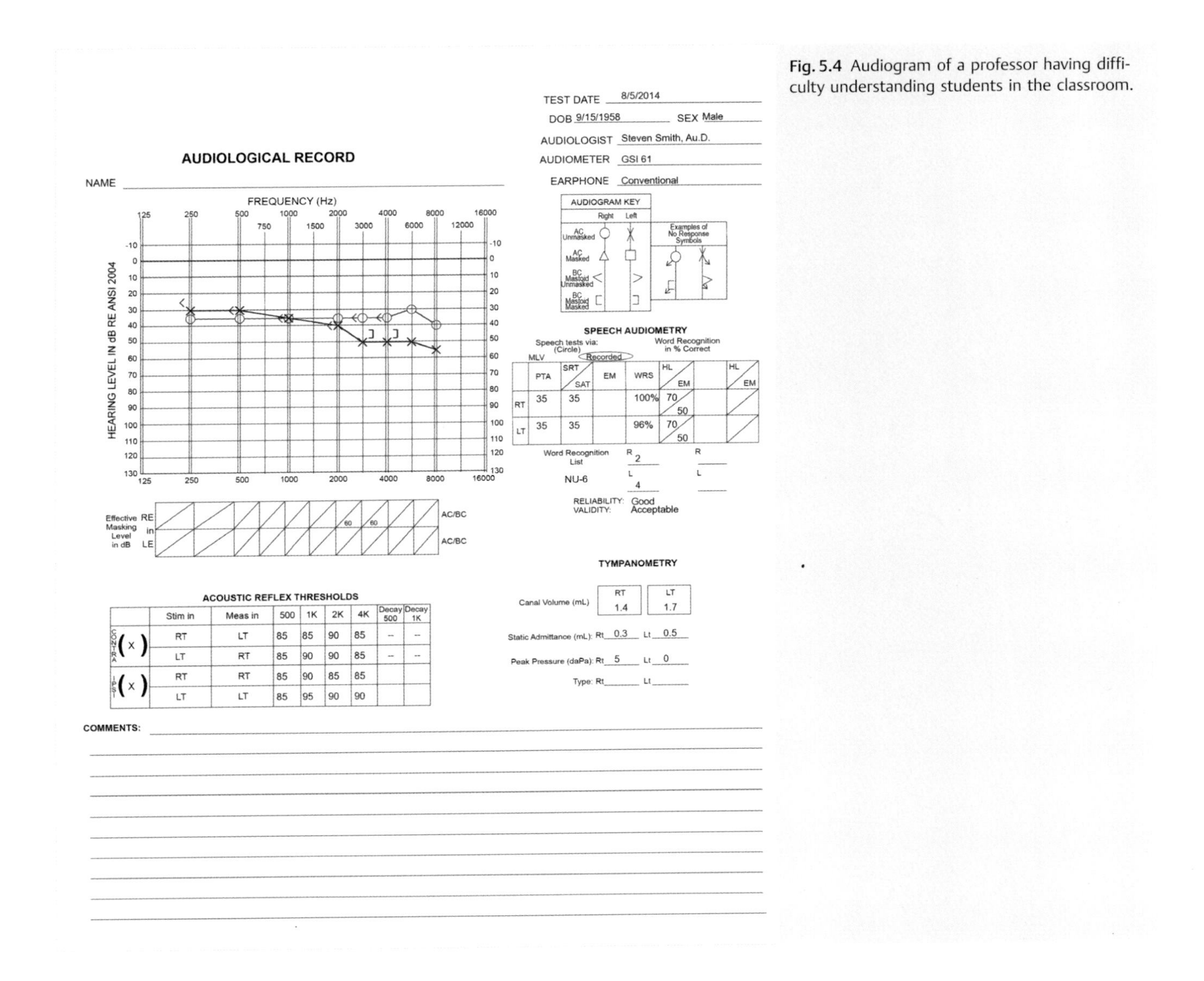

AUDIOLOGICAL RECORD

NAME

TEST DATE 8/5/2014
DOB 9/15/1958 SEX Male
AUDIOLOGIST Steven Smith, Au.D.
AUDIOMETER GSI 61
EARPHONE Conventional

FREQUENCY (Hz)

HEARING LEVEL IN dB RE ANSI 2004

AUDIOGRAM KEY: Right / Left; AC Unmasked; AC Masked; BC Mastoid Unmasked; BC Mastoid Masked; Examples of No Response Symbols

Effective Masking Level in dB: RE in AC/BC — 60, 60; LE in AC/BC

SPEECH AUDIOMETRY

Speech tests via: (Circle) MLV / Recorded (circled)

Word Recognition in % Correct

	PTA	SRT/SAT	EM	WRS	HL/EM		HL/EM
RT	35	35		100%	70/50		
LT	35	35		96%	70/50		

Word Recognition List: R 2, L 4

NU-6

RELIABILITY: Good
VALIDITY: Acceptable

ACOUSTIC REFLEX THRESHOLDS

	Stim in	Meas in	500	1K	2K	4K	Decay 500	Decay 1K
CONTRA (x)	RT	LT	85	85	90	85	--	--
	LT	RT	85	90	90	85	--	--
IPSI (x)	RT	RT	85	90	85	85		
	LT	LT	85	95	90	90		

TYMPANOMETRY

	RT	LT
Canal Volume (mL)	1.4	1.7

Static Admittance (mL): Rt 0.3 Lt 0.5
Peak Pressure (daPa): Rt 5 Lt 0
Type: Rt ____ Lt ____

COMMENTS:

Fig. 5.4 Audiogram of a professor having difficulty understanding students in the classroom.

5.4.2 Interpretation

Right ear—Mild sensorineural hearing loss from 250 to 8,000 Hz. The SRT revealed a mild loss in the ability to receive speech and was in agreement with the PTA. The WRS was normal. Immittance testing revealed a normal tympanogram. Acoustic reflex thresholds were normal with ipsilateral and contralateral stimulation from 500 to 4,000 Hz. Acoustic reflex decay was negative with contralateral stimulation at 500 and 1,000 Hz.

Left ear—Mild sloping to a moderate sensorineural hearing loss from 250 to 8,000 Hz. The SRT revealed a mild loss in the ability to receive speech and was in agreement with the PTA. The WRS was normal. Immittance testing revealed a normal tympanogram. Acoustic reflex thresholds were normal with ipsilateral and contralateral stimulation from 500 to 4,000 Hz. Acoustic reflex decay was negative with contralateral stimulation at 500 and 1,000 Hz.

5.4.3 Intervention

The patient was referred to an ENT specialist due to the asymmetrical sensorineural hearing loss and increased intensity of bilateral tinnitus. The physician did not determine any medical concerns regarding his hearing loss and tinnitus. The patient returned to audiology for a hearing aid evaluation and obtained amplification.

5.5 Case 5

5.5.1 Case History

The patient reported bilateral hearing loss, with the right ear being poorer than the left ear. The right ear had progressive hearing loss due to Ménière's disease, and the left ear had gradually decreased over time due to presbycusis and a history of noise exposure. He had an MRI in the past that was normal. He was considering a cochlear implant and possibly new hearing aid technology, in particular, new BICROS technology. He did not report other otologic symptoms or history. The patient had a previous audiogram approximately a year ago.

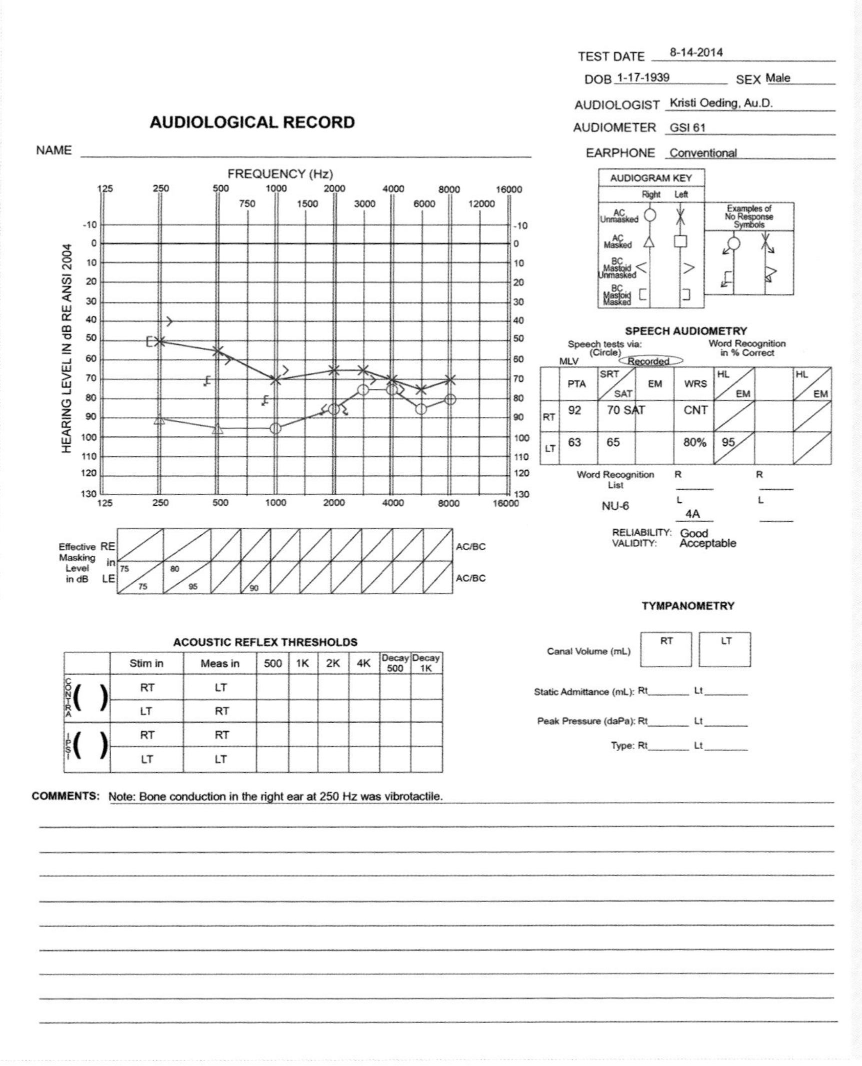

AUDIOLOGICAL RECORD

NAME

TEST DATE 8-14-2014

DOB 1-17-1939 SEX Male

AUDIOLOGIST Kristi Oeding, Au.D.

AUDIOMETER GSI 61

EARPHONE Conventional

SPEECH AUDIOMETRY

Speech tests via: (Circle) MLV Recorded

Word Recognition in % Correct

	PTA	SRT / SAT	EM	WRS	HL / EM	HL / EM
RT	92	70 SAT		CNT		
LT	63	65		80%	95	

Word Recognition List: NU-6, L 4A

RELIABILITY: Good

VALIDITY: Acceptable

Effective Masking Level in dB: RE in LE — 75, 80, 75, 95, 90 (AC/BC)

ACOUSTIC REFLEX THRESHOLDS

	Stim in	Meas in	500	1K	2K	4K	Decay 500	Decay 1K
CONTRA	RT	LT						
	LT	RT						
IPSI	RT	RT						
	LT	LT						

TYMPANOMETRY

Canal Volume (mL): RT ___ LT ___

Static Admittance (mL): Rt ___ Lt ___

Peak Pressure (daPa): Rt ___ Lt ___

Type: Rt ___ Lt ___

COMMENTS: Note: Bone conduction in the right ear at 250 Hz was vibrotactile.

Fig. 5.5 Audiogram of a patient with Ménière's disease in the right ear who was interested in a BICROS or a cochlear implant.

5.5.2 Interpretation

Right ear—Pure-tone thresholds revealed a severe to profound sensorineural hearing loss from 250 to 1,000 Hz, rising to severe from 2,000 to 8,000 Hz. The SAT revealed a moderately severe loss in the ability to detect speech and was in poor agreement with the PTA, which may be due to the rising configuration of the hearing loss. The WRS could not be measured due to the severity of the hearing loss and the patient's ability to detect, but not recognize, speech. Immittance testing was not performed at this follow-up appointment because there were no significant changes.

Left ear—Pure-tone thresholds revealed a moderate sloping to a severe sensorineural hearing loss from 250 to 6,000 Hz and rising to a moderately severe hearing loss at 8,000 Hz. The SRT revealed a moderately severe loss in the ability to receive speech and was in agreement with the PTA. The WRS revealed slight difficulty in the ability to recognize speech. Immittance testing was not performed at this follow-up appointment because there were no significant changes.

5.5.3 Intervention

The otologist discussed the option of a cochlear implant and a hearing aid trial. The patient was fit with new BICROS hearing aid technology and perceived significant benefit with the BICROS. He decided not to pursue a cochlear implant at that time.

5.6 Case 6

5.6.1 Case History

The patient reported bilateral hearing loss for approximately 10 years. She had not had a hearing examination prior to today. There was a significant family history of hearing loss in that the patient's mother, maternal aunt, one sibling, and a son all had varying degrees of hearing loss. The patient denied any tinnitus or dizziness. There was no reported history of ear pathology, ear surgery, or noise exposure. The patient did not report any rapid progression in hearing loss, but reported increased difficulty in understanding soft speech at home and work.

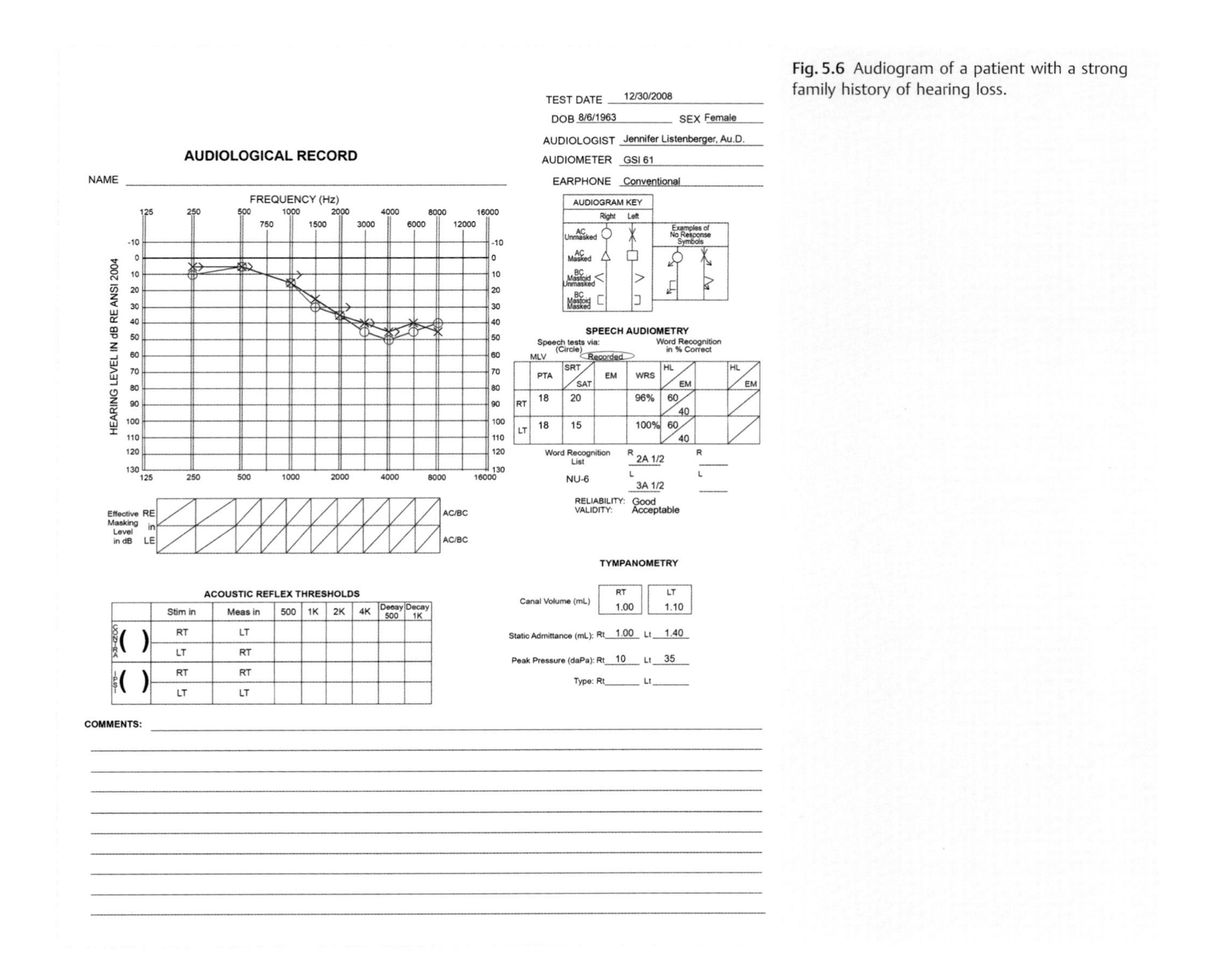

Fig. 5.6 Audiogram of a patient with a strong family history of hearing loss.

5.6.2 Interpretation

Right ear—Normal hearing sensitivity at 250 to 1,000 Hz, sloping to a mild sensorineural hearing loss at 1,500 to 2,000 Hz, sloping to moderate at 3,000 to 6,000 Hz, and rising to mild at 8,000 Hz. The SRT revealed a slight loss in the ability to receive speech and was in agreement with the PTA. The WRS revealed a normal ability to recognize speech. Immittance testing revealed a normal tympanogram. Acoustic reflex threshold and decay testing were not measured.

Left ear—Normal hearing sensitivity at 250 to 1,000 Hz and sloping to slight to mild sensorineural hearing loss at 1,500 to 6,000 Hz, with moderate thresholds at 4,000 and 8,000 Hz. SRT revealed a normal ability to receive speech and was in agreement with the PTA. The WRS revealed a normal ability to recognize speech. Immittance testing revealed a normal tympanogram. Acoustic reflex threshold and decay testing were not measured.

5.6.3 Recommendations/Intervention

An otologic consultation was completed, and the patient was medically cleared for amplification. Audiological recommendations included annual testing to monitor progression of hearing loss, evaluation for amplification and HAT options, and hearing protection in noise.

5.7 Case 7

5.7.1 Case History

A 46-year-old female stated she had a hearing evaluation completed many years ago and, reportedly, revealed a mild high-frequency sensorineural hearing loss in the left ear. She stated that her hearing may have declined in that ear in the last few months. She reported normal hearing in the right ear. She denied tinnitus or dizziness as well as otalgia or aural pressure/fullness.

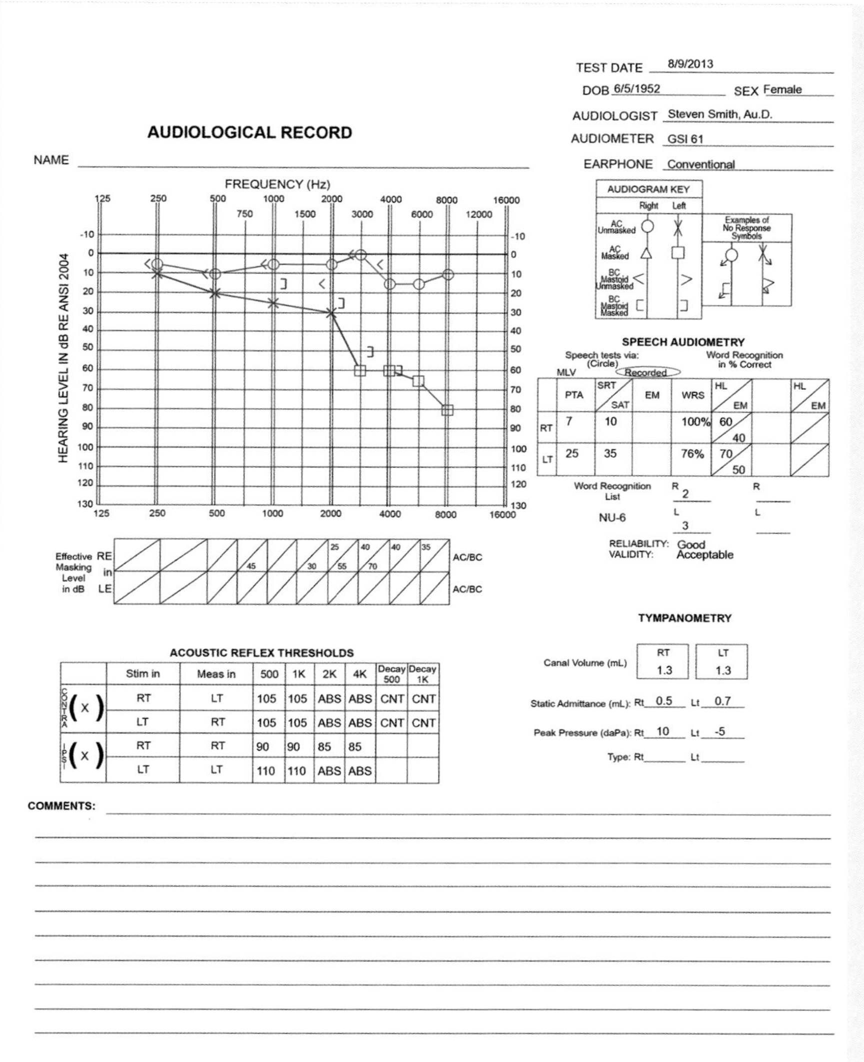

AUDIOLOGICAL RECORD

NAME

TEST DATE 8/9/2013

DOB 6/5/1952 SEX Female

AUDIOLOGIST Steven Smith, Au.D.

AUDIOMETER GSI 61

EARPHONE Conventional

FREQUENCY (Hz)

HEARING LEVEL IN dB RE ANSI 2004

AUDIOGRAM KEY: Right / Left; AC Unmasked; AC Masked; BC Mastoid Unmasked; BC Mastoid Masked; Examples of No Response Symbols

Effective Masking Level in dB: RE 25, 40, 40, 35 (AC/BC); in LE 45, 30, 55, 70 (AC/BC)

SPEECH AUDIOMETRY

Speech tests via: (Circle) MLV Recorded

Word Recognition in % Correct

	PTA	SRT/SAT	EM	WRS	HL/EM	HL/EM
RT	7	10		100%	60/40	
LT	25	35		76%	70/50	

Word Recognition List NU-6: R 2, L 3

RELIABILITY: Good

VALIDITY: Acceptable

ACOUSTIC REFLEX THRESHOLDS

	Stim in	Meas in	500	1K	2K	4K	Decay 500	Decay 1K
CONTRA	RT	LT	105	105	ABS	ABS	CNT	CNT
	LT	RT	105	105	ABS	ABS	CNT	CNT
IPSI	RT	RT	90	90	85	85		
	LT	LT	110	110	ABS	ABS		

TYMPANOMETRY

	RT	LT
Canal Volume (mL)	1.3	1.3

Static Admittance (mL): Rt 0.5 Lt 0.7

Peak Pressure (daPa): Rt 10 Lt -5

Type: Rt Lt

COMMENTS:

Fig. 5.7 Audiogram of a patient with hearing loss in the left ear and normal hearing in the right.

5.7.2 Interpretation

Right ear—Normal hearing sensitivity from 250 Hz through 8,000 Hz. The SRT revealed a normal ability to receive speech and was in agreement with the PTA. The WRS was normal. Immittance testing revealed a normal tympanogram with normal acoustic reflex thresholds with ipsilateral stimulation. Contralateral stimulation revealed present, but elevated acoustic reflex thresholds at 500 and 1,000 Hz and absent acoustic reflex thresholds at 2,000 and 4,000 Hz. Acoustic reflex decay with contralateral stimulation at 500 and 1,000 Hz could not be measured due to the elevated contralateral acoustic reflex thresholds.

Left ear—Normal hearing sensitivity sloping to mild sensorineural hearing loss at 250 through 2,000 Hz, steeply sloping to moderately severe to severe at 3,000 through 8,000 Hz. The SRT revealed a mild loss in the ability to receive speech and was in agreement with the PTA. The WRS revealed slight difficulty in the ability to recognize speech. Immittance testing revealed a normal tympanogram with present, but elevated acoustic reflex thresholds with ipsilateral and contralateral stimulation at 500 and 1,000 Hz. Acoustic reflex thresholds were absent at 2,000 and 4,000 Hz with ipsilateral and contralateral stimulation. Acoustic reflex decay with contralateral stimulation at 500 and 1,000 Hz could not be measured due to the elevated contralateral acoustic reflex thresholds.

5.7.3 Intervention

The patient was referred to an ENT specialist due to the sensorineural hearing loss in the left ear. She was evaluated by the physician and referred for an MRI. A cerebellopontine angle tumor was found on the left side. She was counseled that she could have the tumor removed through a translabyrinthine approach or have gamma knife surgery. She opted for gamma knife surgery for management of the cerebellopontine angle tumor. Postsurgical follow-up hearing testing was recommended.

5.8 Case 8

5.8.1 Case History

The patient reported bilateral hearing loss for several years that had been progressive. She reported a family history of hearing loss with her mother and grandmother having hearing loss. She was noticing difficulty hearing the students that she taught and wanted to hear better in the classroom. She also had difficulty hearing her husband and soft voices. She did not report other otologic symptoms or history.

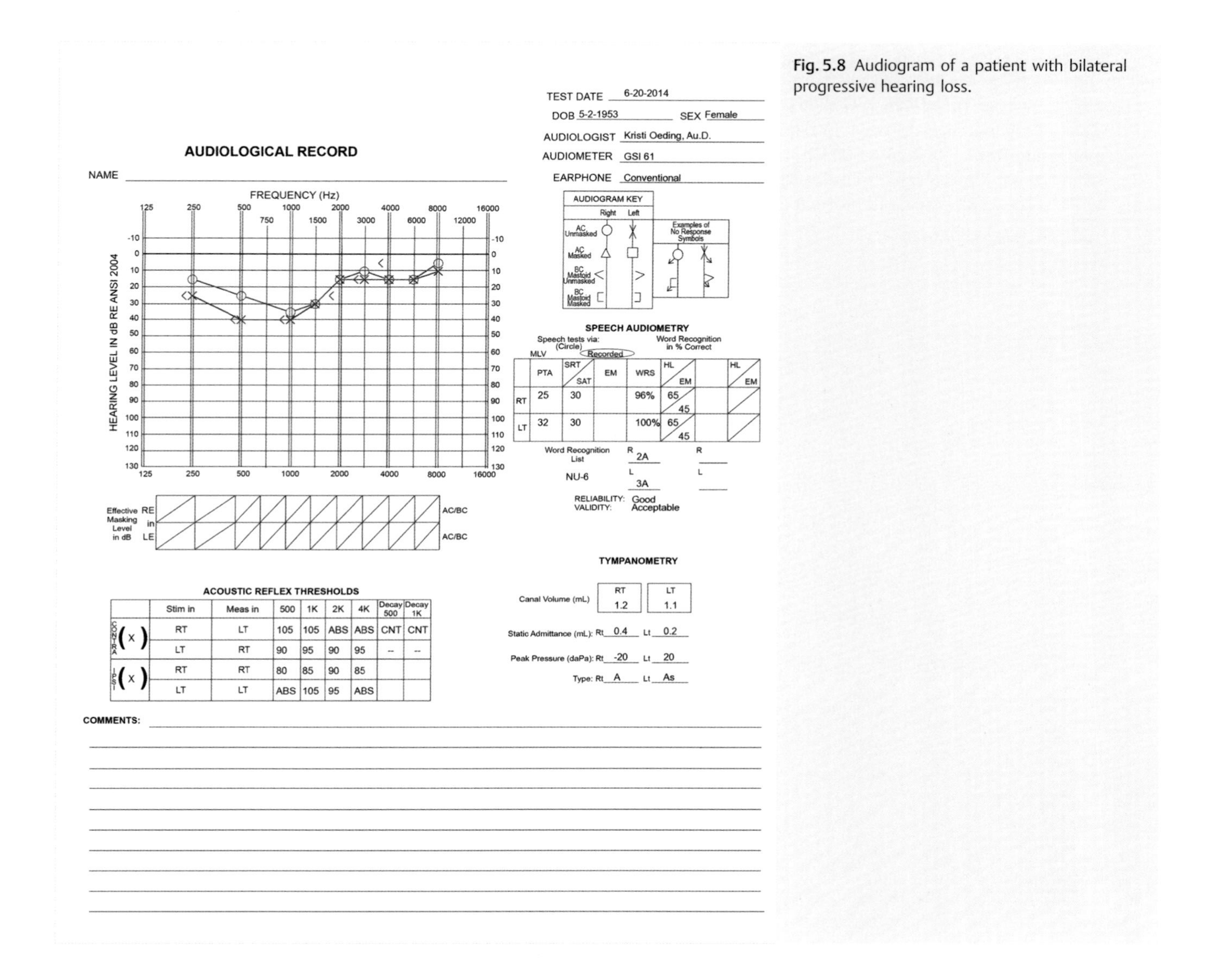

AUDIOLOGICAL RECORD

NAME

TEST DATE 6-20-2014

DOB 5-2-1953 SEX Female

AUDIOLOGIST Kristi Oeding, Au.D.

AUDIOMETER GSI 61

EARPHONE Conventional

SPEECH AUDIOMETRY

Speech tests via: (Circle) MLV Recorded (circled)

Word Recognition in % Correct

	PTA	SRT/SAT	EM	WRS	HL/EM		HL/EM
RT	25	30		96%	65/45		
LT	32	30		100%	65/45		

Word Recognition List NU-6: R 2A; L 3A

RELIABILITY: Good
VALIDITY: Acceptable

TYMPANOMETRY

Canal Volume (mL): RT 1.2 LT 1.1

Static Admittance (mL): Rt 0.4 Lt 0.2

Peak Pressure (daPa): Rt -20 Lt 20

Type: Rt A Lt As

ACOUSTIC REFLEX THRESHOLDS

	Stim in	Meas in	500	1K	2K	4K	Decay 500	Decay 1K
CONTRA (X)	RT	LT	105	105	ABS	ABS	CNT	CNT
	LT	RT	90	95	90	95	--	--
IPSI (X)	RT	RT	80	85	90	85		
	LT	LT	ABS	105	95	ABS		

COMMENTS:

Fig. 5.8 Audiogram of a patient with bilateral progressive hearing loss.

5.8.2 Interpretation

Right ear—Pure-tone thresholds were within normal limits at 250 Hz, sloping to a slight to mild sensorineural hearing loss from 500 to 1,500 Hz, and rising to within normal limits from 2,000 to 8,000 Hz. The SRT revealed a mild loss in the ability to receive speech and was in agreement with the PTA. The WRS revealed a normal ability to recognize speech. Immittance testing revealed a normal tympanogram. The ipsilateral and contralateral acoustic reflex thresholds were within normal limits from 500 to 4,000 Hz. Acoustic reflex decay was negative at 500 Hz and 1,000 Hz.

Left ear—Pure-tone thresholds revealed a slight to mild sensorineural hearing loss from 250 to 1,500 Hz and rising to within normal limits from 2,000 to 8,000 Hz. The SRT revealed a mild loss in the ability to receive speech and was in agreement with the PTA. The WRS revealed a normal ability to recognize speech. Immittance testing revealed a hypocompliant tympanogram. The ipsilateral acoustic reflex thresholds were within normal limits at 2,000 Hz, elevated at 1,000 Hz, and absent at 500 and 4,000 Hz, and the contralateral acoustic reflex thresholds were elevated from 500 to 1,000 Hz and absent from 2,000 to 4,000 Hz. Acoustic reflex decay could not be measured at 500 Hz and 1,000 Hz due to elevated contralateral acoustic reflex thresholds.

5.8.3 Intervention

According to the otologist the cause of her hearing loss was due to genetics. She was fit with bilateral receiver-in-the-canal hearing aids and was able to hear her students well with amplification.

5.9 Case 9

5.9.1 Case History

A 75-year-old male reported sudden hearing loss and sudden onset of facial paralysis on the left side approximately 2 years ago. He reported a diagnosis of Bell's palsy. There had been no reported improvement in facial paralysis or hearing loss. He denied any tinnitus or dizziness. The patient reported communication difficulty due to hearing loss, and he had not had a hearing test prior to today's visit. He reported a significant history of noise exposure in that he worked in an automotive plant for 37 years, and hearing protection was used consistently later in his career. There was no reported familial hearing loss or otosurgery. The patient did report a significant health history of, what was described as, multiple ministrokes for a 1-year period. The last set of known strokes had occurred 5 years ago.

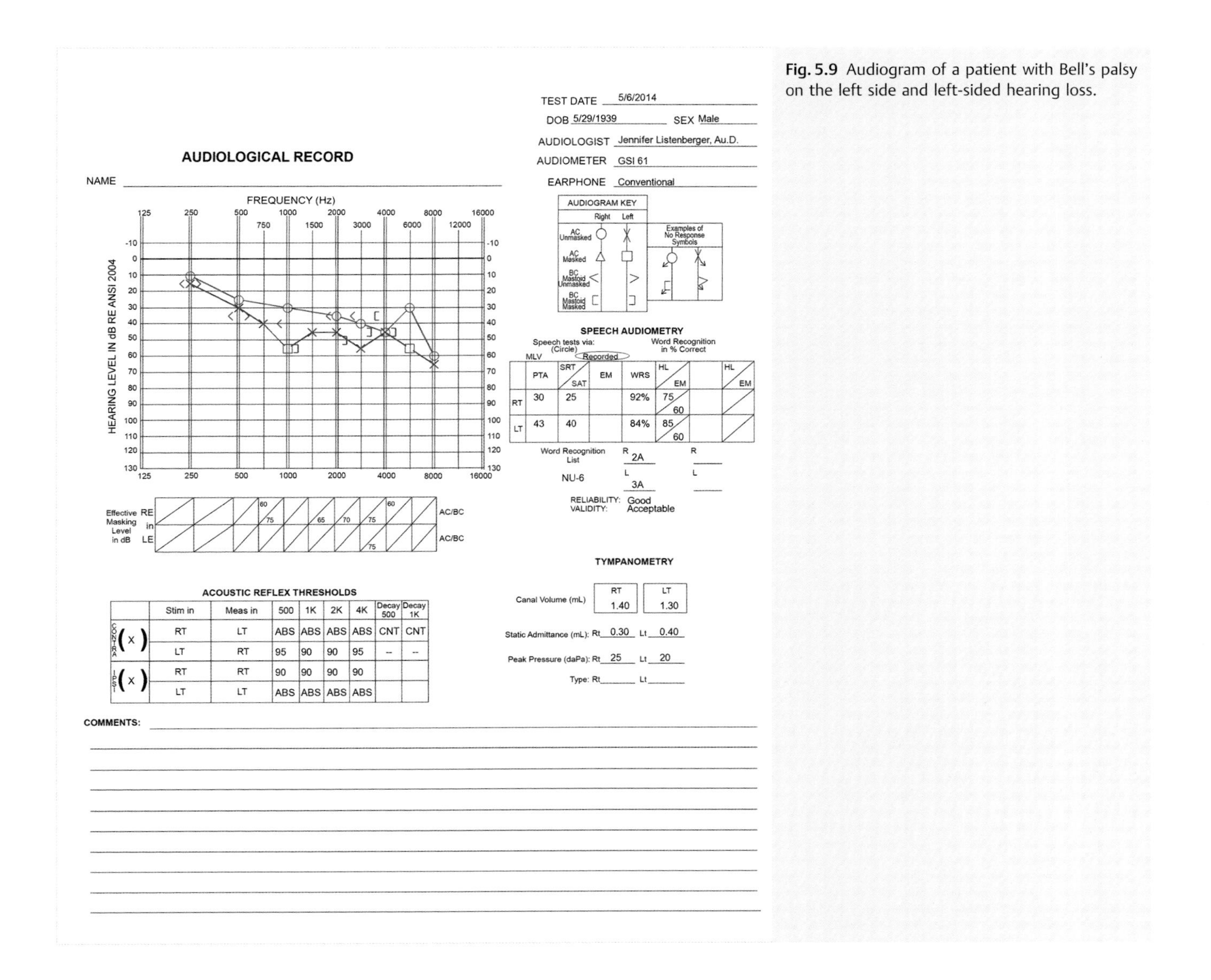

AUDIOLOGICAL RECORD

NAME

TEST DATE 5/6/2014
DOB 5/29/1939 SEX Male
AUDIOLOGIST Jennifer Listenberger, Au.D.
AUDIOMETER GSI 61
EARPHONE Conventional

Effective Masking Level in dB

RE				60 / 75		65	70	75	60		AC/BC
LE								75			AC/BC

SPEECH AUDIOMETRY

Speech tests via: (Circle) MLV Recorded (circled)

Word Recognition in % Correct

	PTA	SRT / SAT	EM	WRS	HL / EM		HL / EM
RT	30	25		92%	75 / 60		
LT	43	40		84%	85 / 60		

Word Recognition List: R 2A, L 3A; R ___, L ___

NU-6

RELIABILITY: Good
VALIDITY: Acceptable

ACOUSTIC REFLEX THRESHOLDS

	Stim in	Meas in	500	1K	2K	4K	Decay 500	Decay 1K
CONTRA (X)	RT	LT	ABS	ABS	ABS	ABS	CNT	CNT
	LT	RT	95	90	90	95	--	--
IPSI (X)	RT	RT	90	90	90	90		
	LT	LT	ABS	ABS	ABS	ABS		

TYMPANOMETRY

	RT	LT
Canal Volume (mL)	1.40	1.30

Static Admittance (mL): Rt 0.30 Lt 0.40
Peak Pressure (daPa): Rt 25 Lt 20
Type: Rt ___ Lt ___

COMMENTS:

Fig. 5.9 Audiogram of a patient with Bell's palsy on the left side and left-sided hearing loss.

5.9.2 Interpretation

Right ear—Pure-tone air and bone conduction threshold testing revealed normal hearing sensitivity at 250 Hz, sloping to a slight to moderate sensorineural hearing loss at 500 to 4,000 Hz, rising to mild at 6,000 Hz, and sloping to moderately severe at 8,000 Hz. The SRT revealed a slight loss in the ability to receive speech and was in agreement with the PTA. The WRS revealed a normal ability to recognize speech. Immittance testing revealed a normal tympanogram and normal acoustic reflex thresholds for ipsilateral and contralateral stimulation at 500 through 4,000 Hz. Acoustic reflex decay was negative at 500 and 1,000 Hz.

Left ear—Pure-tone air and bone conduction threshold testing revealed normal hearing sensitivity at 250 Hz, sloping to mild sensorineural hearing loss at 500 and 750 Hz, sloping to moderate at 1,000 through 6,000 Hz, and sloping to moderately severe at 8,000 Hz. The SRT revealed a mild loss in the ability to receive speech and was in agreement with the PTA. The WRS revealed a slight difficulty in the ability to recognize speech. Immittance testing revealed a normal tympanogram and absent acoustic reflex thresholds for ipsilateral and contralateral stimulation at 500 through 4,000 Hz. Acoustic reflex decay was not measured at 500 Hz or 1,000 Hz due to absent contralateral acoustic reflex thresholds.

5.9.3 Intervention

Patient was referred to an otologist for a medical evaluation due to asymmetric hearing loss. Per the otologist's report, annual follow-up was recommended for cerumen removal and evaluation of symptoms. An annual hearing test was recommended as well as follow-up with audiology for a hearing aid evaluation.

5.10 Case 10

5.10.1 Case History

The patient reported successful use of hearing aids bilaterally for the past 2 years. She stated the hearing in her right ear was slightly worse than the hearing in her left ear. Seemingly, she was not hearing as well as she was previously and was not sure if her hearing aids were malfunctioning or if her hearing had changed. She reported long-standing tinnitus. She denied dizziness, otalgia, and aural pressure or fullness. There was no reported history of loud noise exposure. Previous hearing tests were available for comparison.

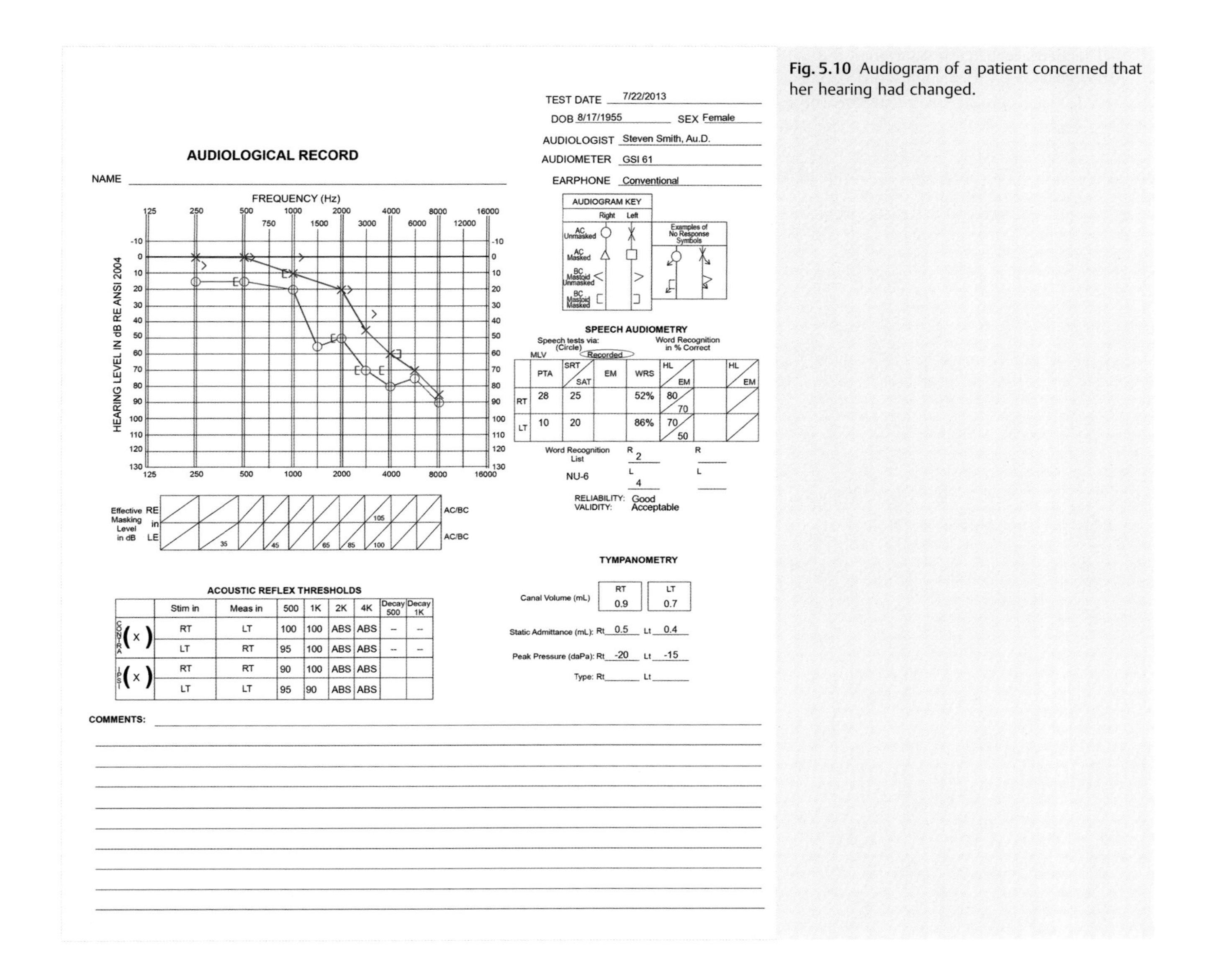

AUDIOLOGICAL RECORD

TEST DATE 7/22/2013
DOB 8/17/1955 SEX Female
AUDIOLOGIST Steven Smith, Au.D.
AUDIOMETER GSI 61
EARPHONE Conventional
NAME

Effective Masking Level in dB

RE								105		AC/BC
LE	35		45		65	85	100			AC/BC

SPEECH AUDIOMETRY

Speech tests via: (Circle) MLV Recorded (circled)

Word Recognition in % Correct

	PTA	SRT/SAT	EM	WRS	HL/EM		HL/EM
RT	28	25		52%	80/70		
LT	10	20		86%	70/50		

Word Recognition List NU-6: R 2, L 4; R ___, L ___

RELIABILITY: Good
VALIDITY: Acceptable

ACOUSTIC REFLEX THRESHOLDS

	Stim in	Meas in	500	1K	2K	4K	Decay 500	Decay 1K
CONTRA (X)	RT	LT	100	100	ABS	ABS	--	--
	LT	RT	95	100	ABS	ABS	--	--
IPSI (X)	RT	RT	90	100	ABS	ABS		
	LT	LT	95	90	ABS	ABS		

TYMPANOMETRY

	RT	LT
Canal Volume (mL)	0.9	0.7

Static Admittance (mL): Rt 0.5 Lt 0.4
Peak Pressure (daPa): Rt -20 Lt -15
Type: Rt ___ Lt ___

COMMENTS:

Fig. 5.10 Audiogram of a patient concerned that her hearing had changed.

5.10.2 Interpretation

Right ear—Normal to a slight sensorineural hearing loss from 250 to 1,000 Hz, steeply sloping to a moderate sensorineural hearing loss at 1,500 to 2,000 Hz, sloping to moderately severe and severe at 3,000 to 8,000 Hz. The SRT revealed a slight loss in the ability to receive speech and was in agreement with the PTA. The WRS was poor. Immittance testing revealed a normal tympanogram. Acoustic reflex thresholds were present at 500 and 1,000 Hz and absent at 2,000 and 4,000 Hz with ipsilateral and contralateral stimulation. Acoustic reflex decay was negative with contralateral stimulation at 500 and 1,000 Hz.

Left ear—Normal to a slight sensorineural hearing loss from 250 to 2,000 Hz, sloping to a moderate and severe sensorineural hearing loss at 3,000 to 8,000 Hz. The SRT revealed a slight loss in the ability to receive speech and was in agreement with the PTA. The WRS revealed a slight difficulty. Immittance testing revealed a normal tympanogram. Acoustic reflex thresholds were present at 500 and 1,000 Hz and absent at 2,000 and 4,000 Hz with ipsilateral and contralateral stimulation. Acoustic reflex decay was negative with contralateral stimulation at 500 and 1,000 Hz.

5.10.3 Intervention

Comparison between test results from the previous and current hearing tests revealed a slight decrease at 2,000 and 3,000 Hz in the right ear and a significant decrease in the WRS in the right. The previous WRS was 88%, and the current WRS was 56%. The patient was referred to an ENT specialist due to a significant change in the right ear WRS. The ENT then referred the patient for an ABR to rule out a retrocochlear pathology.

5.11 Case 11

5.11.1 Case History

The patient returned for monthly ototoxic monitoring. She had been taking large doses of amikacin for a lung infection and reported she may take the antibiotics for 1 year. She had a family history of hearing loss—her brother and two uncles on her father's side had hearing loss. She had a minimal history of noise exposure from attending a few concerts. She was on dialysis. Her baseline hearing test revealed normal hearing sensitivity from 250 to 8,000 Hz bilaterally. High-frequency audiometry revealed a slight to moderate hearing loss from 9,000 to 16,000 Hz and no response from 18,000 to 20,000 Hz in the right ear and within normal limits to a moderately severe hearing loss from 9,000 to 14,000 Hz and no response from 16,000 to 20,000 Hz in the left ear. She did not report other otologic symptoms or history.

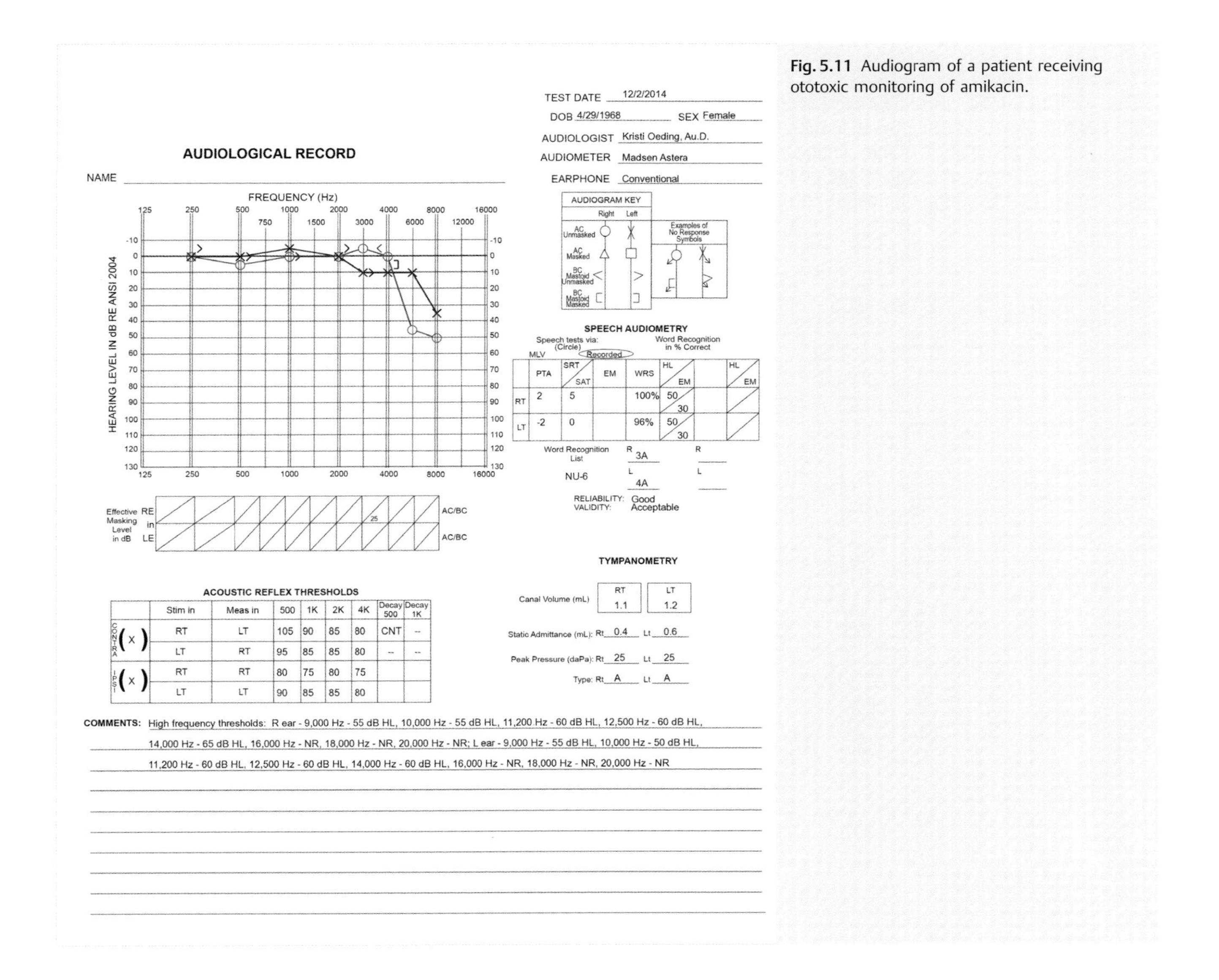

AUDIOLOGICAL RECORD

NAME

TEST DATE 12/2/2014
DOB 4/29/1968 SEX Female
AUDIOLOGIST Kristi Oeding, Au.D.
AUDIOMETER Madsen Astera
EARPHONE Conventional

FREQUENCY (Hz)
HEARING LEVEL IN dB RE ANSI 2004

AUDIOGRAM KEY (Right / Left): AC Unmasked; AC Masked; BC Mastoid Unmasked; BC Mastoid Masked; Examples of No Response Symbols

Effective Masking Level in dB: RE / LE — AC/BC

SPEECH AUDIOMETRY

Speech tests via: (Circle) MLV Recorded

Word Recognition in % Correct

	PTA	SRT/SAT	EM	WRS	HL/EM		HL/EM
RT	2	5		100%	50/30		
LT	-2	0		96%	50/30		

Word Recognition List: NU-6 — R 3A; L 4A

RELIABILITY: Good
VALIDITY: Acceptable

ACOUSTIC REFLEX THRESHOLDS

	Stim in	Meas in	500	1K	2K	4K	Decay 500	Decay 1K
CONTRA (X)	RT	LT	105	90	85	80	CNT	--
	LT	RT	95	85	85	80	--	--
IPSI (X)	RT	RT	80	75	80	75		
	LT	LT	90	85	85	80		

TYMPANOMETRY

	RT	LT
Canal Volume (mL)	1.1	1.2

Static Admittance (mL): Rt 0.4 Lt 0.6
Peak Pressure (daPa): Rt 25 Lt 25
Type: Rt A Lt A

COMMENTS: High frequency thresholds: R ear - 9,000 Hz - 55 dB HL, 10,000 Hz - 55 dB HL, 11,200 Hz - 60 dB HL, 12,500 Hz - 60 dB HL, 14,000 Hz - 65 dB HL, 16,000 Hz - NR, 18,000 Hz - NR, 20,000 Hz - NR; L ear - 9,000 Hz - 55 dB HL, 10,000 Hz - 50 dB HL, 11,200 Hz - 60 dB HL, 12,500 Hz - 60 dB HL, 14,000 Hz - 60 dB HL, 16,000 Hz - NR, 18,000 Hz - NR, 20,000 Hz - NR

Fig. 5.11 Audiogram of a patient receiving ototoxic monitoring of amikacin.

5.11.2 Interpretation

Right ear—Pure-tone thresholds were within normal limits at 250 to 4,000 Hz and sloping to a moderate likely sensorineural hearing loss from 6,000 to 8,000 Hz. She had a moderate to moderately severe hearing loss from 9,000 to 14,000 Hz and no response from 16,000 to 20,000 Hz. Compared to baseline, thresholds were decreased by 20 dB HL at 11,200 Hz, by 30 dB HL at 9,000 and 10,000 Hz, by 35 dB HL at 6,000 Hz, by 45 dB HL at 8,000 Hz, and to NR at 16,000 Hz. The SRT revealed a normal ability to receive speech and was in agreement with the PTA. The WRS revealed a normal ability to recognize speech. Immittance testing revealed a normal tympanogram. Ipsilateral and contralateral acoustic reflex thresholds were within normal limits from 500 to 4,000 Hz. Acoustic reflex decay was negative at 500 and 1,000 Hz.

Left ear—Pure-tone thresholds were within normal limits from 250 to 6,000 Hz and sloping to a mild likely sensorineural hearing loss at 8,000 Hz. She had a moderate to moderately severe hearing loss from 9,000 to 14,000 Hz and no response from 16,000 to 20,000 Hz. Compared to baseline, thresholds were decreased by 25 dB HL at 11,200 Hz, by 30 dB HL at 10,000 Hz, by 35 dB HL at 9,000 Hz, and by 40 dB HL at 8,000 Hz. The SRT revealed a normal ability to receive speech and was in agreement with the PTA. The WRS revealed a normal ability to recognize speech. Immittance testing revealed a normal tympanogram. The ipsilateral acoustic reflex thresholds were within normal limits from 500 to 4,000 Hz, and the contralateral acoustic reflex thresholds were within normal limits from 1,000 to 4,000 Hz and elevated at 500 Hz. Acoustic reflex decay was negative at 1,000 Hz and could not be measured at 500 Hz due to an elevated contralateral acoustic reflex threshold.

5.11.3 Intervention

The physicians overseeing her treatment decided to switch from amikacin to another antibiotic due to her hearing loss and because the lung infection was not improving. Her hearing was tested 1 month later and was stable. Hearing protection was recommended.

5.12 Case 12

5.12.1 Case History

The patient reported a sudden deterioration in hearing in the left ear and a sudden onset of aural fullness, tinnitus, and hyperacusis, all in the left ear after hearing a "pop" in her left ear after shooting a pistol 5 months prior. She reported having completed a course of oral steroids 2 months after the incident and then having a hearing test after treatment. There had been no noticeable improvements in any symptoms. The patient reported the tinnitus to be a high-pitched and constant ringing sound that was extremely distracting. The patient reported difficulty understanding speech in groups and many other different communication situations. There was no report of ear pathology, otosurgery, familial hearing loss, or other significant noise exposure. There was no significant health history reported.

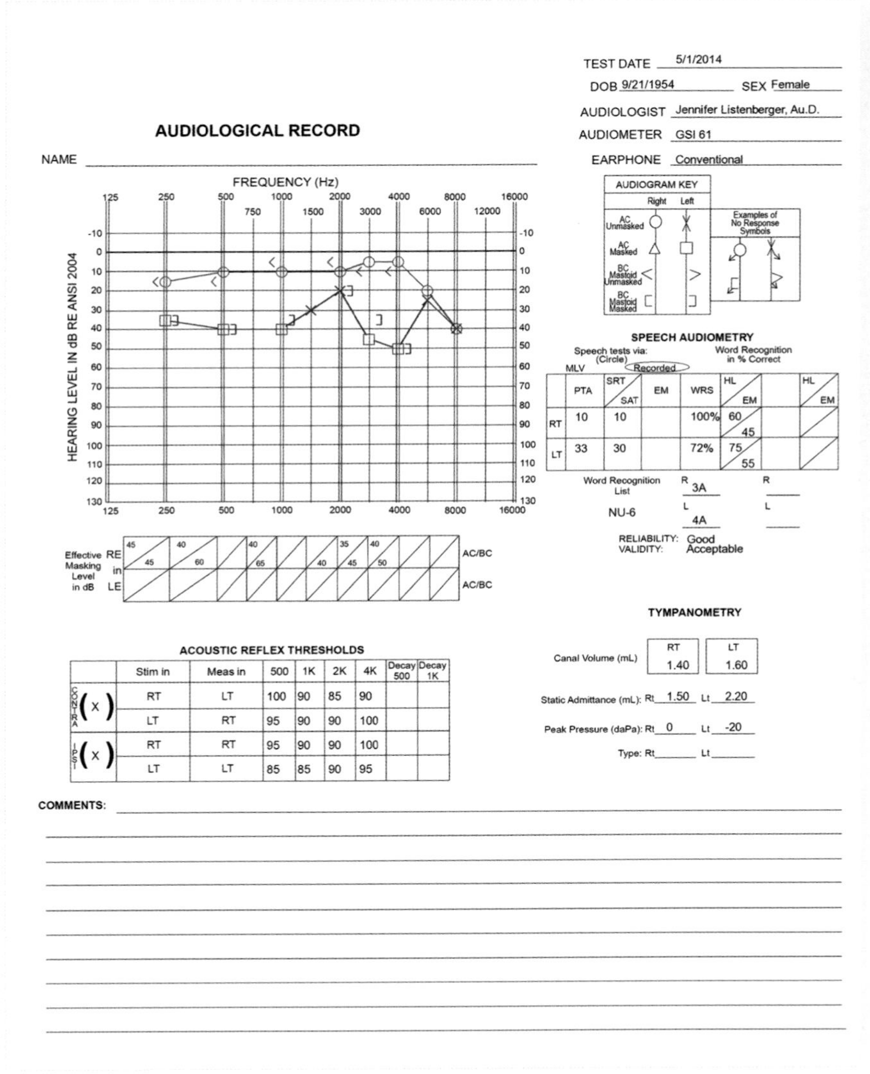

AUDIOLOGICAL RECORD

TEST DATE 5/1/2014
DOB 9/21/1954 SEX Female
AUDIOLOGIST Jennifer Listenberger, Au.D.
AUDIOMETER GSI 61
NAME
EARPHONE Conventional

SPEECH AUDIOMETRY

Speech tests via: (Circle) MLV Recorded

	PTA	SRT/SAT	EM	WRS	HL/EM
RT	10	10		100%	60/45
LT	33	30		72%	75/55

Word Recognition List: R 3A, L 4A
NU-6

RELIABILITY: Good
VALIDITY: Acceptable

TYMPANOMETRY

	RT	LT
Canal Volume (mL)	1.40	1.60

Static Admittance (mL): Rt 1.50 Lt 2.20
Peak Pressure (daPa): Rt 0 Lt -20
Type: Rt Lt

ACOUSTIC REFLEX THRESHOLDS

	Stim in	Meas in	500	1K	2K	4K	Decay 500	Decay 1K
CONTRA	RT	LT	100	90	85	90		
	LT	RT	95	90	90	100		
IPSI	RT	RT	95	90	90	100		
	LT	LT	85	85	90	95		

COMMENTS:

Fig. 5.12 Audiogram of a patient having decreased hearing in the left ear due to possible acoustic trauma.

5.12.2 Interpretation

Right ear—Pure-tone air and bone conduction thresholds revealed normal hearing sensitivity at 250 through 4,000 Hz and sloping to slight sloping to mild likely sensorineural hearing loss at 6,000 and 8,000 Hz. The SRT revealed a normal ability to receive speech and was in agreement with the PTA. The WRS revealed a normal ability to recognize speech. Immittance testing revealed a normal tympanogram and normal acoustic reflex thresholds at 500 through 4,000 Hz with ipsilateral and contralateral stimulation. Acoustic reflex decay was not measured.

Left ear—Pure-tone air and bone conduction thresholds revealed a mild sensorineural hearing loss at 250 through 1,500 Hz, rising to slight at 2,000 Hz, sloping to moderate at 3,000 and 4,000 Hz, and rising to slight and mild at 6,000 and 8,000 Hz. The SRT revealed a mild loss in the ability to receive speech and was in agreement with the PTA. The WRS revealed moderate difficulty in the ability to recognize speech. Immittance testing revealed a hypercompliant tympanogram and normal acoustic reflex thresholds at 500 through 4,000 Hz with ipsilateral and contralateral stimulation. Acoustic reflex decay was not measured.

5.12.3 Intervention

The patient proceeded with the scheduled otologic consultation. Per the otologist's report, medical clearance for amplification was provided and no further medical intervention was recommended. The patient was recommended to follow up with the Audiology department for a hearing aid evaluation, evaluation for HAT, evaluation for management of tinnitus and hyperacusis, annual hearing testing, and use of hearing protection in noise.

5.13 Case 13

5.13.1 Case History

The patient was a 34-year-old woman who reported she woke up one morning with decreased hearing in her left ear about 2 years ago. She noted that, prior to this, she had not had concerns about her hearing. She was seen by an otologist, and oral steroids were prescribed, but no perceived improvement was noted. The patient was also treated with a series of steroid injections in her ear, but the symptoms remained unchanged. She reported that she had tinnitus in the left ear and that she could not hear much from the left ear. There were no balance difficulties reported. She was a teacher and reported difficulty hearing in the classroom and in many social situations.

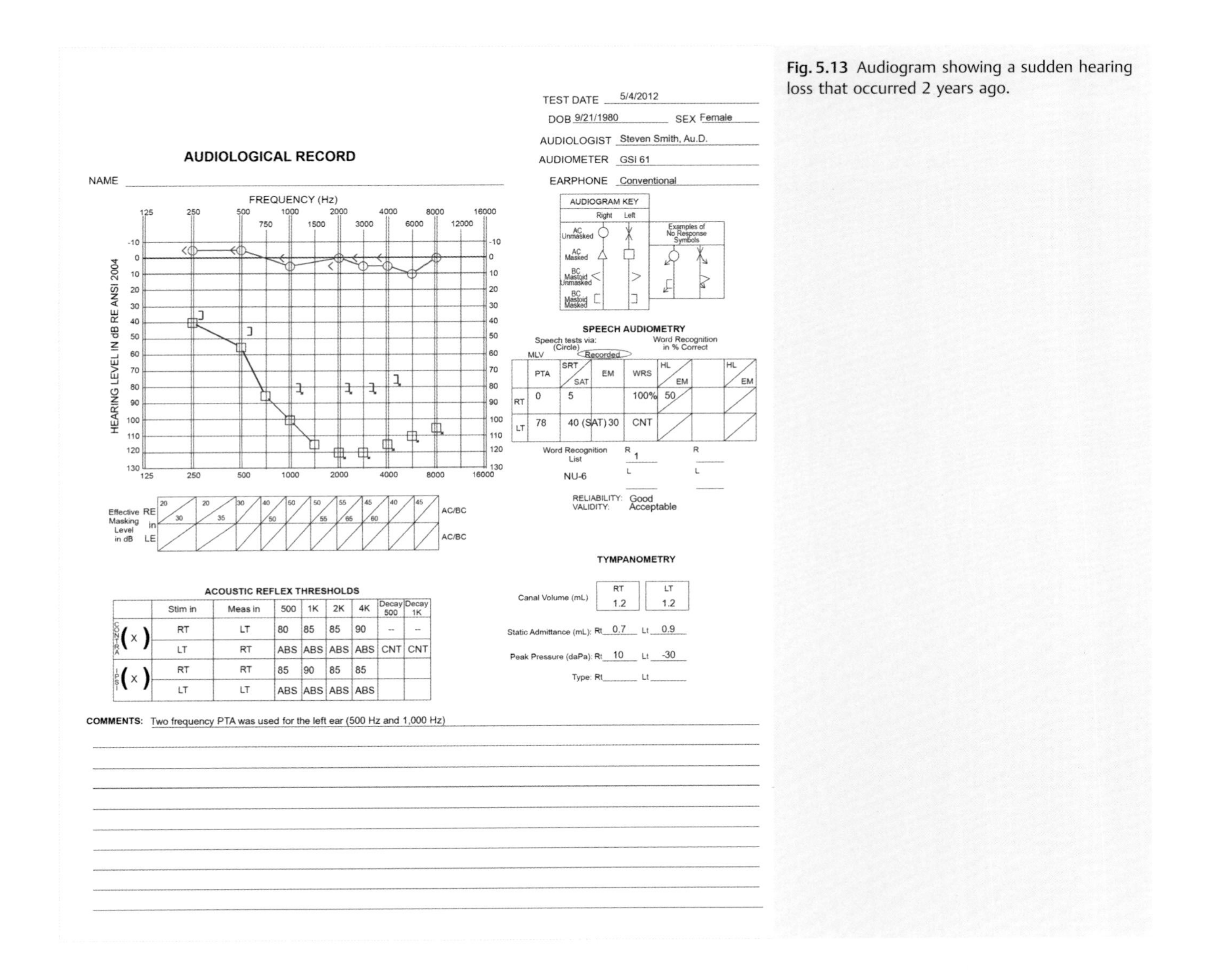

AUDIOLOGICAL RECORD

NAME

TEST DATE 5/4/2012
DOB 9/21/1980 SEX Female
AUDIOLOGIST Steven Smith, Au.D.
AUDIOMETER GSI 61
EARPHONE Conventional

Effective Masking Level in dB

	250	500	750	1000	1500	2000	3000	4000	6000	8000	
RE	20 / 30	20 / 35	30 /	40 / 50	50 /	50 / 55	55 / 65	45 / 60	40 /	45 /	AC/BC
LE											AC/BC

SPEECH AUDIOMETRY

Speech tests via: (Circle) MLV Recorded (circled)

Word Recognition in % Correct

	PTA	SRT / SAT	EM	WRS	HL / EM		HL / EM
RT	0	5		100%	50		
LT	78	40 (SAT)	30	CNT			

Word Recognition List: NU-6 R 1 L

RELIABILITY: Good
VALIDITY: Acceptable

ACOUSTIC REFLEX THRESHOLDS

	Stim in	Meas in	500	1K	2K	4K	Decay 500	Decay 1K
CONTRA (X)	RT	LT	80	85	85	90	--	--
	LT	RT	ABS	ABS	ABS	ABS	CNT	CNT
IPSI (X)	RT	RT	85	90	85	85		
	LT	LT	ABS	ABS	ABS	ABS		

TYMPANOMETRY

	RT	LT
Canal Volume (mL)	1.2	1.2

Static Admittance (mL): Rt 0.7 Lt 0.9
Peak Pressure (daPa): Rt 10 Lt -30
Type: Rt ____ Lt ____

COMMENTS: Two frequency PTA was used for the left ear (500 Hz and 1,000 Hz)

Fig. 5.13 Audiogram showing a sudden hearing loss that occurred 2 years ago.

5.13.2 Interpretation

Right ear—Normal hearing. The SRT was within normal limits for the ability to receive speech and was in agreement with the PTA. The WRS was normal. Immittance testing revealed a normal tympanogram with normal ipsilateral acoustic reflex thresholds at 500 through 4,000 Hz and absent contralateral acoustic reflex thresholds at 500 through 4,000 Hz. Contralateral acoustic reflex decay could not be measured due to absent contralateral acoustic reflex thresholds.

Left ear—Mild and moderate sensorineural hearing loss at 250 to 500 Hz, sloping to severe sloping to profound at 750 to 8,000 Hz, with no measurable response within the limits of the audiometer at 2,000 to 8,000 Hz. The SAT revealed a mild loss in the ability to detect speech and was in poor agreement with the PTA, likely due to the steeply sloping hearing loss. The WRS could not be measured due to a lack of speech reception. Immittance testing revealed a normal tympanogram with absent ipsilateral acoustic reflex thresholds at 500 through 4,000 Hz and normal contralateral acoustic reflex thresholds at 500 through 4,000 Hz. Negative acoustic reflex decay was obtained with contralateral stimulation at 500 and 1,000 Hz.

5.13.3 Intervention

The patient was counseled that a conventional hearing aid would not assist her with hearing from the left ear. She was counseled on appropriate devices to help her improve her ability to hear from the left side, such as osseointegrated implants. This was demonstrated to her with the processor on a headband. A demonstration was also provided for the CROS hearing aid. She determined that she would pursue right CROS technology and has been satisfied with the results.

5.14 Case 14

5.14.1 Case History

The patient reported difficulty hearing in the left ear for 10 months. The initial decrease in hearing was sudden, but had not progressed since the onset. She initially had bilateral pulsatile tinnitus, but this had subsided, and now she had intermittent tinnitus in the left ear. She flew on an airplane prior to the onset of her symptoms. She saw her primary care physician and was told she had fluid in her ears. Several years ago she was in a car accident and her head hit the windshield, but she did not have any long-term injuries due to the accident. She did not report other otologic symptoms or history.

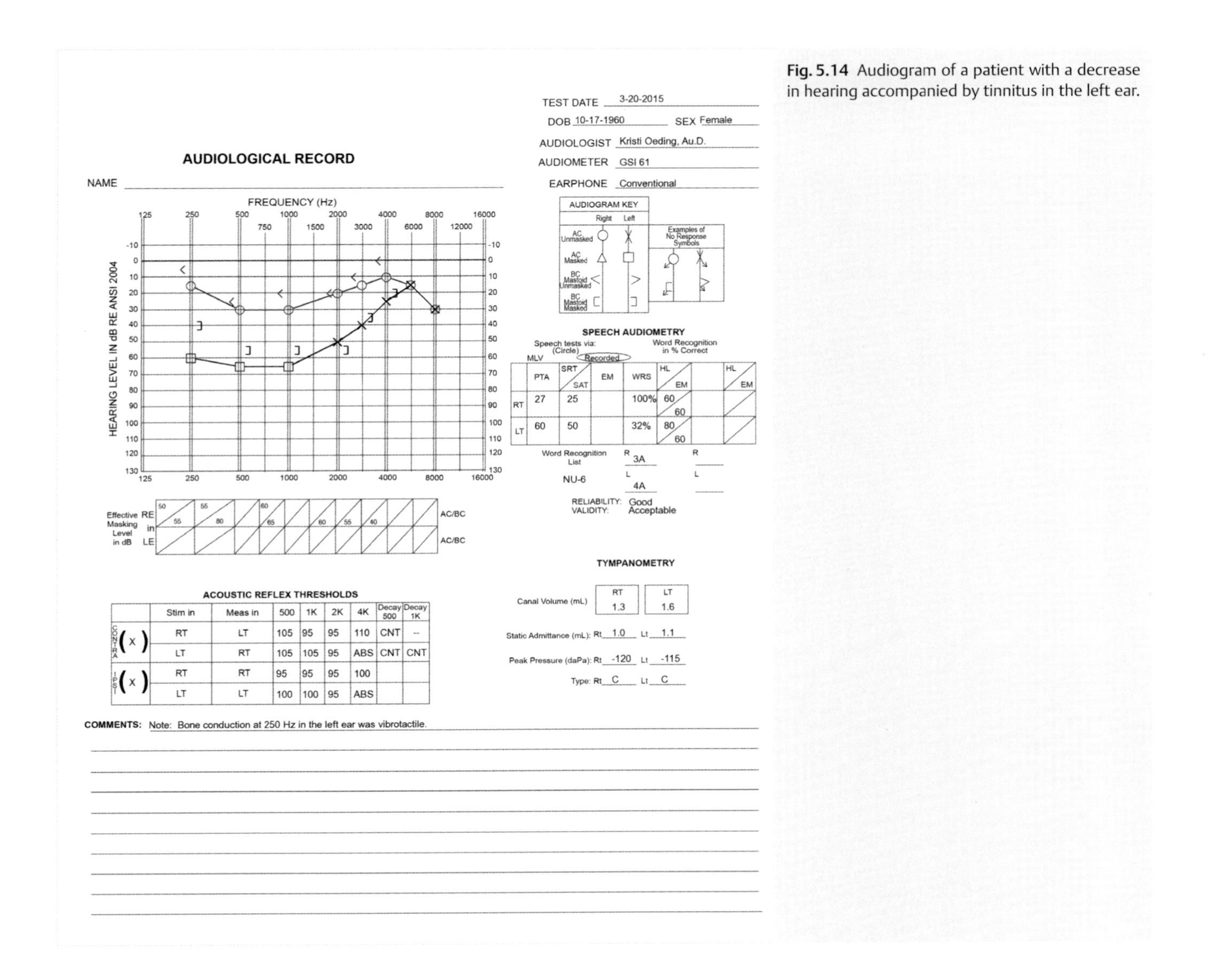

	Stim in	Meas in	500	1K	2K	4K	Decay 500	Decay 1K
CONTRA (x)	RT	LT	105	95	95	110	CNT	--
	LT	RT	105	105	95	ABS	CNT	CNT
IPSI (x)	RT	RT	95	95	95	100		
	LT	LT	100	100	95	ABS		

Fig. 5.14 Audiogram of a patient with a decrease in hearing accompanied by tinnitus in the left ear.

5.14.2 Interpretation

Right ear—Pure-tone thresholds were within normal limits at 250 Hz, sloping to a mild sensorineural hearing loss from 500 to 1,000 Hz, rising to a slight sensorineural hearing loss at 2,000 Hz to within normal limits from 3,000 to 6,000 Hz, and sloping to a mild hearing loss at 8,000 Hz. The SRT revealed a slight loss in the ability to receive speech and was in agreement with the PTA. The WRS revealed a normal ability to recognize speech. Immittance testing revealed excessive negative pressure on the tympanogram. Ipsilateral acoustic reflex thresholds were within normal limits from 500 to 4,000 Hz. Contralateral acoustic reflex thresholds were within normal limits at 2,000 Hz, elevated from 500 to 1,000 Hz, and absent at 4,000 Hz. Acoustic reflex decay could not be measured at 500 and 1,000 Hz due to elevated contralateral acoustic reflex thresholds.

Left ear—Pure-tone thresholds revealed a moderately severe sensorineural hearing loss from 250 to 1,000 Hz, rising from a moderate sensorineural hearing loss to within normal limits from 2,000 to 6,000 Hz, and sloping to a mild hearing loss at 8,000 Hz. The SRT revealed a moderate loss in the ability to receive speech and was in agreement with the PTA. The WRS revealed a very poor ability to recognize speech. Immittance testing revealed excessive negative pressure on the tympanogram. The ipsilateral acoustic reflex thresholds were within normal limits at 500 to 2,000 Hz and absent at 4,000 Hz. The contralateral acoustic reflex thresholds were within normal limits from 1,000 to 2,000 Hz and elevated at 500 and 4,000 Hz. Acoustic reflex decay was negative at 1,000 Hz and could not be measured at 500 Hz due to an elevated contralateral acoustic reflex threshold.

5.14.3 Intervention

An MRI was performed and revealed a small, left-sided basal turn cochlear schwannoma with internal auditory canal fundus involvement. Options were presented to the patient, and it was decided to wait and watch the tumor. Audiological recommendations included annual hearing tests, a hearing aid evaluation, HAT, and hearing protection in noise.

5.15 Case 15

5.15.1 Case History

A 33-year-old male reported a long-standing history of constant bilateral tinnitus and perceived hearing loss. The patient described the tinnitus as a steady, low-level, high-pitched ringing sound. The patient stated that there had been a relatively sudden change in the tinnitus in only the right ear over the past 3 months in that the tinnitus had become louder and much more noticeable for short periods of time. He related the changes in tinnitus to recent aural and head pressure. The hearing in the right ear seemed to be poorer and the patient reported difficulty understanding speech in noisy situations. He did not perceive much difficulty in a quiet office setting. He reported a significant history of firearms use without hearing protection as a young child and continued to use firearms, but now he consistently used hearing protection. He reported using various calibers and of being a left-handed shooter. There was some familial hearing loss, but the history of noise exposure was similar. There was no report of ear pathology. There were no significant health incidences reported.

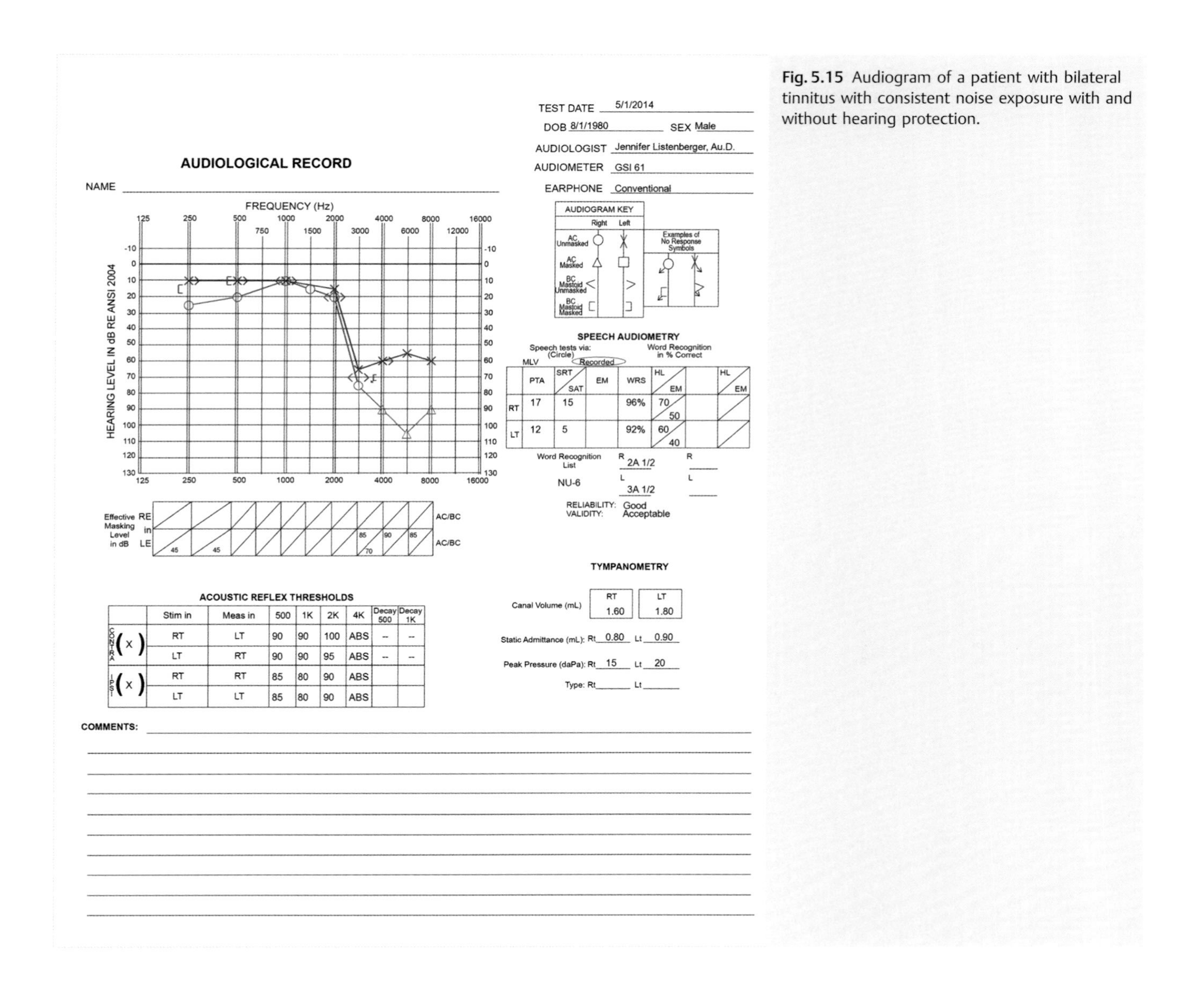

Fig. 5.15 Audiogram of a patient with bilateral tinnitus with consistent noise exposure with and without hearing protection.

5.15.2 Interpretation

Right ear—Pure-tone air and bone conduction threshold testing revealed an essentially flat slight sensorineural hearing loss at 250 through 2,000 Hz, with the exception of normal hearing sensitivity at 1,000 and 1,500 Hz, and steeply sloping to severe at 3,000 through 8,000 Hz, with a profound notch at 6,000 Hz. The SRT revealed a normal ability to receive speech and was in agreement with the PTA. The WRS revealed a normal ability to recognize speech. Immittance testing revealed a normal tympanogram and normal acoustic reflex thresholds for ipsilateral and contralateral stimulation at 500 through 2,000 Hz and absent thresholds at 4,000 Hz. Acoustic reflex decay was negative for contralateral stimulation at 500 and 1,000 Hz.

Left ear—Pure-tone air and bone conduction threshold testing revealed normal hearing sensitivity at 250 through 2,000 Hz and steeply sloping to moderately severe sensorineural hearing loss at 3,000 through 8,000 Hz, with a rise to moderate at 6,000 Hz. The SRT revealed a normal ability to receive speech and was in agreement with the PTA. The WRS revealed a normal ability to recognize speech. Immittance testing revealed a normal tympanogram and normal acoustic reflex thresholds for ipsilateral and contralateral stimulation at 500 through 2,000 Hz and absent thresholds at 4,000 Hz. Acoustic reflex decay was negative for contralateral stimulation at 500 and 1,000 Hz.

5.15.3 Intervention

The patient was referred to an ENT specialist regarding the sudden change in tinnitus and asymmetric hearing loss. Audiological recommendations included continued use of hearing protection with an emphasis on custom earplugs, annual hearing testing to monitor hearing sensitivity, and evaluation with an audiologist to discuss HAT or amplification when the patient was ready and perceived changes in communication abilities.

5.16 Case 16

5.16.1 Case History

The patient was a 56-year-old male who had hearing loss and tinnitus for many years. He stated that, for many years, he was not bothered by his hearing loss or tinnitus. He stated that he had multiple health issues over the last year, including chemotherapy and radiation therapy. Since some of these health issues and treatments, he had noted an increased difficulty with hearing, especially in noise, and the tinnitus seemed louder. He described the tinnitus as "out of control." He was a musician and had been around music the majority of his life. He had completed annual hearing tests for the last 3 years. The patient was unable to recall the chemotherapy medications that were used to treat his cancer.

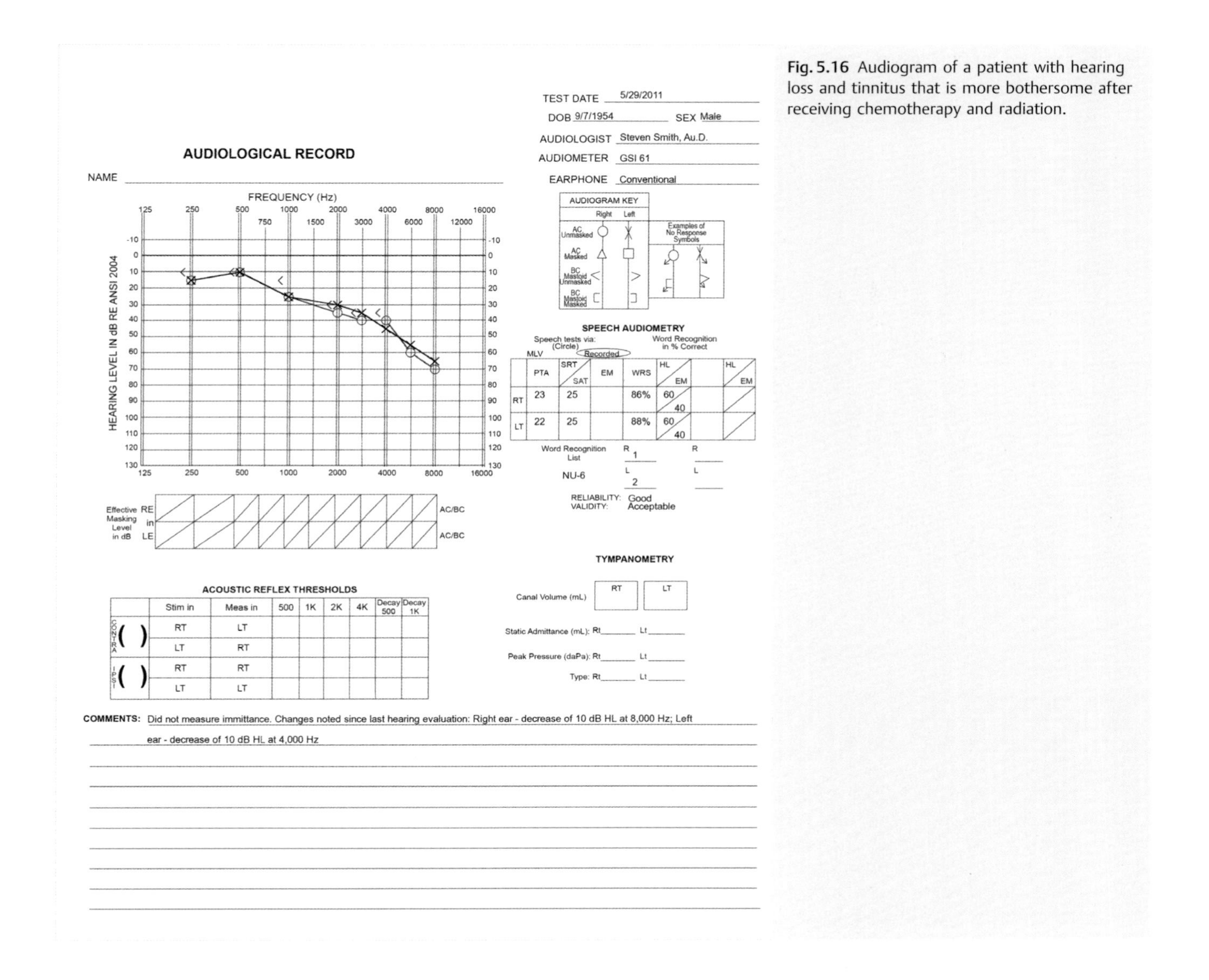

AUDIOLOGICAL RECORD

NAME

TEST DATE 5/29/2011

DOB 9/7/1954 SEX Male

AUDIOLOGIST Steven Smith, Au.D.

AUDIOMETER GSI 61

EARPHONE Conventional

SPEECH AUDIOMETRY

Speech tests via: (Circle) MLV Recorded

Word Recognition in % Correct

	PTA	SRT/SAT	EM	WRS	HL/EM		HL/EM
RT	23	25		86%	60/40		
LT	22	25		88%	60/40		

Word Recognition List: R 1, L 2

NU-6

RELIABILITY: Good

VALIDITY: Acceptable

TYMPANOMETRY

Canal Volume (mL): RT ___ LT ___

Static Admittance (mL): Rt ___ Lt ___

Peak Pressure (daPa): Rt ___ Lt ___

Type: Rt ___ Lt ___

ACOUSTIC REFLEX THRESHOLDS

	Stim in	Meas in	500	1K	2K	4K	Decay 500	Decay 1K
CONTRA	RT	LT						
	LT	RT						
IPSI	RT	RT						
	LT	LT						

COMMENTS: Did not measure immittance. Changes noted since last hearing evaluation: Right ear - decrease of 10 dB HL at 8,000 Hz; Left ear - decrease of 10 dB HL at 4,000 Hz

Fig. 5.16 Audiogram of a patient with hearing loss and tinnitus that is more bothersome after receiving chemotherapy and radiation.

5.16.2 Interpretation

Right ear—Normal hearing at 250 to 500 Hz, sloping to a slight and mild sensorineural hearing loss at 1,000 to 4,000 Hz, sloping to moderately severe at 6,000 and 8,000 Hz. The SRT revealed a slight loss in the ability to receive speech and was in agreement with the PTA. The WRS was obtained and revealed a slight difficulty. Immittance testing was not measured. A decrease of 10 dB HL was noted at 8,000 Hz. No other changes were obtained for threshold testing or the WRS.

Left ear—Normal hearing at 250 to 500 Hz, sloping to a slight and mild sensorineural hearing loss at 1,000 to 3,000 Hz, sloping to moderate and moderately severe at 4,000 to 8,000 Hz. The SRT revealed a slight loss in the ability to receive speech and was in agreement with the PTA. The WRS was obtained and revealed a slight difficulty. Immittance testing was not measured. A decrease of 10 dB HL was noted at 4,000 Hz. No other changes were obtained for threshold testing or the WRS.

5.16.3 Intervention

The patient was referred to an ENT specialist for the increase in tinnitus. He was advised of hearing aid technology and tinnitus retraining therapy. He will consider the use of hearing aids and tinnitus retraining therapy and will follow up with an ENT specialist.

5.17 Case 17

5.17.1 Case History

The patient reported hearing loss in the right ear and was uncertain of the onset of hearing loss. He thought he had always had hearing loss in the right ear, possibly since birth. The hearing loss had decreased over the past 6 months. He reported a constant, non-bothersome tinnitus in the right ear and a recent onset of episodes of vertigo and nausea. He did not have increased tinnitus, changes in hearing, or a sensation of fullness during an episode of vertigo. He stated that the episodes could last for minutes to hours, and if he took meclizine it seemed to help. He did not report other otologic symptoms or history.

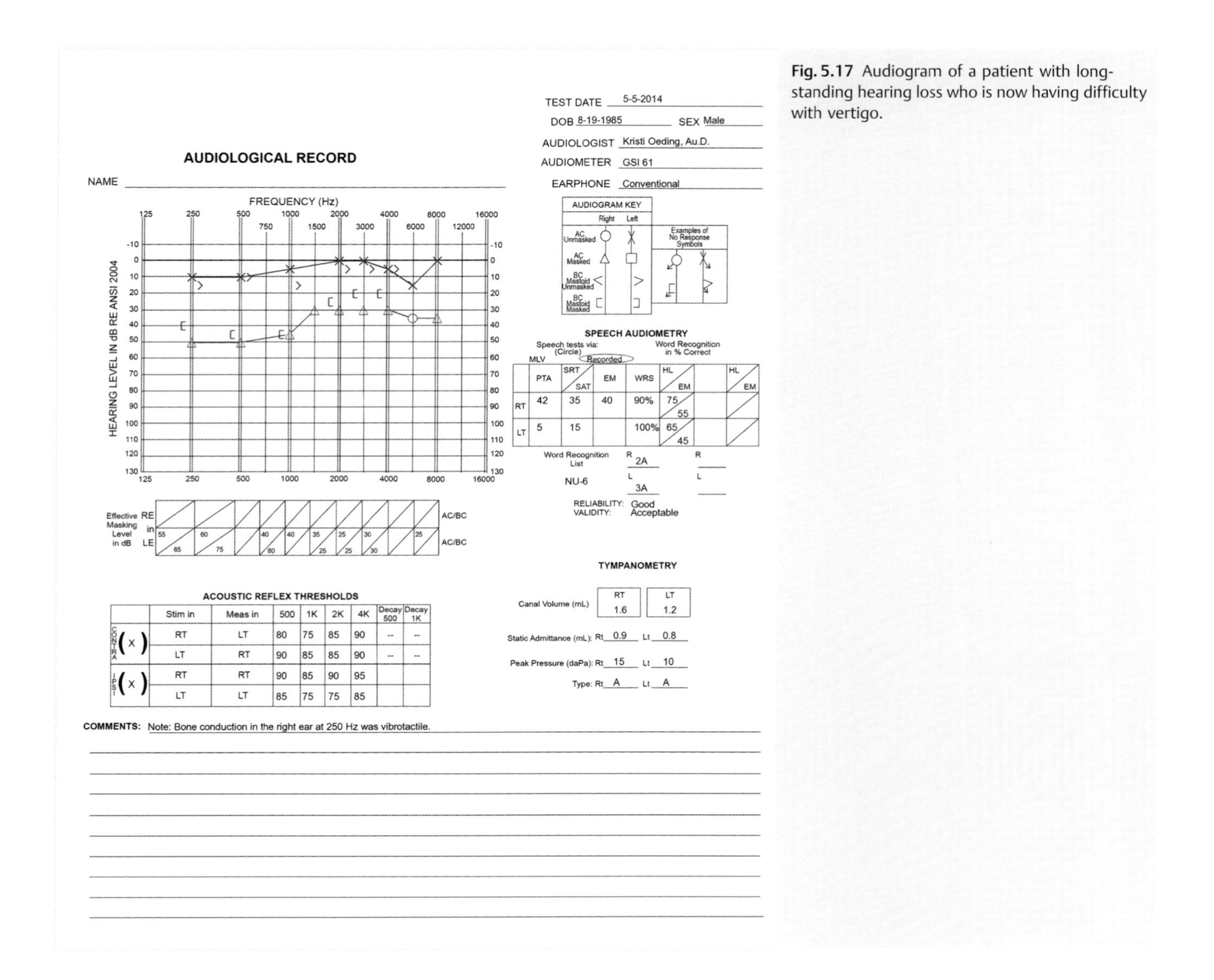

AUDIOLOGICAL RECORD

NAME

TEST DATE 5-5-2014
DOB 8-19-1985 SEX Male
AUDIOLOGIST Kristi Oeding, Au.D.
AUDIOMETER GSI 61
EARPHONE Conventional

FREQUENCY (Hz): 125, 250, 500, 750, 1000, 1500, 2000, 3000, 4000, 6000, 8000, 12000, 16000

HEARING LEVEL IN dB RE ANSI 2004: -10 to 130

AUDIOGRAM KEY (Right / Left): AC Unmasked; AC Masked; BC Mastoid Unmasked; BC Mastoid Masked. Examples of No Response Symbols

Effective Masking Level in dB
RE in AC/BC
LE in AC/BC: 55/65, 60/75, 40/80, 40, 35/25, 25/25, 30/30, 25

SPEECH AUDIOMETRY

Speech tests via: (Circle) MLV Recorded (circled)

Word Recognition in % Correct

	PTA	SRT/SAT	EM	WRS	HL/EM		HL/EM
RT	42	35	40	90%	75/55		
LT	5	15		100%	65/45		

Word Recognition List NU-6: R 2A, L 3A

RELIABILITY: Good
VALIDITY: Acceptable

TYMPANOMETRY

Canal Volume (mL): RT 1.6, LT 1.2
Static Admittance (mL): Rt 0.9 Lt 0.8
Peak Pressure (daPa): Rt 15 Lt 10
Type: Rt A Lt A

ACOUSTIC REFLEX THRESHOLDS

	Stim in	Meas in	500	1K	2K	4K	Decay 500	Decay 1K
CONTRA (X)	RT	LT	80	75	85	90	--	--
	LT	RT	90	85	85	90	--	--
IPSI (X)	RT	RT	90	85	90	95		
	LT	LT	85	75	75	85		

COMMENTS: Note: Bone conduction in the right ear at 250 Hz was vibrotactile.

Fig. 5.17 Audiogram of a patient with long-standing hearing loss who is now having difficulty with vertigo.

5.17.2 Interpretation

Right ear—Pure-tone thresholds revealed a moderate sensorineural hearing loss from 250 to 1,000 Hz and rising to a mild sensorineural hearing loss from 1,500 to 8,000 Hz. The SRT revealed a mild loss in the ability to receive speech and was in agreement with the PTA. The WRS revealed a normal ability to recognize speech. Immittance testing revealed a normal tympanogram. Ipsilateral and contralateral acoustic reflex thresholds were within normal limits from 500 to 4,000 Hz. Acoustic reflex decay was negative at 500 and 1,000 Hz.

Left ear—Pure-tone thresholds were within normal limits from 250 to 8,000 Hz. The SRT revealed a normal ability to receive speech and was in agreement with the PTA. The WRS revealed a normal ability to recognize speech. Immittance testing revealed a normal tympanogram. The ipsilateral and contralateral acoustic reflex thresholds were within normal limits from 500 to 4,000 Hz. Acoustic reflex decay was negative at 500 and 1,000 Hz.

5.17.3 Intervention

The otologist was uncertain if the patient had labyrinthitis or Ménière's disease. The patient was placed on a high dose of oral steroids and had an intratympanic dexamethasone injection. MRI and CT scans were performed and were normal. At the follow-up visit a slight improvement was noted in hearing, and three more intratympanic dexamethasone injections were completed. The patient continued to have episodes of vertigo, and electrocochleography was performed and revealed a positive result for right-sided cochlear hydrops (Ménière's disease). He was placed on a diuretic and a low-salt diet.

5.18 Case 18

5.18.1 Case History

The patient was diagnosed with cystic fibrosis at approximately 5 years old. He received intravenous tobramycin and nebulized gentamicin intermittently for approximately 10 years. There was no reported familial hearing loss, ear pathology, or noise exposure. The patient denied any tinnitus or dizziness. He had a lung transplant in 1998 and a kidney transplant in 2005. The patient also reported a supraventricular tachycardia that was treated successfully with medication. He reported no significant communication difficulties, but said the hearing in the left ear had been poor for as long as he could remember. In fact, the patient stated that he had no memory of ever having normal hearing in the left ear.

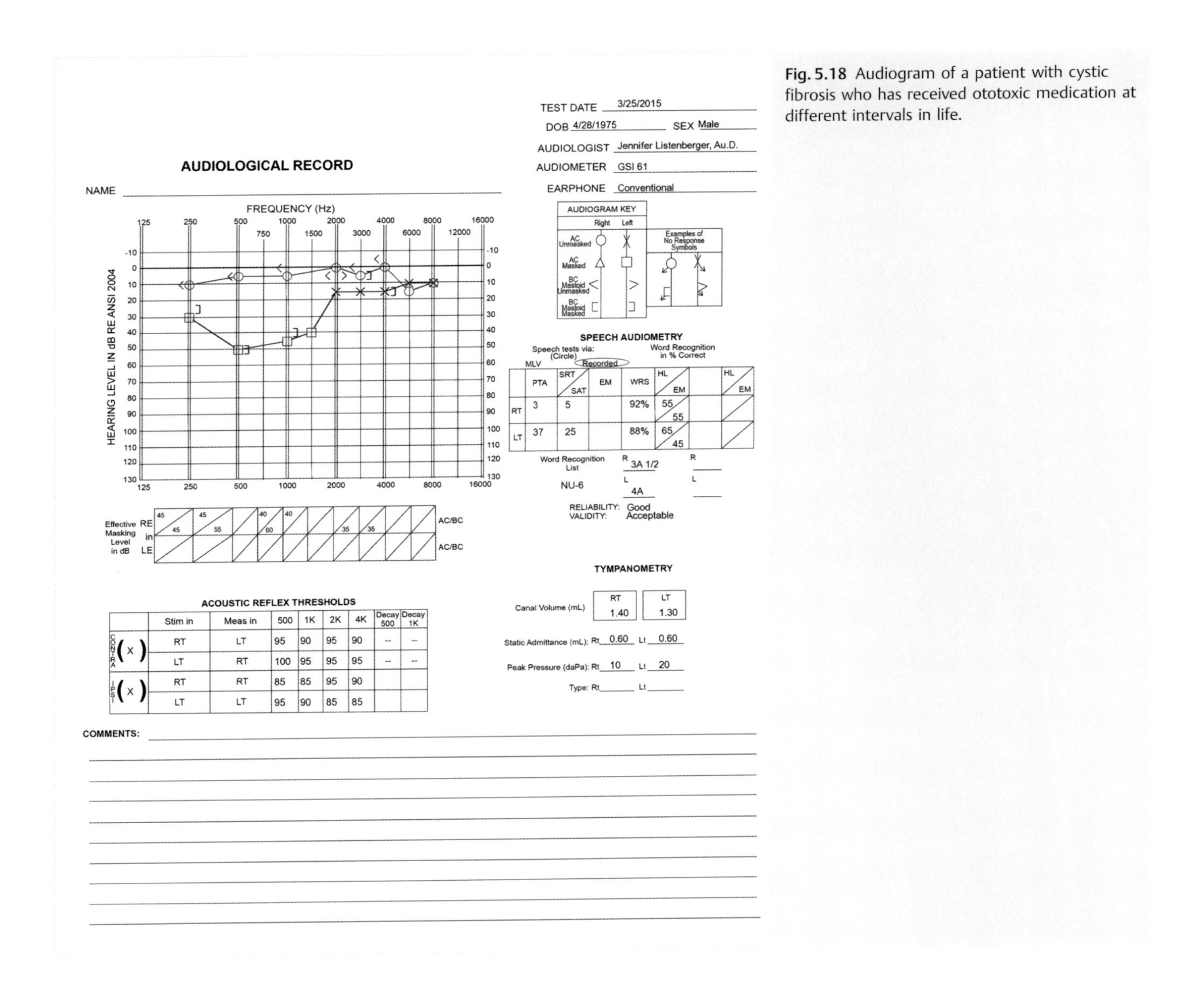

AUDIOLOGICAL RECORD

TEST DATE 3/25/2015
DOB 4/28/1975 SEX Male
AUDIOLOGIST Jennifer Listenberger, Au.D.
AUDIOMETER GSI 61
EARPHONE Conventional

NAME

SPEECH AUDIOMETRY

Speech tests via: (Circle) MLV Recorded

Word Recognition in % Correct

	PTA	SRT / SAT	EM	WRS	HL / EM		HL / EM
RT	3	5		92%	55 / 55		
LT	37	25		88%	65 / 45		

Word Recognition List NU-6: R 3A 1/2; L 4A

RELIABILITY: Good
VALIDITY: Acceptable

Effective Masking Level in dB

	250	500	750	1000	1500	2000	3000	4000	6000	8000
RE in (AC/BC)	45 / 45	45 / 55		40 / 60	40		35	35		
LE in (AC/BC)										

TYMPANOMETRY

	RT	LT
Canal Volume (mL)	1.40	1.30
Static Admittance (mL)	0.60	0.60
Peak Pressure (daPa)	10	20
Type		

ACOUSTIC REFLEX THRESHOLDS

	Stim in	Meas in	500	1K	2K	4K	Decay 500	Decay 1K
CONTRA (X)	RT	LT	95	90	95	90	--	--
	LT	RT	100	95	95	95	--	--
IPSI (X)	RT	RT	85	85	95	90		
	LT	LT	95	90	85	85		

COMMENTS:

Fig. 5.18 Audiogram of a patient with cystic fibrosis who has received ototoxic medication at different intervals in life.

5.18.2 Interpretation

Right ear—Pure-tone air and bone conduction threshold testing revealed normal hearing sensitivity at 250 through 8,000 Hz. The SRT revealed a normal ability to receive speech and was in agreement with the PTA. The WRS revealed a normal ability to recognize speech. Immittance testing revealed a normal tympanogram and normal acoustic reflex thresholds for ipsilateral and contralateral stimulation at 500 through 4,000 Hz. Acoustic reflex decay was negative at 500 and 1,000 Hz.

Left ear—Pure-tone air and bone conduction threshold testing revealed a mild and moderate sloping and rising low-frequency sensorineural hearing loss at 250 through 1,500 Hz and rising to normal at 2,000 through 8,000 Hz. The SRT revealed a slight loss in the ability to receive speech and was in agreement with the PTA. The WRS revealed a slight difficulty in the ability to recognize speech. Immittance testing revealed a normal tympanogram and normal acoustic reflex thresholds for ipsilateral and contralateral stimulation at 500 through 4,000 Hz. Acoustic reflex decay was negative at 500 and 1,000 Hz.

5.18.3 Intervention

The patient will follow up with an ENT specialist as scheduled. Audiological recommendations included annual testing to monitor the stability of the hearing loss, hearing protection in noise, and to follow up with an audiologist regarding HAT and amplification if the patient notices difficulty with communication.

5.19 Case 19

5.19.1 Case History

The patient was a 38-year-old female who started to notice difficulty with her hearing approximately 14 years ago. She reported having her hearing evaluated, and this showed some hearing loss bilaterally. Her mother reported hearing loss at a younger age as well. The patient also reported having tinnitus. She denied otalgia or pressure as well as dizziness or loud noise exposure. She started using amplification approximately 9 years ago, and her most recent set of hearing aids were 2 years old. In the last 6 months, she noticed a decrease in her hearing and an increase in tinnitus in her right ear. The patient stopped using the hearing aid in the right ear due to a perceived lack of benefit and an inability to have the hearing aid adjusted for the changes in her hearing.

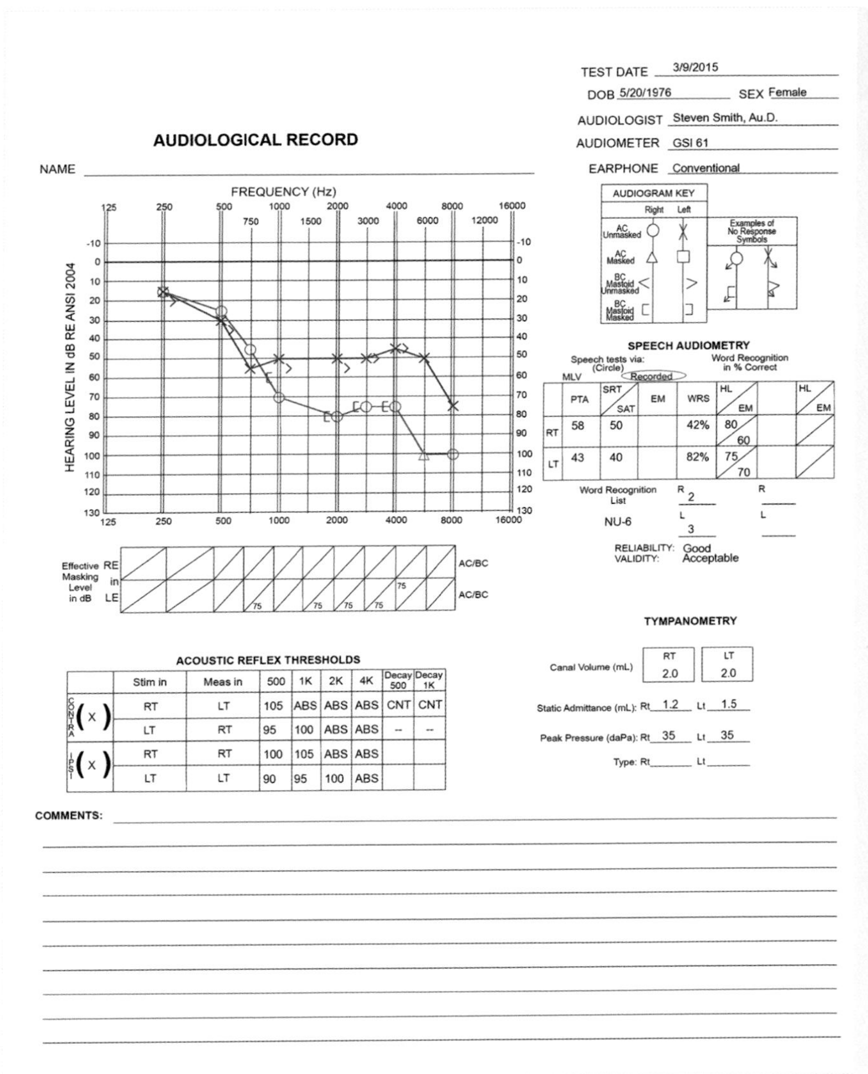

AUDIOLOGICAL RECORD

TEST DATE 3/9/2015
DOB 5/20/1976 SEX Female
AUDIOLOGIST Steven Smith, Au.D.
AUDIOMETER GSI 61
EARPHONE Conventional

NAME

Effective Masking Level in dB												
RE												AC/BC
LE				75		75	75	75	75			AC/BC

SPEECH AUDIOMETRY

Speech tests via: (Circle) MLV Recorded (circled)

Word Recognition in % Correct

	PTA	SRT / SAT	EM	WRS	HL / EM		HL / EM
RT	58	50		42%	80 / 60		
LT	43	40		82%	75 / 70		

Word Recognition List NU-6: R 2, L 3; R ___, L ___

RELIABILITY: Good
VALIDITY: Acceptable

TYMPANOMETRY

	RT	LT
Canal Volume (mL)	2.0	2.0

Static Admittance (mL): Rt 1.2 Lt 1.5
Peak Pressure (daPa): Rt 35 Lt 35
Type: Rt ___ Lt ___

ACOUSTIC REFLEX THRESHOLDS

	Stim in	Meas in	500	1K	2K	4K	Decay 500	Decay 1K
CONTRA (X)	RT	LT	105	ABS	ABS	ABS	CNT	CNT
	LT	RT	95	100	ABS	ABS	--	--
IPSI (X)	RT	RT	100	105	ABS	ABS		
	LT	LT	90	95	100	ABS		

COMMENTS:

Fig. 5.19 Audiogram of a patient with progressive hearing loss starting approximately 14 years ago.

5.19.2 Interpretation

Right ear—Normal hearing sensitivity at 250 Hz, sloping to slight and moderate sensorineural hearing loss at 500 to 750 Hz, sloping to moderately severe and severe at 1,000 to 4,000 Hz, and sloping to profound at 6,000 to 8,000 Hz. The SRT revealed a moderate loss in the ability to receive speech and was in agreement with the PTA. The WRS was very poor. Immittance testing revealed a normal tympanogram. Acoustic reflex thresholds with ipsilateral stimulation were normal at 500 Hz, elevated at 1,000 Hz, and absent at 2,000 and 4,000 Hz. Acoustic reflex thresholds with contralateral stimulation were normal at 500 Hz and 1,000 Hz, and absent at 2,000 Hz and 4,000 Hz. Acoustic reflex decay with contralateral stimulation was negative at 500 Hz and 1,000 Hz.

Left ear—Normal hearing sloping to mild sensorineural hearing loss at 250 to 500 Hz, sloping to moderate from 750 to 6,000 Hz, and sloping to severe at 8,000 Hz. The SRT revealed a mild loss in the ability to receive speech and was in agreement with the PTA. The WRS revealed a slight difficulty. Immittance testing revealed a normal tympanogram. Acoustic reflex thresholds with ipsilateral stimulation were normal at 500 through 2,000 Hz and absent at 4,000 Hz. Acoustic reflex thresholds with contralateral stimulation were elevated at 500 Hz and absent for 1,000 through 4,000 Hz. Acoustic reflex decay could not be measured due to elevated and absent contralateral acoustic reflex thresholds.

5.19.3 Intervention

The patient was referred to an ENT specialist due to the asymmetric hearing loss and WRS. The physician referred the patient for an MRI to rule out any retrocochlear pathology. It was recommended that the patient follow up with an audiologist for hearing aid programming and HAT pending the results of the MRI.

5.20 Case 20

5.20.1 Case History

The patient reported a long-standing bilateral hearing loss for several years that had been progressive. The hearing loss was attributed to his family history of hearing loss as well as the fact that he had fallen when he was water skiing and had trauma to his right ear. He wore bilateral BTE hearing aids that were more than 10 years old, and he did well conversing one-on-one in quiet. He owned his own business and tried to conduct business in quiet areas due to his hearing loss. He did not report other otologic symptoms or history.

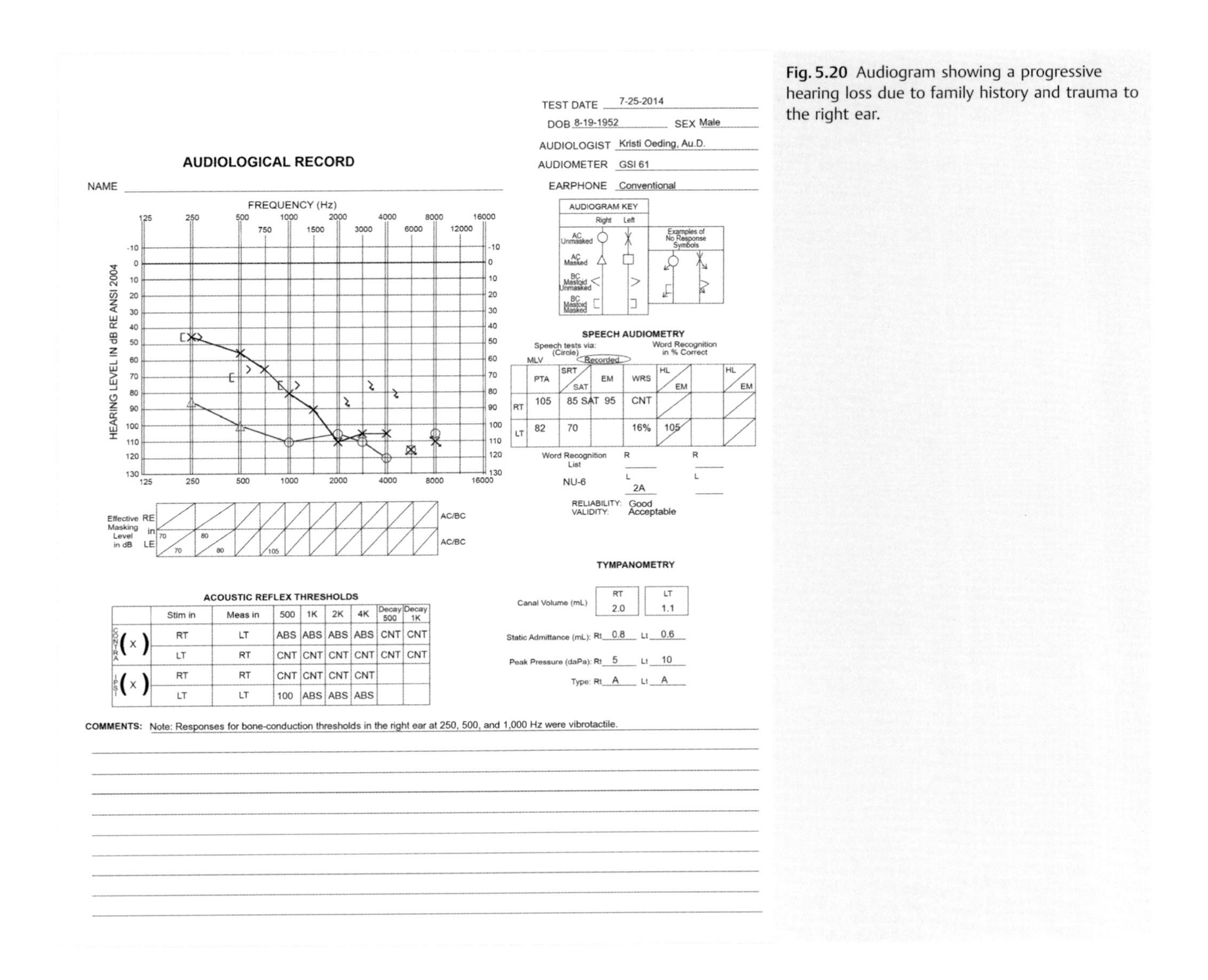

AUDIOLOGICAL RECORD

NAME

TEST DATE 7-25-2014

DOB 8-19-1952 SEX Male

AUDIOLOGIST Kristi Oeding, Au.D.

AUDIOMETER GSI 61

EARPHONE Conventional

SPEECH AUDIOMETRY

Speech tests via: (Circle) MLV Recorded

Word Recognition in % Correct

	PTA	SRT / SAT	EM	WRS	HL / EM		HL / EM
RT	105	85 SAT	95	CNT			
LT	82	70		16%	105		

Word Recognition List: NU-6; R ___ L 2A; R ___ L ___

RELIABILITY: Good

VALIDITY: Acceptable

Effective Masking Level in dB: RE (AC/BC); LE 70/70, 80/80, 105 (AC/BC)

ACOUSTIC REFLEX THRESHOLDS

	Stim in	Meas in	500	1K	2K	4K	Decay 500	Decay 1K
CONTRA (X)	RT	LT	ABS	ABS	ABS	ABS	CNT	CNT
	LT	RT	CNT	CNT	CNT	CNT	CNT	CNT
IPSI (X)	RT	RT	CNT	CNT	CNT	CNT		
	LT	LT	100	ABS	ABS	ABS		

TYMPANOMETRY

	RT	LT
Canal Volume (mL)	2.0	1.1
Static Admittance (mL)	0.8	0.6
Peak Pressure (daPa)	5	10
Type	A	A

COMMENTS: Note: Responses for bone-conduction thresholds in the right ear at 250, 500, and 1,000 Hz were vibrotactile.

Fig. 5.20 Audiogram showing a progressive hearing loss due to family history and trauma to the right ear.

5.20.2 Interpretation

Right ear—Pure-tone thresholds revealed a severe sloping to a profound sensorineural hearing loss from 250 to 8,000 Hz, with no measurable responses within the limits of the audiometer at 6,000 and 8,000 Hz. The SAT revealed a severe loss in the ability to detect speech and was in poor agreement with the PTA, which may be due to the sloping hearing loss. The WRS could not be tested because only an SAT could be obtained. Immittance testing revealed a normal tympanogram. The ipsilateral and contralateral acoustic reflex thresholds and reflex decay could not be measured due to artifact.

Left ear—Pure-tone thresholds revealed moderate sloping to a severe sensorineural hearing loss from 250 to 1,500 Hz and sloping to a profound sensorineural hearing loss from 2,000 to 8,000 Hz, with no measurable responses within the limits of the audiometer at 6,000 and 8,000 Hz. The SRT revealed a moderately severe loss in the ability to receive speech and was in agreement with the PTA. The WRS revealed a very poor ability to recognize speech. Immittance testing revealed a normal tympanogram. The ipsilateral acoustic reflex thresholds were within normal limits at 500 Hz and absent from 1,000 to 4,000 Hz, and contralateral acoustic reflex thresholds were absent from 500 to 4,000 Hz. Acoustic reflex decay could not be measured at 500 and 1,000 Hz due to absent contralateral acoustic reflex thresholds and artifact.

5.20.3 Intervention

It was recommended that he consider a cochlear implant evaluation, but he was not interested in a cochlear implant at that time. After this appointment he obtained new hearing aids with a remote control and did well with the hearing aids because he heard more soft sounds. He used a telecoil to communicate on the telephone and also obtained a captioned telephone.

5.21 Case 21

5.21.1 Case History

A 76-year-old female was seen with a long-standing history of asymmetric hearing loss due to gamma knife radiation treatment for a right vestibular schwannoma in 2002. The patient was seen today for follow-up testing to monitor stability of her hearing sensitivity. The last hearing test was completed in 2012. The patient reported that she does very well with left BICROS amplification using a hearing aid for the left and a transmitter for the right side. She stated she travels frequently on bus trips and said she does well with amplification in this communication situation.

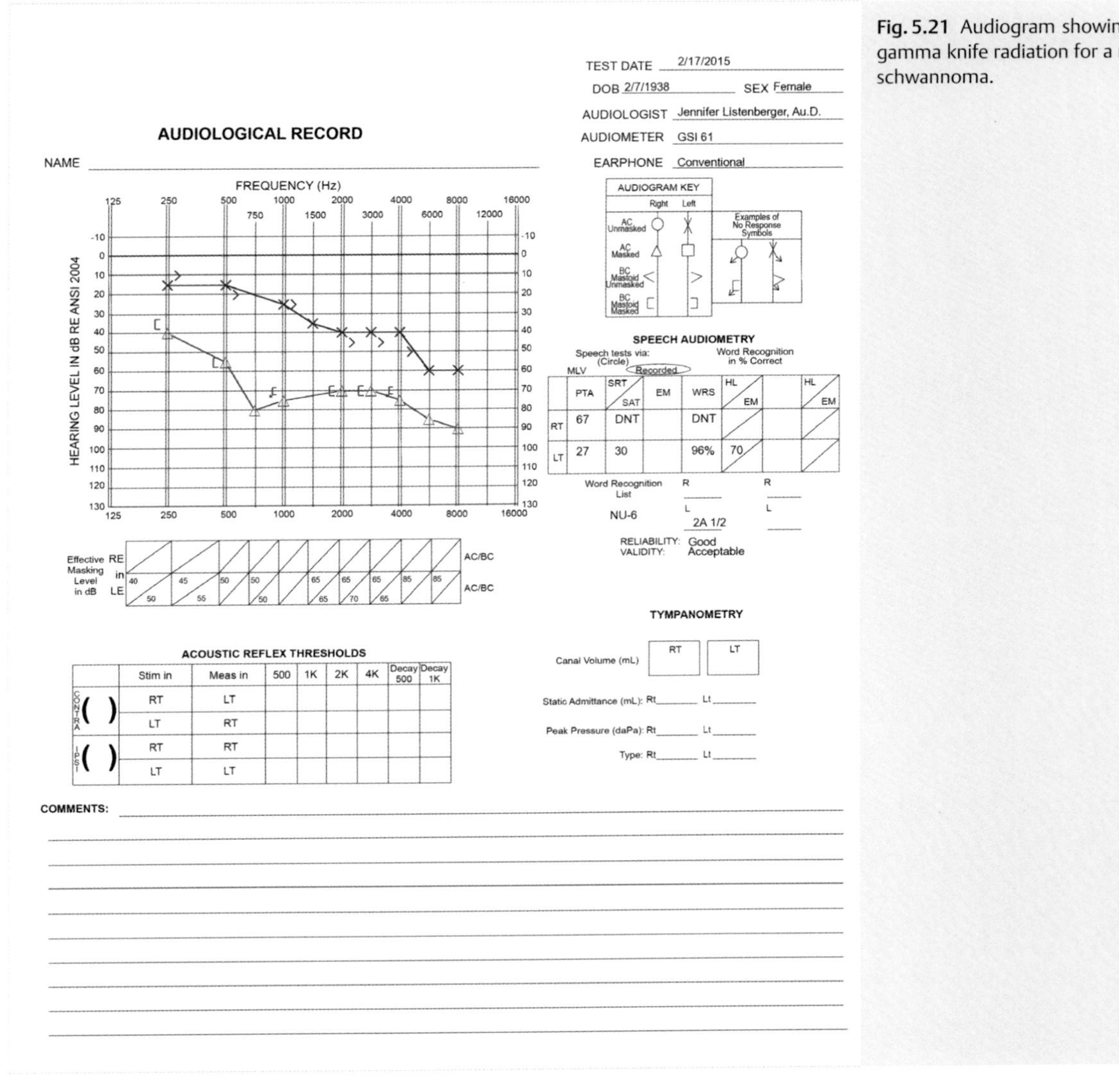

Fig. 5.21 Audiogram showing the results of gamma knife radiation for a right-sided vestibular schwannoma.

5.21.2 Interpretation

Right ear—Pure-tone air and bone conduction threshold testing revealed a mild sloping to moderate sensorineural hearing loss at 250 through 500 Hz, sloping and rising to severe and moderately severe at 750 through 3,000 Hz, and sloping to severe at 4,000 through 8,000 Hz. Speech testing and immittance testing were not measured. Previous tests revealed no measurable speech scores for SRT or WRS.

Left ear—Pure-tone air and bone conduction threshold testing revealed normal hearing sensitivity at 250 through 500 Hz, sloping to slight to mild sensorineural hearing loss at 1,000 through 4,000 Hz, and sloping to moderately severe at 6,000 through 8,000 Hz. The SRT revealed a mild loss in the ability to receive speech and was in agreement with the PTA. The WRS revealed a normal ability to recognize speech. Immittance testing was not measured. Thresholds and WRS remained unchanged in comparison to previous hearing tests.

5.21.3 Intervention

The patient returned to an ENT specialist as scheduled. Audiological recommendations included annual testing to monitor hearing sensitivity and testing after medical management as needed, continued use of amplification, and use of HAT.

5.22 Case 22

5.22.1 Case History

The patient was an 82-year-old male who had bilateral hearing loss in the high frequencies for many years. He reported a sudden decrease in his hearing approximately 6 weeks ago. He denied any increase in tinnitus or any dizziness. The patient reported a significant increase in difficulty hearing those around him. He reported trying hearing aids several years ago and, having perceived little benefit, returned the hearing aids.

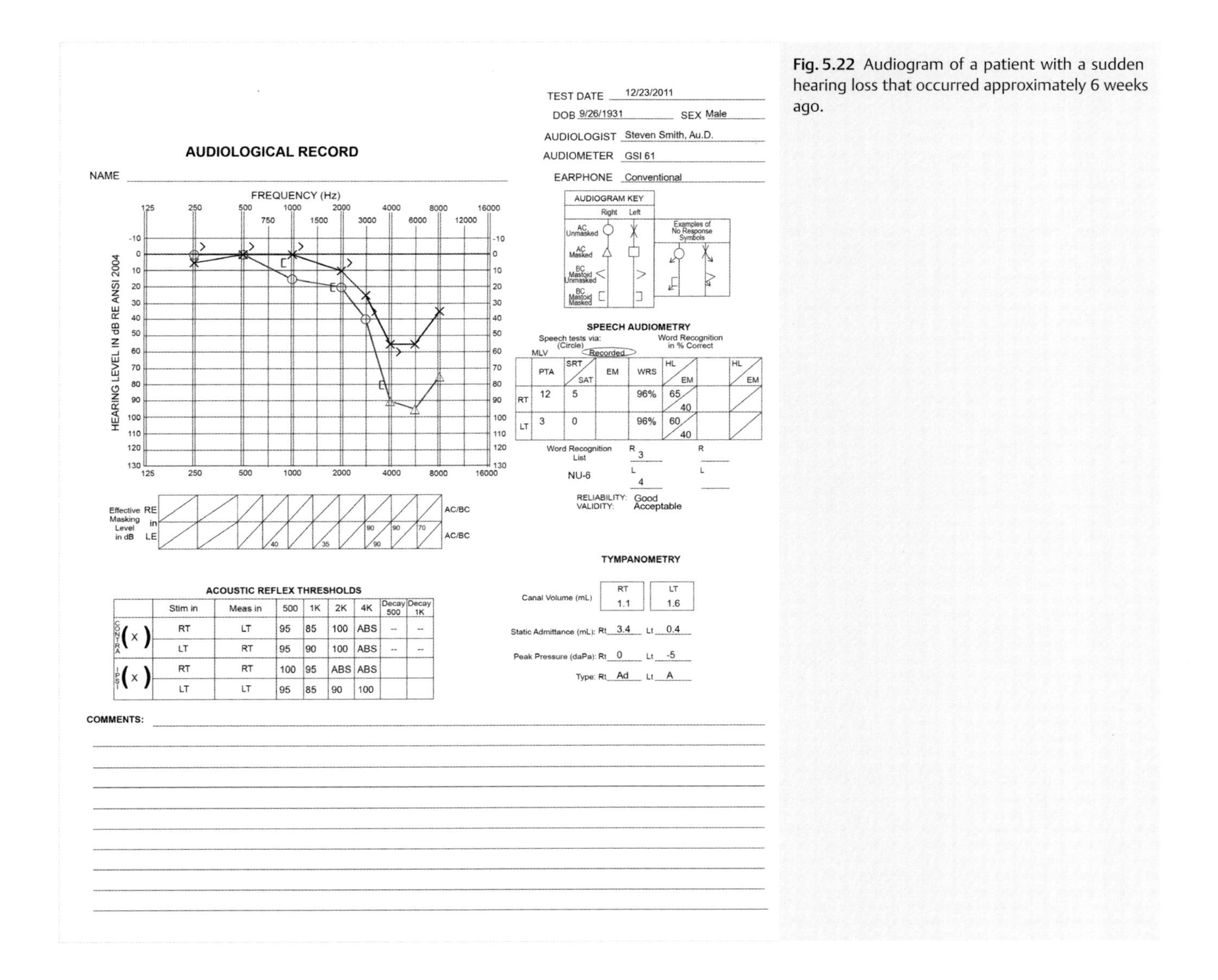

AUDIOLOGICAL RECORD

NAME

TEST DATE 12/23/2011
DOB 9/26/1931 SEX Male
AUDIOLOGIST Steven Smith, Au.D.
AUDIOMETER GSI 61
EARPHONE Conventional

SPEECH AUDIOMETRY

Speech tests via: (Circle) MLV Recorded — Word Recognition in % Correct

	PTA	SRT/SAT	EM	WRS	HL/EM		HL/EM
RT	12	5		96%	65/40		
LT	3	0		96%	60/40		

Word Recognition List: R 3, L 4 — NU-6

RELIABILITY: Good
VALIDITY: Acceptable

Effective Masking Level in dB: LE 40, 35, 90, 90, 90, 70

ACOUSTIC REFLEX THRESHOLDS

	Stim in	Meas in	500	1K	2K	4K	Decay 500	Decay 1K
CONTRA (x)	RT	LT	95	85	100	ABS	--	--
	LT	RT	95	90	100	ABS	--	--
IPSI (x)	RT	RT	100	95	ABS	ABS		
	LT	LT	95	85	90	100		

TYMPANOMETRY

	RT	LT
Canal Volume (mL)	1.1	1.6
Static Admittance (mL)	3.4	0.4
Peak Pressure (daPa)	0	-5
Type	Ad	A

COMMENTS:

Fig. 5.22 Audiogram of a patient with a sudden hearing loss that occurred approximately 6 weeks ago.

5.22.2 Interpretation

Right ear—Normal sloping to mild sensorineural hearing loss at 250 to 3,000 Hz, steeply sloping to severe and profound at 4,000 to 6,000 Hz, rising to severe at 8,000 Hz. The SRT was normal and was in agreement with the PTA. The WRS was obtained and was normal. Immittance testing revealed a hypercompliant tympanogram. Acoustic reflex thresholds with ipsilateral stimulation were normal at 500 and 1,000 Hz and absent at 2,000 and 4,000 Hz. Acoustic reflex thresholds with contralateral stimulation were normal at 500, 1,000, and 2,000 Hz and absent at 4,000 Hz. Contralateral acoustic reflex decay was negative at 500 and 1,000 Hz.

Left ear—Normal hearing at 250 to 2,000 Hz, sloping to slight and moderate sensorineural hearing loss 3,000 to 6,000 Hz, rising to a mild at 8,000 Hz. The SRT was normal and was in agreement with the PTA. The WRS was obtained and was normal. Immittance testing revealed a normal tympanogram. Acoustic reflex thresholds for ipsilateral stimulation were normal at 500 through 4,000 Hz. Acoustic reflex thresholds with contralateral stimulation were normal at 500, 1,000, and 2,000 Hz and absent at 4,000 Hz. Contralateral acoustic reflex decay was negative at 500 and 1,000 Hz.

5.22.3 Intervention

The patient visited with an otologist who prescribed oral steroids for 5 days in an attempt to restore his hearing. He was scheduled for an MRI to determine if an acoustic neuroma was present. The MRI was negative, and the steroids did not help with hearing restoration. He scheduled a hearing aid evaluation and purchased bilateral hearing aids that he perceived to be beneficial.

5.23 Case 23

5.23.1 Case History

The patient reported bilateral hearing loss for several years that had progressed over the last 12 years compared to his last hearing test. The patient currently wore CIC hearing aids from another clinic, but did not notice as much benefit as he would like in meetings and at church. He had intermittent bilateral tinnitus that was not bothersome. He had some imbalance, which he attributed to his heart because he had recently had a stent placed. He had a family history of hearing loss in that his sister had hearing loss. He did not report other otologic symptoms or history.

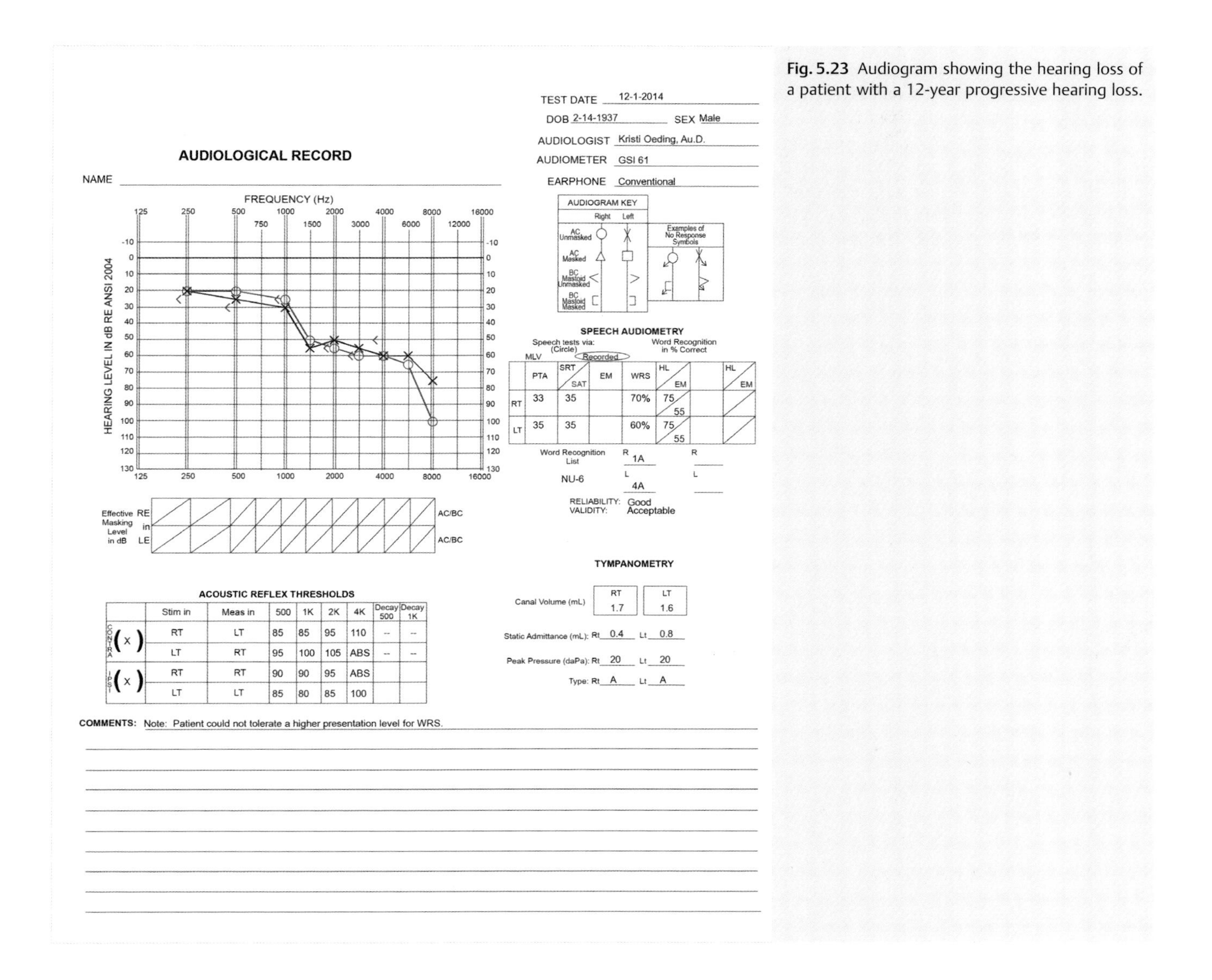

AUDIOLOGICAL RECORD

NAME

TEST DATE 12-1-2014
DOB 2-14-1937 SEX Male
AUDIOLOGIST Kristi Oeding, Au.D.
AUDIOMETER GSI 61
EARPHONE Conventional

SPEECH AUDIOMETRY

Speech tests via: (Circle) MLV Recorded

	PTA	SRT/SAT	EM	WRS	HL/EM	HL/EM
RT	33	35		70%	75 / 55	
LT	35	35		60%	75 / 55	

Word Recognition List NU-6: R 1A; L 4A

RELIABILITY: Good
VALIDITY: Acceptable

TYMPANOMETRY

	RT	LT
Canal Volume (mL)	1.7	1.6
Static Admittance (mL)	0.4	0.8
Peak Pressure (daPa)	20	20
Type	A	A

ACOUSTIC REFLEX THRESHOLDS

	Stim in	Meas in	500	1K	2K	4K	Decay 500	Decay 1K
CONTRA (X)	RT	LT	85	85	95	110	--	--
	LT	RT	95	100	105	ABS	--	--
IPSI (X)	RT	RT	90	90	95	ABS		
	LT	LT	85	80	85	100		

COMMENTS: Note: Patient could not tolerate a higher presentation level for WRS.

Fig. 5.23 Audiogram showing the hearing loss of a patient with a 12-year progressive hearing loss.

5.23.2 Interpretation

Right ear—Pure-tone thresholds revealed a slight sensorineural hearing loss from 250 to 1,000 Hz, sloping to a moderate to moderately severe sensorineural hearing loss from 1,500 to 6,000 Hz, and further sloping to a profound hearing loss at 8,000 Hz. The SRT revealed a mild loss in the ability to receive speech and was in agreement with the PTA. The WRS revealed moderate difficulty in the ability to recognize speech. Immittance testing revealed a normal tympanogram. Ipsilateral acoustic reflex thresholds were within normal limits from 500 to 2,000 Hz and absent at 4,000 Hz. Contralateral acoustic reflex thresholds were within normal limits from 500 to 1,000 Hz, elevated at 2,000 Hz, and absent at 4,000 Hz. Acoustic reflex decay was negative at 500 and 1,000 Hz.

Left ear—Pure-tone thresholds revealed a slight to mild sensorineural hearing loss from 250 to 1,000 Hz, sloping to a moderate to moderately severe sensorineural hearing loss from 1,500 to 6,000 Hz, and further sloping to a severe hearing loss at 8,000 Hz. The SRT revealed a mild loss in the ability to receive speech and was in agreement with the PTA. The WRS revealed moderate difficulty in the ability to recognize speech. Immittance testing revealed a normal tympanogram. Ipsilateral acoustic reflex thresholds were within normal limits from 500 to 4,000 Hz. Contralateral acoustic reflex thresholds were within normal limits from 500 to 2,000 Hz and elevated at 4,000 Hz. Acoustic reflex decay was negative at 500 and 1,000 Hz.

5.23.3 Intervention

Compared to the last hearing test, his hearing had decreased 15 to 35 dB HL at most frequencies. The otologist ordered tests to rule out an autoimmune inner ear disease. Results revealed a positive Western Blot for inner ear antigen antibodies. He was medically cleared for new hearing aids and followed up 4 months later to determine how quickly his hearing loss was progressing.

5.24 Case 24

5.24.1 Case History

The patient was a 95-year-old female who reported being diagnosed with hearing loss over 25 years ago. She did not report having hearing loss as a child or as a young adult. There was a significant familial history of hearing loss reported with her maternal grandmother, sister, and two children having hearing loss. There was no report of ear pathology or noise exposure. The patient denied tinnitus and dizziness. She had used amplification for 25 years, and her latest pair of hearing aids were 7-year-old digital BTE hearing aids with custom standard earmolds. The patient reported having difficulty hearing music when line dancing. She reported using an amplified telephone, but did not receive much benefit with speech understanding when listening to telephone conversations.

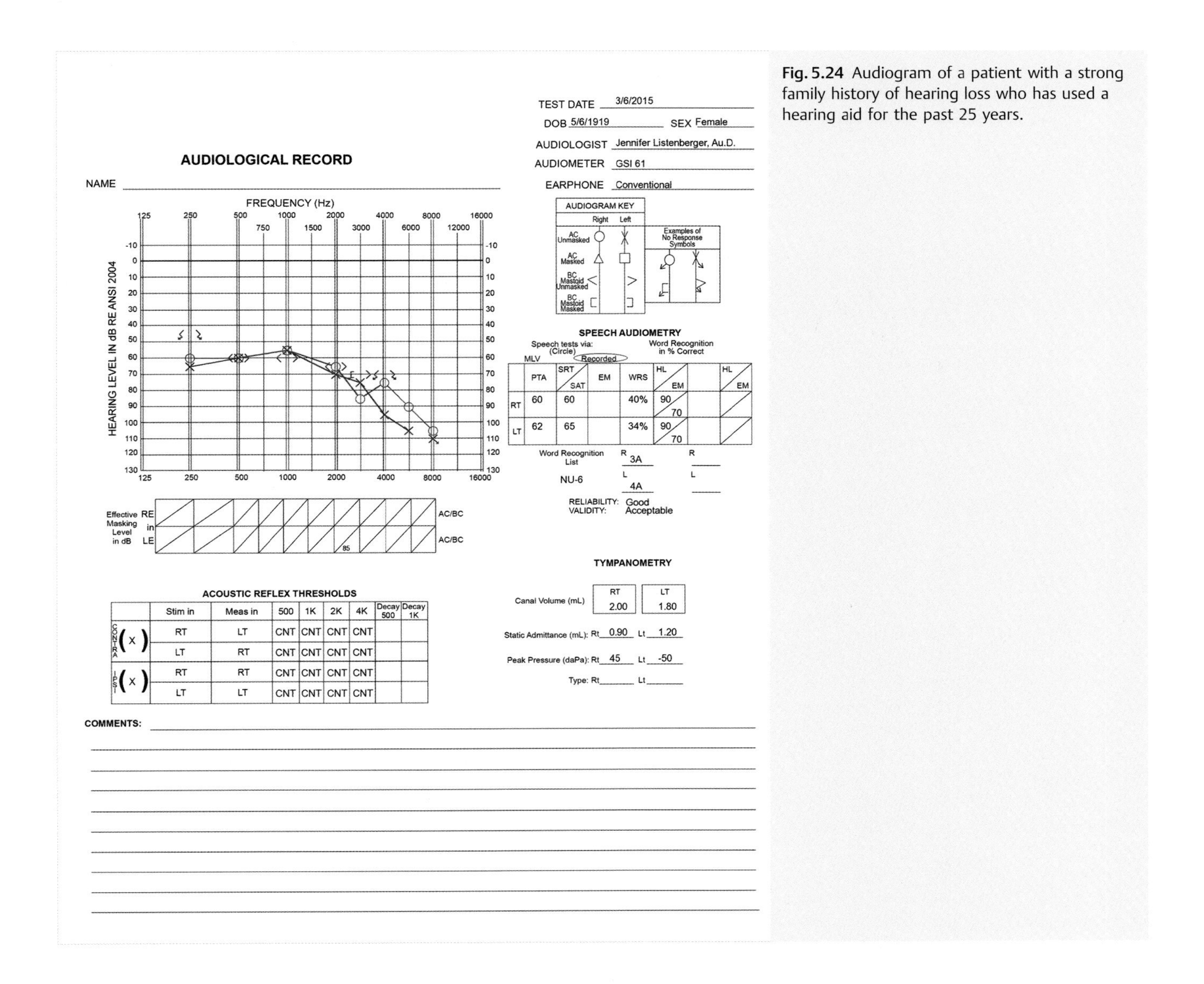

Fig. 5.24 Audiogram of a patient with a strong family history of hearing loss who has used a hearing aid for the past 25 years.

5.24.2 Interpretation

Right ear—Pure-tone air and bone conduction threshold testing revealed a moderately severe sensorineural hearing loss at 250 through 2,000 Hz, except for a moderate hearing loss at 1,000 Hz, sloping to severe at 3,000 through 6,000 Hz, and sloping to profound at 8,000 Hz. The SRT revealed a moderately severe loss in the ability to receive speech and was in agreement with the PTA. The WRS revealed very poor ability to recognize speech. Immittance testing revealed a normal tympanogram. Acoustic reflex threshold and decay testing could not be measured due to excessive artifact.

Left ear—Pure-tone air and bone conduction threshold testing revealed a moderately severe sensorineural hearing loss at 250 through 2,000 Hz, except for a moderate hearing loss at 1,000 Hz, and sloping to severe to profound at 3,000 through 8,000 Hz with no measurable response within the limits of the audiometer at 8,000 Hz. The SRT revealed a moderately severe loss in the ability to receive speech and was in agreement with the PTA. The WRS revealed a very poor ability to recognize speech. Immittance testing revealed a normal tympanogram. Acoustic reflex threshold and decay testing could not be measured due to excessive artifact.

5.24.3 Intervention

It was recommended that the patient consider a different type of HAT, such as captioning for the television and telephone. New amplification was also recommended. Communication strategies were discussed and encouraged. Annual hearing testing to monitor her hearing sensitivity was also encouraged.

5.25 Case 25

5.25.1 Case History

The patient was a 73-year-old male who stated he began to notice hearing loss in his left ear many years ago. Reportedly, this was examined, and he was told that there was nothing concerning at that time. He reported that his hearing continued to decline in the left ear. He noted a hissing tinnitus in the left ear. He perceived relatively good hearing in the right ear. He stated that intermittent dizziness had started in the last few months.

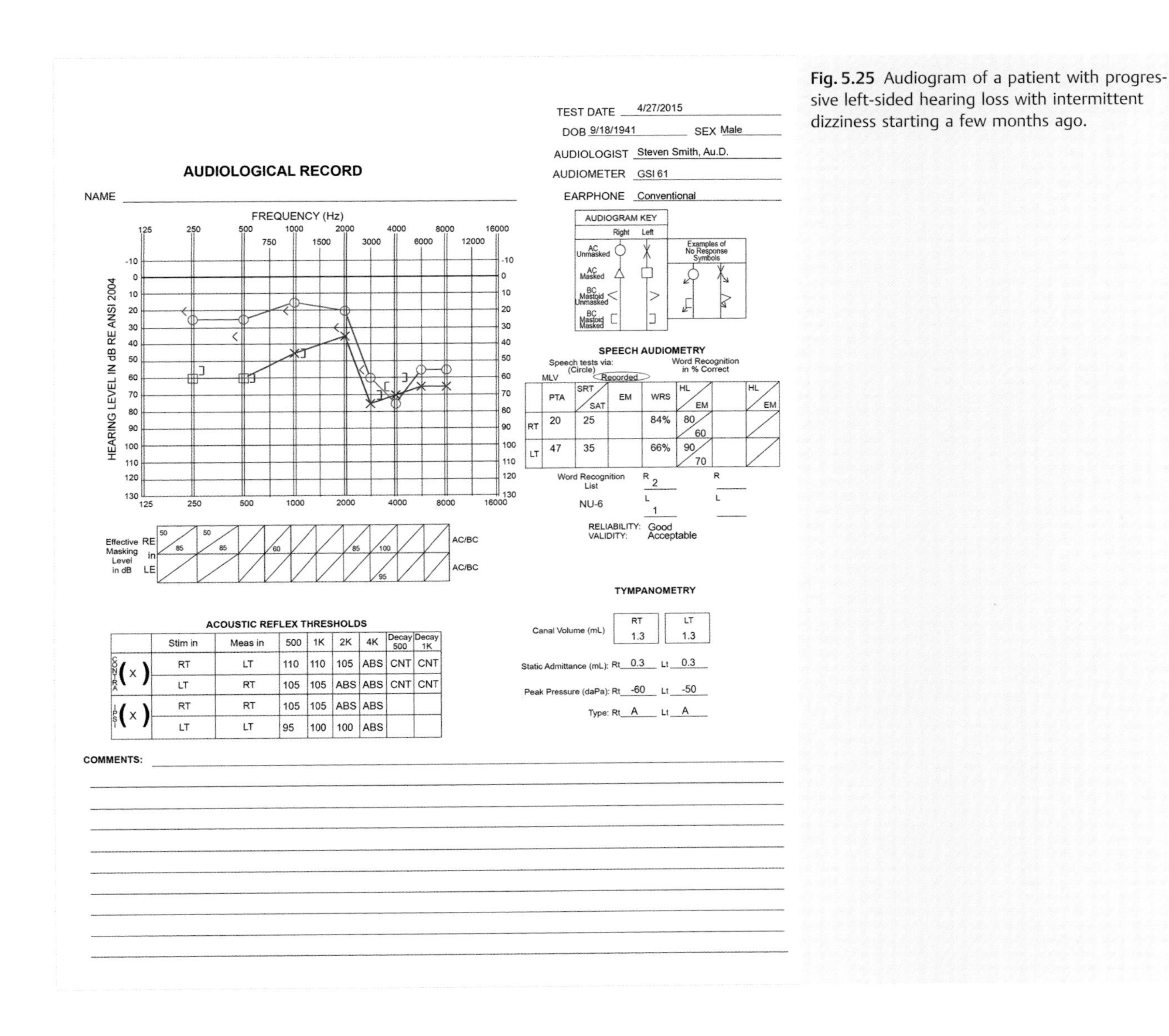

AUDIOLOGICAL RECORD

TEST DATE 4/27/2015
DOB 9/18/1941 SEX Male
AUDIOLOGIST Steven Smith, Au.D.
AUDIOMETER GSI 61
EARPHONE Conventional
NAME

SPEECH AUDIOMETRY

Speech tests via: (Circle) MLV Recorded (circled)
Word Recognition in % Correct

	PTA	SRT/SAT	EM	WRS	HL/EM		HL/EM
RT	20	25		84%	80/60		
LT	47	35		66%	90/70		

Word Recognition List NU-6: R 2, L 1

RELIABILITY: Good
VALIDITY: Acceptable

TYMPANOMETRY

	RT	LT
Canal Volume (mL)	1.3	1.3
Static Admittance (mL)	0.3	0.3
Peak Pressure (daPa)	-60	-50
Type	A	A

Effective Masking Level in dB: RE 50/85, 50/85, 60, 85, 100; LE 95

ACOUSTIC REFLEX THRESHOLDS

	Stim in	Meas in	500	1K	2K	4K	Decay 500	Decay 1K
CONTRA (X)	RT	LT	110	110	105	ABS	CNT	CNT
	LT	RT	105	105	ABS	ABS	CNT	CNT
IPSI (X)	RT	RT	105	105	ABS	ABS		
	LT	LT	95	100	100	ABS		

COMMENTS:

Fig. 5.25 Audiogram of a patient with progressive left-sided hearing loss with intermittent dizziness starting a few months ago.

5.25.2 Interpretation

Right ear—Slight sensorineural hearing loss at 250 to 2,000 Hz, with a rise to normal at 1,000 Hz, sloping to moderately severe to severe at 3,000 to 4,000 Hz, rising to moderate at 6,000 to 8,000 Hz. The SRT demonstrated a slight loss and was in agreement with the PTA. The WRS was obtained and showed a slight difficulty. Immittance testing revealed a normal tympanogram. Acoustic reflex thresholds for ipsilateral and contralateral stimulation were present, but elevated at 500 and 1,000 Hz and absent at 2,000 and 4,000 Hz. The contralateral acoustic reflex decay could not be measured.

Left ear—Moderately severe rising to mild sensorineural hearing loss at 250 to 2,000 Hz, sloping to severe at 3,000 Hz, rising to moderately severe at 4,000 to 8,000 Hz. The SRT demonstrated a mild loss and was relatively in agreement with the PTA. The WRS was obtained and showed moderate difficulty. Immittance testing revealed a normal tympanogram. Acoustic reflex thresholds for ipsilateral stimulation were normal at 500 through 2,000 Hz and absent at 4,000 Hz. Acoustic reflex thresholds for contralateral stimulation were present, but elevated at 500 through 2,000 Hz and absent at 4,000 Hz. The contralateral acoustic reflex decay could not be measured.

5.25.3 Intervention

The patient was referred to an ENT specialist for follow-up due to the asymmetry of his hearing and WRS. He was referred for an MRI to rule out a retrocochlear pathology, and it was recommended that he follow up for a hearing aid evaluation, pending medical clearance.

5.26 Case 26

5.26.1 Case History

The patient reported a long-standing history of bilateral profound sensorineural hearing loss. The hearing loss in the right ear occurred suddenly and was gradual in the left ear. Over the last year she had noticed a decrease in hearing with her left BTE hearing aid compared to her last hearing test. She could no longer hear anything with the left hearing aid. She had extreme difficulty hearing during the appointment, and all communication was completed by writing to her. She noted intermittent clicking and other noises in her left ear when she watched TV at night. She had occasional otalgia in the left ear. She had previously been evaluated for a cochlear implant, but did not qualify at the time because her heart was not able to handle anesthesia. She did not report other otologic symptoms or history.

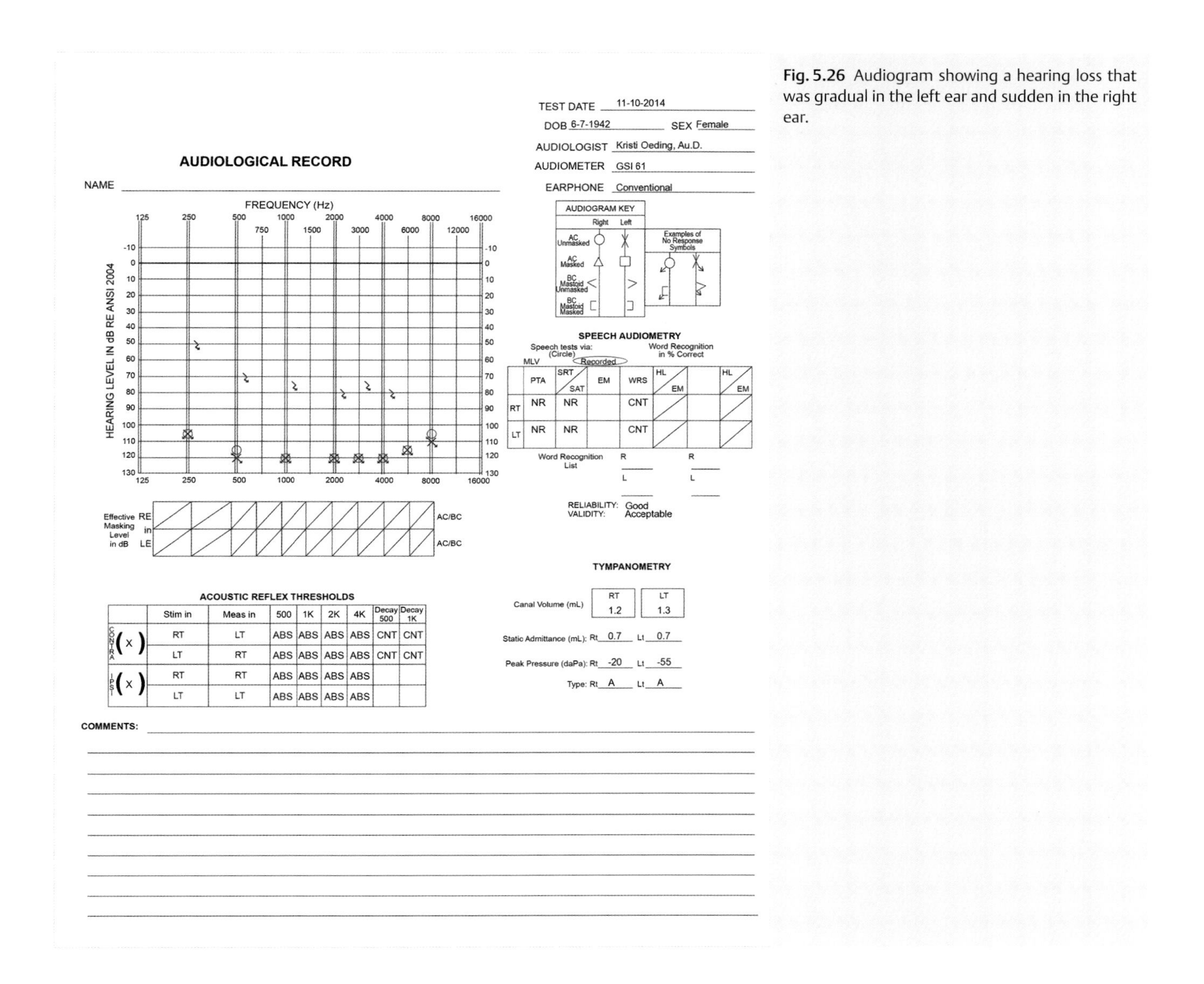

AUDIOLOGICAL RECORD

TEST DATE 11-10-2014
DOB 6-7-1942 SEX Female
AUDIOLOGIST Kristi Oeding, Au.D.
AUDIOMETER GSI 61
EARPHONE Conventional

NAME

SPEECH AUDIOMETRY
Speech tests via: (Circle) MLV Recorded

	PTA	SRT/SAT	EM	WRS	HL/EM	HL/EM
RT	NR	NR		CNT		
LT	NR	NR		CNT		

Word Recognition List R L

RELIABILITY: Good
VALIDITY: Acceptable

TYMPANOMETRY

	RT	LT
Canal Volume (mL)	1.2	1.3
Static Admittance (mL)	0.7	0.7
Peak Pressure (daPa)	-20	-55
Type	A	A

ACOUSTIC REFLEX THRESHOLDS

	Stim in	Meas in	500	1K	2K	4K	Decay 500	Decay 1K
CONTRA	RT	LT	ABS	ABS	ABS	ABS	CNT	CNT
	LT	RT	ABS	ABS	ABS	ABS	CNT	CNT
IPSI	RT	RT	ABS	ABS	ABS	ABS		
	LT	LT	ABS	ABS	ABS	ABS		

COMMENTS:

Fig. 5.26 Audiogram showing a hearing loss that was gradual in the left ear and sudden in the right ear.

5.26.2 Interpretation

Right ear—Pure-tone thresholds revealed a profound sensorineural hearing loss with no measurable response within the limits of the audiometer at 250 to 8,000 Hz. The SAT revealed an inability to detect speech at the limits of the audiometer and was in agreement with the PTA. The WRS could not be tested because an SAT could not be obtained. Immittance testing revealed a normal tympanogram. Ipsilateral and contralateral acoustic reflex thresholds were absent from 500 to 4,000 Hz. Acoustic reflex decay could not be measured at 500 and 1,000 Hz due to absent contralateral acoustic reflex thresholds.

Left ear—Pure-tone thresholds revealed a profound sensorineural hearing loss with no measurable response within the limits of the audiometer at 250 to 8,000 Hz. The SAT revealed an inability to detect speech at the limits of the audiometer and was in agreement with the PTA. The WRS could not be tested because an SAT could not be obtained. Immittance testing revealed a normal tympanogram. The ipsilateral and contralateral acoustic reflex thresholds were absent from 500 to 4,000 Hz. Acoustic reflex decay could not be measured at 500 and 1,000 Hz due to absent contralateral acoustic reflex thresholds.

5.26.3 Intervention

The pure-tone air conduction thresholds had decreased to no response in the left ear from 250 to 4,000 Hz compared to her last hearing test. The otologist could not see a reason why she could not undergo surgery because her most recent cardiology report was good. She was scheduled for a CI evaluation and a CT scan, and the otologist planned to talk with her cardiologist about surgery.

5.27 Case 27

5.27.1 Case History

The patient was diagnosed with unilateral sensorineural hearing loss in the right ear approximately 6 years ago. She had since used amplification in the right ear and stated that there was a significant benefit; however, she was noticing an increased need for repetition and felt she was struggling more in group settings. She was seen for a follow-up hearing test to monitor stability of hearing due to concerns that her hearing had deteriorated. The last hearing test was completed 2 years ago. An MRI was completed when the patient was first diagnosed with hearing loss, and the results were negative for a vestibular schwannoma. She had continued medical follow-up since then.

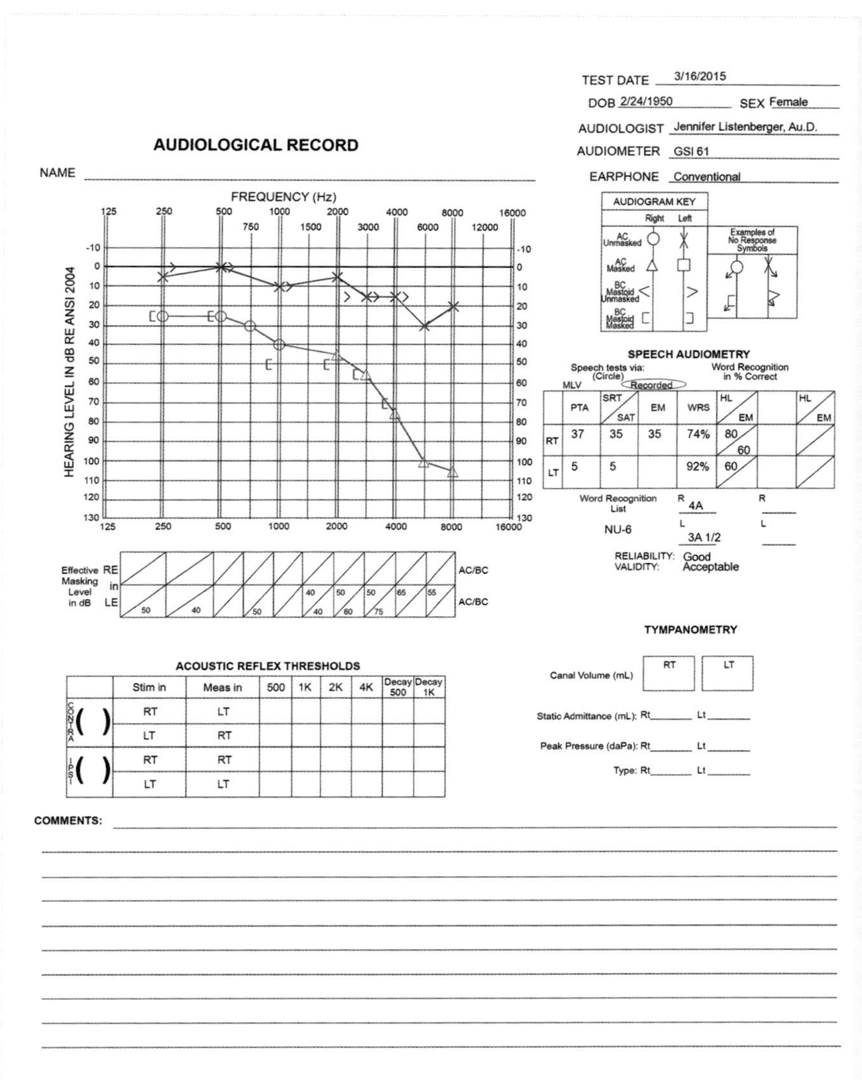

Fig. 5.27 Audiogram showing a long-standing hearing loss in the right ear and the patient is having more difficulty hearing in noise.

5.27.2 Interpretation

Right ear—Pure-tone air and bone conduction threshold testing revealed a slight sloping to moderate sensorineural hearing loss at 250 to 3,000 Hz, sloping to severe at 4,000 Hz, and sloping to profound at 6,000 to 8,000 Hz. The SRT revealed a mild loss in the ability to receive speech and was in agreement with the PTA. The WRS revealed moderate difficulty in the ability to recognize speech. Immittance testing was not measured.

Left ear—Pure-tone air and bone conduction threshold testing revealed normal hearing sensitivity at 250 to 4,000 Hz and sloping to mild and rising to a slight, presumably sensorineural, hearing loss at 6,000 to 8,000 Hz. The SRT revealed a normal ability to receive speech and was in agreement with the PTA. The WRS revealed a normal ability to recognize speech. Immittance testing was not measured.

5.27.3 Intervention

The test results were reviewed with the patient and remained relatively unchanged since the last test, but comparison to the original test revealed a significant progression in thresholds at 2,000 to 8,000 Hz and a decrease in the WRS from normal to moderate difficulty in the ability to recognize speech in the right ear. The patient was referred to an otologist for follow-up regarding progression of hearing loss and changes in WRS. The audiological recommendations were to return for a hearing test annually to monitor hearing stability, continued use of amplification, use of HAT, and hearing protection in noise.

5.28 Case 28

5.28.1 Case History

The patient was a 54-year-old male who reported difficulties with dizziness for the last few months. He reported that the dizziness occurred when he turned over in bed or looked up. He reported normal hearing bilaterally. He reported some pain at times bilaterally as well as itchiness.

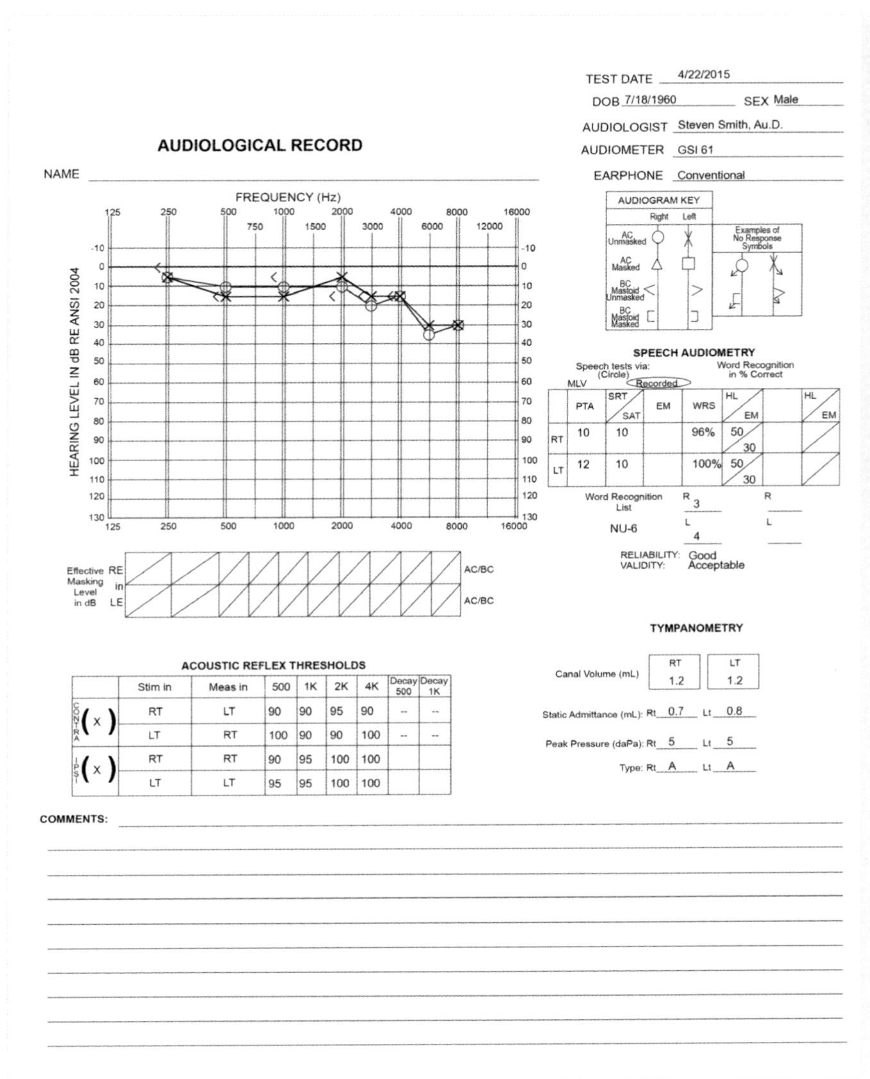

AUDIOLOGICAL RECORD

NAME

TEST DATE 4/22/2015

DOB 7/18/1960 SEX Male

AUDIOLOGIST Steven Smith, Au.D.

AUDIOMETER GSI 61

EARPHONE Conventional

SPEECH AUDIOMETRY

Speech tests via: (Circle) MLV Recorded

Word Recognition in % Correct

	PTA	SRT / SAT	EM	WRS	HL / EM		HL / EM
RT	10	10		96%	50 / 30		
LT	12	10		100%	50 / 30		

Word Recognition List: R 3, L 4; R ___, L ___

NU-6

RELIABILITY: Good

VALIDITY: Acceptable

TYMPANOMETRY

	RT	LT
Canal Volume (mL)	1.2	1.2

Static Admittance (mL): Rt 0.7 Lt 0.8

Peak Pressure (daPa): Rt 5 Lt 5

Type: Rt A Lt A

ACOUSTIC REFLEX THRESHOLDS

	Stim in	Meas in	500	1K	2K	4K	Decay 500	Decay 1K
CONTRA (x)	RT	LT	90	90	95	90	--	--
	LT	RT	100	90	90	100	--	--
IPSI (x)	RT	RT	90	95	100	100		
	LT	LT	95	95	100	100		

COMMENTS:

Fig. 5.28 Audiogram of a patient who has been having dizziness.

5.28.2 Interpretation

Right ear—Normal hearing at 250 to 4,000 Hz, with a slight sensorineural hearing loss notch at 3,000 Hz, sloping to mild at 6,000 to 8,000 Hz. The SRT was normal and was in agreement with the PTA. The WRS was normal. Immittance testing revealed a normal tympanogram with normal acoustic reflex thresholds at 500 to 4,000 Hz with ipsilateral and contralateral stimulation. Negative acoustic reflex decay was obtained with contralateral stimulation at 500 and 1,000 Hz.

Left ear—Normal hearing at 250 to 4,000 Hz, sloping to mild at 6,000 to 8,000 Hz. The SRT was normal and was in agreement with the PTA. The WRS was normal. Immittance testing revealed a normal tympanogram with normal acoustic reflex thresholds at 500 to 4,000 Hz with ipsilateral and contralateral stimulation. Negative acoustic reflex decay was obtained with contralateral stimulation at 500 and 1,000 Hz.

5.28.3 Intervention

The patient was referred to an ENT specialist for follow-up regarding the dizziness. The Dix–Hallpike maneuver determined that he had BPPV. An Epley procedure was performed, which resolved his dizziness.

5.29 Case 29

5.29.1 Case History

The patient attended a loud concert 1 month ago. Afterward he noted constant bilateral tinnitus, decreased hearing, increased sensitivity to loud sounds such as sirens and the seat belt alert signal in the car, and distorted sound quality, particularly for music. After 2 weeks his hearing seemed to improve, and the sensitivity and distortion improved, but he still noted bilateral constant tinnitus. The tinnitus was not bothersome and could increase in intensity for a few seconds. He reported he may have bilateral hearing loss because he had worked around loud music for many years. He noticed difficulty hearing in background noise. He did not wear hearing protection prior to attending the concert, but he did now. He had a family history of hearing loss, with his grandfather acquiring hearing loss later in life, possibly due to noise exposure. He did not report other otologic symptoms or history.

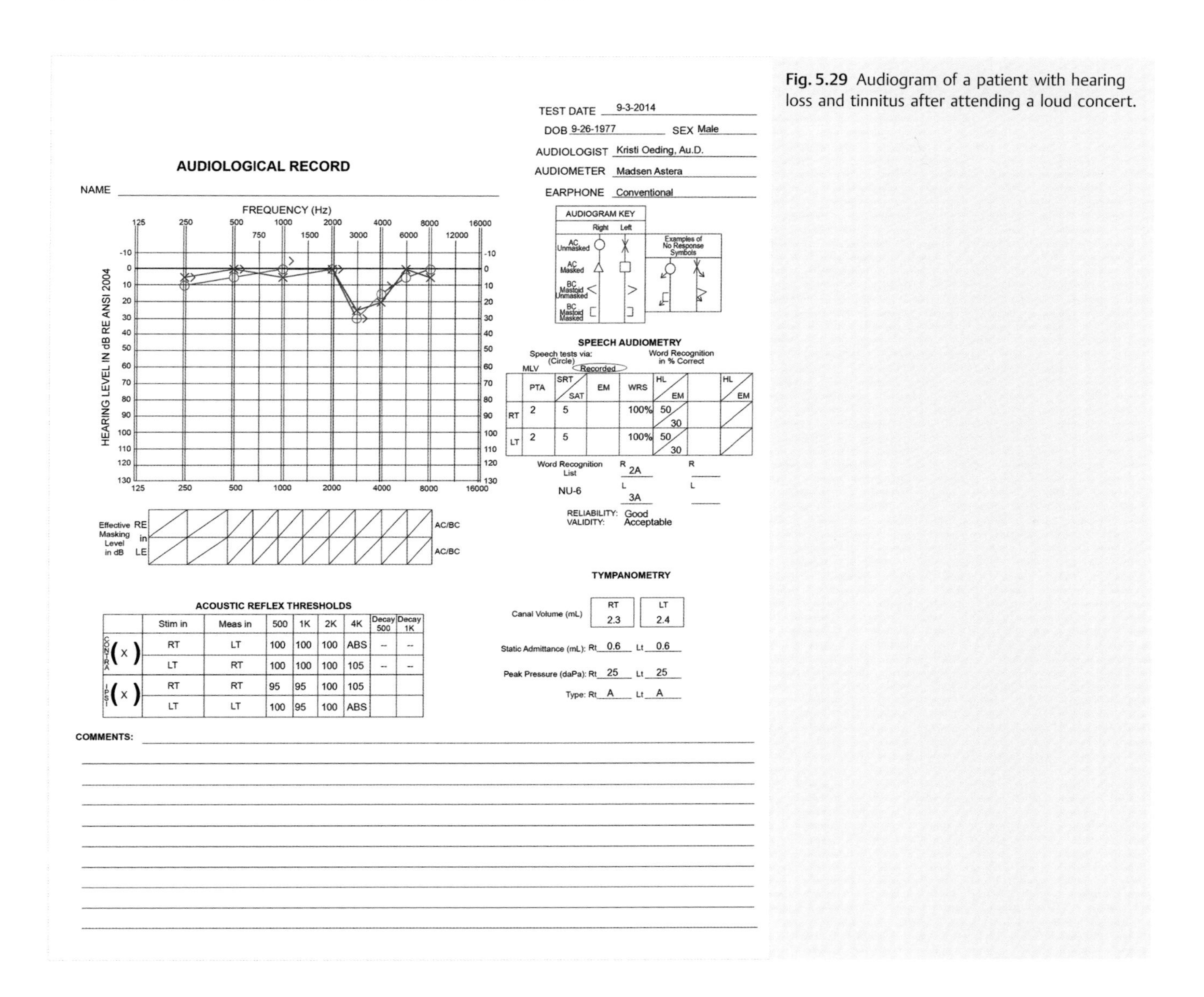

AUDIOLOGICAL RECORD

NAME

TEST DATE 9-3-2014
DOB 9-26-1977 SEX Male
AUDIOLOGIST Kristi Oeding, Au.D.
AUDIOMETER Madsen Astera
EARPHONE Conventional

SPEECH AUDIOMETRY

Speech tests via: (Circle) MLV Recorded

Word Recognition in % Correct

	PTA	SRT/SAT	EM	WRS	HL/EM		HL/EM
RT	2	5		100%	50/30		
LT	2	5		100%	50/30		

Word Recognition List NU-6: R 2A, L 3A

RELIABILITY: Good
VALIDITY: Acceptable

ACOUSTIC REFLEX THRESHOLDS

	Stim in	Meas in	500	1K	2K	4K	Decay 500	Decay 1K
CONTRA	RT	LT	100	100	100	ABS	--	--
CONTRA	LT	RT	100	100	100	105	--	--
IPSI	RT	RT	95	95	100	105		
IPSI	LT	LT	100	95	100	ABS		

TYMPANOMETRY

	RT	LT
Canal Volume (mL)	2.3	2.4
Static Admittance (mL)	0.6	0.6
Peak Pressure (daPa)	25	25
Type	A	A

COMMENTS:

Fig. 5.29 Audiogram of a patient with hearing loss and tinnitus after attending a loud concert.

5.29.2 Interpretation

Right ear—Pure-tone thresholds were within normal limits from 250 to 2,000 Hz, sloping to a mild sensorineural hearing loss at 3,000 Hz, and rising to within normal limits from 4,000 to 8,000 Hz. The SRT revealed a normal ability to receive speech and was in agreement with the PTA. The WRS revealed a normal ability to recognize speech. Immittance testing revealed a normal tympanogram. Ipsilateral and contralateral acoustic reflex thresholds were within normal limits from 500 to 2,000 Hz and elevated at 4,000 Hz. Acoustic reflex decay was negative at 500 and 1,000 Hz.

Left ear—Pure-tone thresholds were within normal limits from 250 to 2,000 Hz, sloping to a slight sensorineural hearing loss from 3,000 to 4,000 Hz, and rising to within normal limits from 6,000 to 8,000 Hz. The SRT revealed a normal ability to receive speech and was in agreement with the PTA. The WRS revealed a normal ability to recognize speech. Immittance testing revealed a normal tympanogram. The ipsilateral and contralateral acoustic reflex thresholds were within normal limits from 500 to 2,000 Hz and absent at 4,000 Hz. Acoustic reflex decay was negative at 500 and 1,000 Hz.

5.29.3 Intervention

The otologist reported that the hearing loss was due to his history of noise exposure. The patient was encouraged to continue using hearing protection when around loud sounds.

5.30 Case 30

5.30.1 Case History

The patient was seen annually for a hearing test to monitor hearing sensitivity after being diagnosed with a right-sided vestibular schwannoma in 2007. The patient had constant low-level bilateral tinnitus that he reported had not changed, except that it had recently seemed to become a little louder in the right. He had an asymmetric high-frequency sensorineural hearing loss that he perceived to have remained stable. There was no significant history of noise exposure.

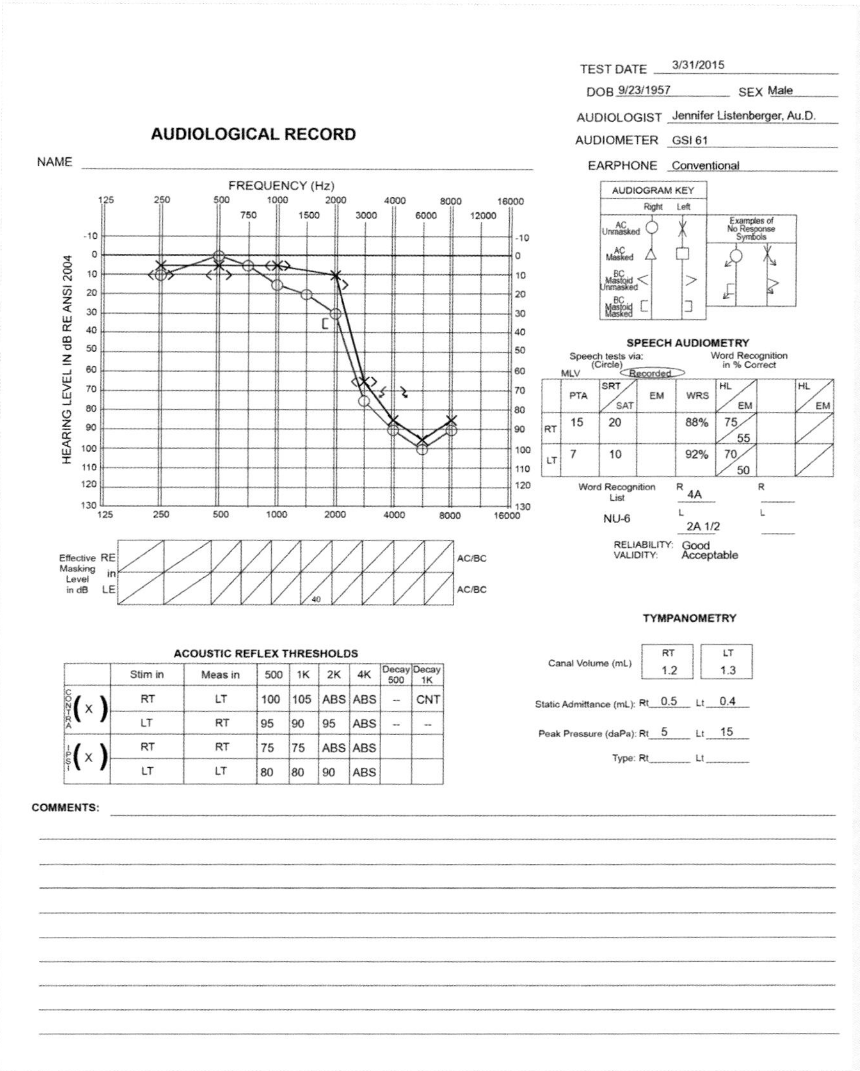

AUDIOLOGICAL RECORD

NAME ______

TEST DATE 3/31/2015
DOB 9/23/1957 SEX Male
AUDIOLOGIST Jennifer Listenberger, Au.D.
AUDIOMETER GSI 61
EARPHONE Conventional

SPEECH AUDIOMETRY

Speech tests via: (Circle) MLV Recorded (circled)

Word Recognition in % Correct

	PTA	SRT / SAT	EM	WRS	HL / EM		HL / EM
RT	15	20		88%	75 / 55		
LT	7	10		92%	70 / 50		

Word Recognition List: R 4A; L 2A 1/2; R ___; L ___

NU-6

RELIABILITY: Good
VALIDITY: Acceptable

TYMPANOMETRY

	RT	LT
Canal Volume (mL)	1.2	1.3

Static Admittance (mL): Rt 0.5 Lt 0.4

Peak Pressure (daPa): Rt 5 Lt 15

Type: Rt ___ Lt ___

ACOUSTIC REFLEX THRESHOLDS

	Stim in	Meas in	500	1K	2K	4K	Decay 500	Decay 1K
CONTRA (X)	RT	LT	100	105	ABS	ABS	--	CNT
	LT	RT	95	90	95	ABS	--	--
IPSI (X)	RT	RT	75	75	ABS	ABS		
	LT	LT	80	80	90	ABS		

COMMENTS:

Fig. 5.30 Audiogram of a patient who received an annual hearing evaluation to monitor a right-sided vestibular schwannoma.

5.30.2 Interpretation

Right ear—Pure-tone air and bone conduction threshold testing revealed normal hearing sensitivity at 250 through 1,000 Hz, sloping to a slight to mild sensorineural hearing loss at 1,500 through 2,000 Hz, and steeply sloping to severe at 3,000 through 8,000 Hz, with a profound notch at 6,000 Hz. The SRT revealed a slight loss in the ability to receive speech and was in agreement with the PTA. The WRS revealed a slight difficulty in the ability to recognize speech. Immittance testing revealed a normal tympanogram and normal acoustic reflex thresholds for ipsilateral stimulation at 500 and 1,000 Hz, and thresholds were absent at 2,000 and 4,000 Hz. Acoustic reflex thresholds for contralateral stimulation were within normal limits at 500 through 2,000 Hz and absent at 4,000 Hz. Acoustic reflex decay was negative for contralateral stimulation at 500 and 1,000 Hz.

Left ear—Pure-tone air and bone conduction threshold testing revealed normal hearing sensitivity at 250 through 2,000 Hz, steeply sloping to a moderately severe sensorineural hearing loss at 3,000 Hz, and sloping to severe at 4,000 through 8,000 Hz, with a profound notch at 6,000 Hz. The SRT revealed a normal ability to receive speech and was in agreement with the PTA. The WRS revealed a normal ability to recognize speech. Immittance testing revealed a normal tympanogram, and acoustic reflex thresholds for ipsilateral stimulation were within normal limits at 500 through 2,000 Hz and absent at 4,000 Hz. The acoustic reflex thresholds for contralateral stimulation were within normal limits at 500 Hz, elevated at 1,000 Hz, and absent at 2,000 and 4,000 Hz. Acoustic reflex decay was negative for contralateral stimulation at 500 Hz and could not be measured at 1,000 Hz due to an elevated contralateral acoustic reflex threshold.

5.30.3 Intervention

The test results revealed stable pure-tone thresholds and WRS. Test results were compared with the original test and no clinically significant changes were noted. The patient will follow up with an otologist as recommended. The audiological recommendations were to return annually for hearing testing, use HAT for TV, and use hearing protection in noise as well as to consider using amplification.

5.31 Case 31

5.31.1 Case History

A 24-year-old female scheduled an appointment for a hearing evaluation. She reported she was diagnosed with hearing loss at the age of 3 and reported consistent use of amplification since that time. She used an FM system in conjunction with a hearing aid until the eighth grade. She reported using hearing aids alone throughout high school and college. She enrolled in graduate school and was looking to upgrade her hearing aids because her current aids were approximately 7 years old. She was interested in new technology that would allow her to connect directly to her cell phone without any additional accessories. She reported tinnitus bilaterally and denied any problems with dizziness or fullness in her ears.

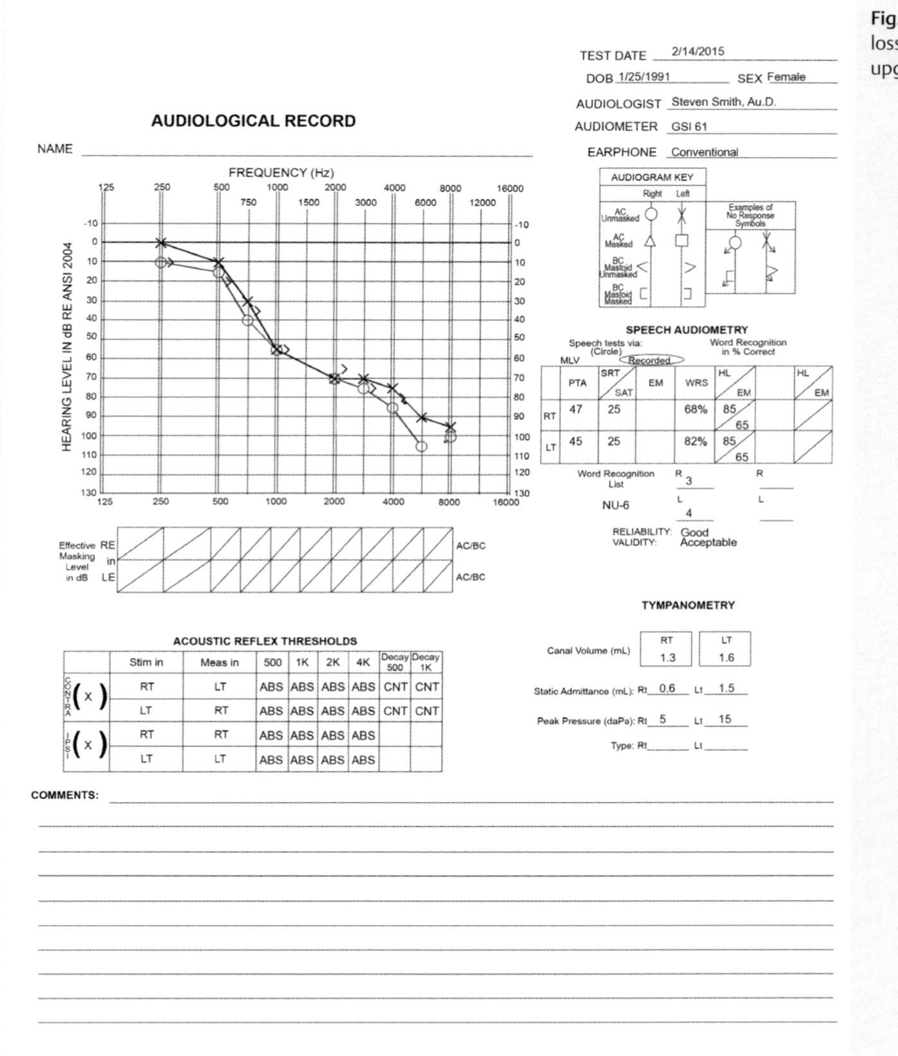

AUDIOLOGICAL RECORD

TEST DATE 2/14/2015
DOB 1/25/1991 SEX Female
AUDIOLOGIST Steven Smith, Au.D.
AUDIOMETER GSI 61
EARPHONE Conventional

NAME

Effective Masking Level in dB: RE AC/BC; LE AC/BC

SPEECH AUDIOMETRY

Speech tests via: (Circle) MLV Recorded

Word Recognition in % Correct

	PTA	SRT / SAT	EM	WRS	HL / EM		HL / EM
RT	47	25		68%	85 / 65		
LT	45	25		82%	85 / 65		

Word Recognition List: NU-6 R 3, L 4; R ___, L ___

RELIABILITY: Good
VALIDITY: Acceptable

TYMPANOMETRY

	RT	LT
Canal Volume (mL)	1.3	1.6

Static Admittance (mL): Rt 0.6 Lt 1.5
Peak Pressure (daPa): Rt 5 Lt 15
Type: Rt ___ Lt ___

ACOUSTIC REFLEX THRESHOLDS

	Stim in	Meas in	500	1K	2K	4K	Decay 500	Decay 1K
CONTRA (x)	RT	LT	ABS	ABS	ABS	ABS	CNT	CNT
	LT	RT	ABS	ABS	ABS	ABS	CNT	CNT
IPSI (x)	RT	RT	ABS	ABS	ABS	ABS		
	LT	LT	ABS	ABS	ABS	ABS		

COMMENTS:

Fig. 5.31 Audiogram of a patient with hearing loss diagnosed at the age of 3 who is looking to upgrade hearing aids.

5.31.2 Interpretation

Right ear—Normal sloping to a profound sensorineural hearing loss from 250 to 8,000 Hz. The SRT revealed a slight loss in the ability to receive speech and was not in agreement with the PTA, which is likely due to the steeply sloping hearing loss. The WRS revealed moderate difficulty in speech recognition. Immittance testing revealed a normal tympanogram. Acoustic reflex thresholds with ipsilateral and contralateral stimulation were absent from 500 to 4,000 Hz. Acoustic reflex decay could not be measured.

Left ear—Normal sloping to a profound sensorineural hearing loss from 250 to 8,000 Hz. The SRT revealed a slight loss in the ability to receive speech and was not in agreement with the PTA, which is likely due to the steeply sloping hearing loss. The WRS revealed a slight difficulty in speech recognition. Immittance testing revealed a normal tympanogram. Acoustic reflex thresholds with ipsilateral and contralateral stimulation were absent from 500 to 4,000 Hz. Acoustic reflex decay could not be performed.

5.31.3 Intervention

The patient was counseled on her hearing loss and information regarding updated technology for hearing aids was provided. She decided to purchase new hearing aids. Bilateral receiver-in-the-canal hearing aids with canal molds were made, and she reported receiving significantly improved hearing compared with her older hearing aids. She reported being satisfied with her ability to connect directly to her cell phone.

6 Conductive Hearing Loss Cases

6.1 Case 1

6.1.1 Case History

The patient was a 24-year-old male who reported he was walking down the street and was shot in the head approximately 2 months ago. He reported the bullet entered through his left cheek by his ear and traveled into his neck. At the time, he noted a loud ringing that started in his left ear, and, after being treated, he realized that he had difficulty hearing in that ear. The hearing loss persisted, and he noted that the tinnitus had decreased, but was still present. He reported that sound could be heard in the left ear, but it was muffled and it seemed like he was hearing with his head under water. He denied pain at the time. There was no reported dizziness and no history of noise exposure or other ear problems prior to the incident.

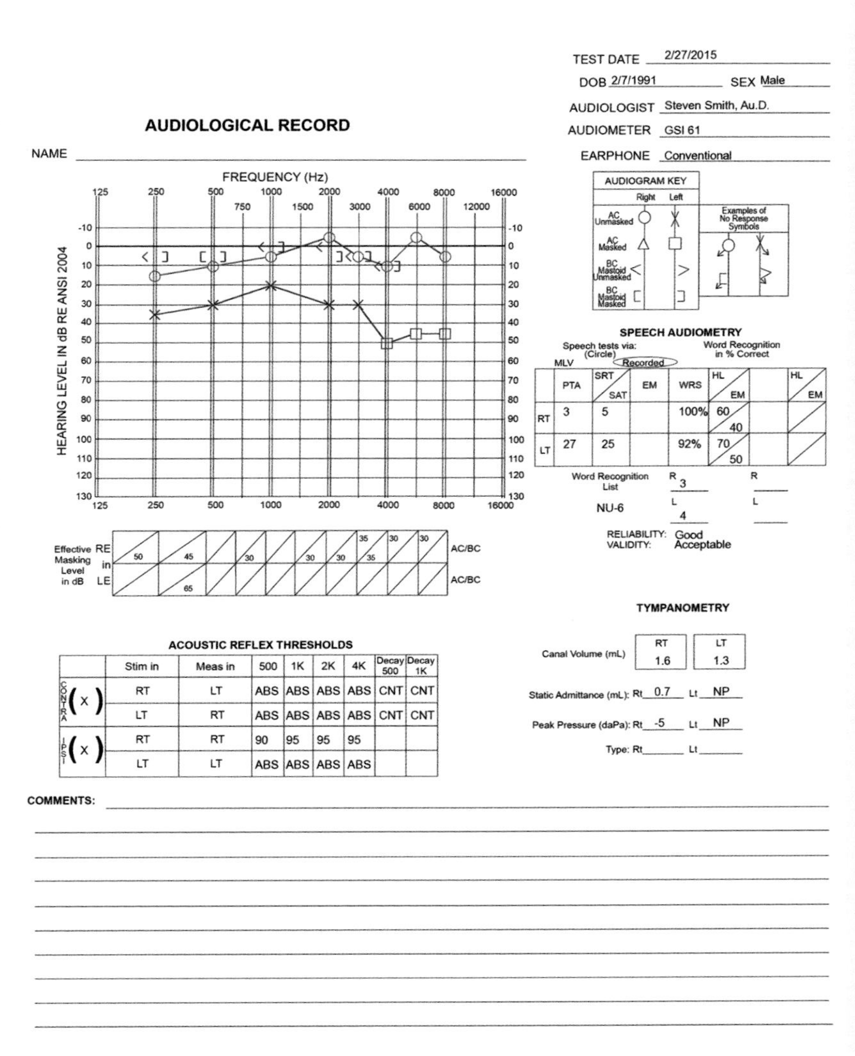

AUDIOLOGICAL RECORD

TEST DATE 2/27/2015
DOB 2/7/1991 SEX Male
AUDIOLOGIST Steven Smith, Au.D.
AUDIOMETER GSI 61
EARPHONE Conventional
NAME

SPEECH AUDIOMETRY

Speech tests via: (Circle) MLV Recorded (circled)
Word Recognition in % Correct

	PTA	SRT/SAT	EM	WRS	HL/EM		HL/EM
RT	3	5		100%	60/40		
LT	27	25		92%	70/50		

Word Recognition List NU-6: R 3, L 4

RELIABILITY: Good
VALIDITY: Acceptable

ACOUSTIC REFLEX THRESHOLDS

	Stim in	Meas in	500	1K	2K	4K	Decay 500	Decay 1K
CONTRA (X)	RT	LT	ABS	ABS	ABS	ABS	CNT	CNT
	LT	RT	ABS	ABS	ABS	ABS	CNT	CNT
IPSI (X)	RT	RT	90	95	95	95		
	LT	LT	ABS	ABS	ABS	ABS		

TYMPANOMETRY

	RT	LT
Canal Volume (mL)	1.6	1.3
Static Admittance (mL)	0.7	NP
Peak Pressure (daPa)	-5	NP
Type		

COMMENTS:

Fig. 6.1 Audiogram of a patient who was shot near his left ear and reported tinnitus and hearing loss in the left ear.

6.1.2 Interpretation

Right ear—Normal hearing sensitivity from 250 to 8,000 Hz. The SRT revealed a normal ability to receive speech and was in agreement with the PTA. The WRS was normal. Immittance testing revealed a normal tympanogram with normal acoustic reflex thresholds with ipsilateral stimulation and absent acoustic reflex thresholds with contralateral stimulation from 500 to 4,000 Hz. Acoustic reflex decay could not be tested due to absent contralateral acoustic reflex thresholds.

Left ear—Mild rising to a slight conductive hearing loss at 250 through 1,000 Hz, sloping to mild and moderate at 2,000 through 8,000 Hz. The SRT revealed a slight loss in the ability to receive speech and was in agreement with the PTA. The WRS was normal. Immittance testing revealed a flat tympanogram. The acoustic reflex thresholds with ipsilateral and contralateral stimulation from 500 to 4,000 Hz were absent. Acoustic reflex decay could not be tested due to absent contralateral acoustic reflex thresholds.

6.1.3 Intervention

The patient was referred to an ENT specialist for the conductive hearing loss in the left ear. Per the ENT specialist's report, he was diagnosed with middle ear effusion, which will be watched to determine if the effusion resolves on its own or if a pressure equalization tube might be needed.

6.2 Case 2

6.2.1 Case History

The patient had recurrent otitis media since childhood in the right ear. Later, he developed a cholesteatoma in the right ear canal that was surgically removed. He had a tympanoplasty to repair the right tympanic membrane. He did not notice hearing loss in the left ear. He noticed greater difficulty hearing and was interested in amplification options. He did not report other otologic symptoms or history.

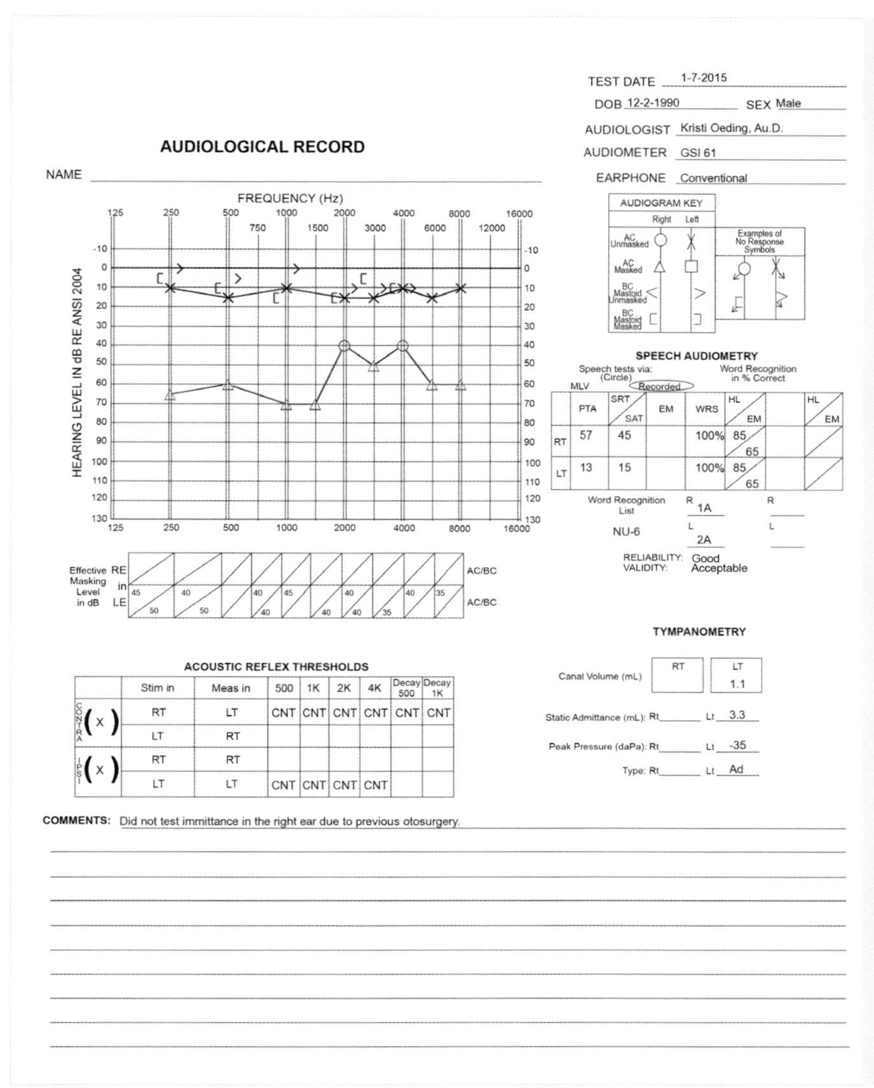

Fig. 6.2 Audiogram of a patient with a history of otitis media, cholesteatoma, and tympanoplasty in the right ear. The patient was diagnosed with otosclerosis.

6.2.2 Interpretation

Right ear—Pure-tone thresholds revealed a moderately severe conductive hearing loss from 250–1,500 Hz, rising to a mild to moderate conductive hearing loss from 2,000–4,000 Hz, and sloping to a moderately severe hearing loss from 6,000–8,000 Hz. The SRT revealed a moderate loss in the ability to receive speech and was in relative agreement with the PTA. The WRS revealed a normal ability to recognize speech. Immittance testing was not measured due to previous otosurgery.

Left ear—Pure-tone thresholds were within normal limits from 250–8,000 Hz. The SRT revealed a normal ability to receive speech and was in agreement with the PTA. The WRS revealed a normal ability to recognize speech. Immittance testing revealed a hypercompliant tympanogram. Acoustic reflex thresholds and decay could not be measured due to artifact from the hypercompliant tympanic membrane.

6.2.3 Intervention

A CT scan revealed an absent malleus and incus, and the stapes was fixed (otosclerosis). The otologist recommended a hearing aid in the right ear or a BAHA, and, if needed, an ossicular chain reconstruction could be considered in the future.

6.3 Case 3

6.3.1 Case History

The patient reported a history of left unilateral hearing loss and multiple ear infections and otosurgeries in that ear. A tympanomastoidectomy was completed in the left ear in 2000. The patient denied any tinnitus or dizziness. She reported not having a hearing test in more than 10 years.

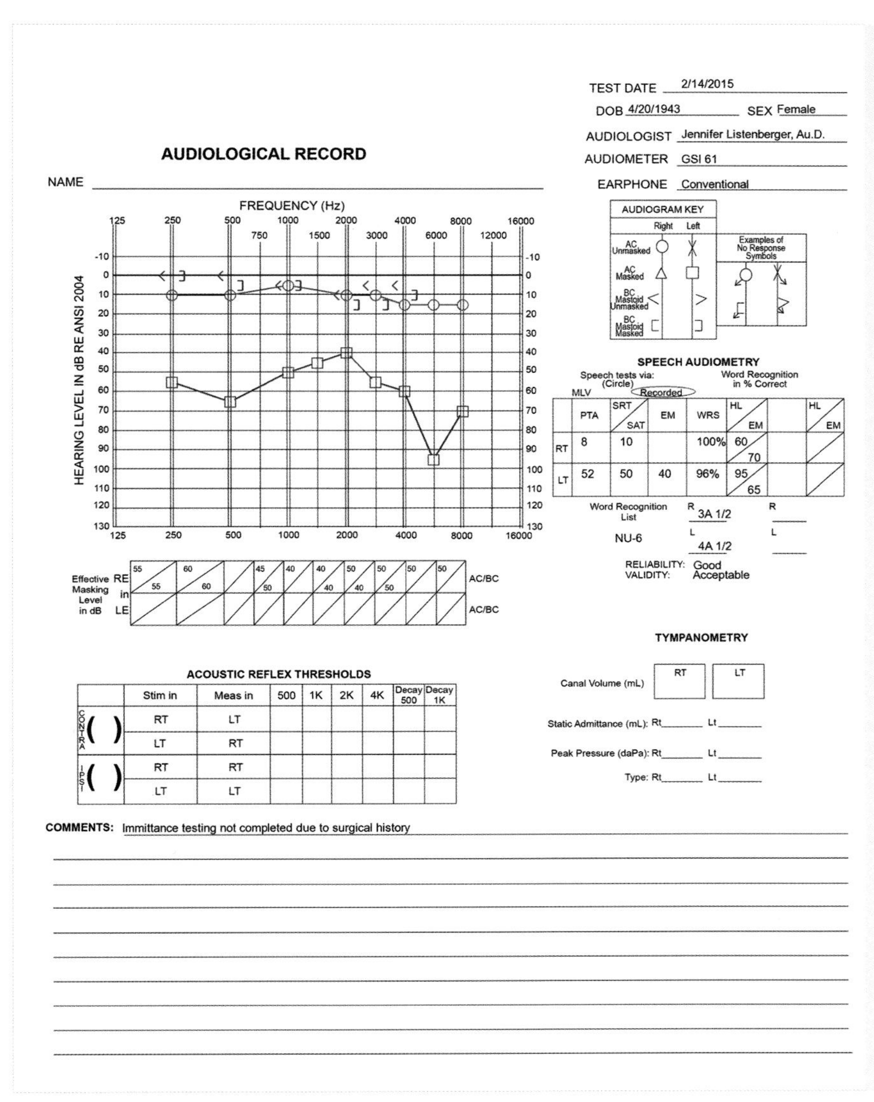

AUDIOLOGICAL RECORD

NAME

TEST DATE 2/14/2015

DOB 4/20/1943 SEX Female

AUDIOLOGIST Jennifer Listenberger, Au.D.

AUDIOMETER GSI 61

EARPHONE Conventional

SPEECH AUDIOMETRY

Speech tests via: (Circle) MLV Recorded

Word Recognition in % Correct

	PTA	SRT / SAT	EM	WRS	HL / EM		HL / EM
RT	8	10		100%	60 / 70		
LT	52	50	40	96%	95 / 65		

Word Recognition List NU-6: R 3A 1/2; L 4A 1/2; R ____; L ____

RELIABILITY: Good

VALIDITY: Acceptable

TYMPANOMETRY

Canal Volume (mL) RT ____ LT ____

Static Admittance (mL): Rt____ Lt____

Peak Pressure (daPa): Rt____ Lt____

Type: Rt____ Lt____

ACOUSTIC REFLEX THRESHOLDS

	Stim in	Meas in	500	1K	2K	4K	Decay 500	Decay 1K
CONTRA ( )	RT	LT						
	LT	RT						
IPSI ( )	RT	RT						
	LT	LT						

COMMENTS: Immittance testing not completed due to surgical history

Fig. 6.3 Audiogram of a patient with a history of unilateral hearing loss, chronic otitis media, and a tympanomastoidectomy in the left ear.

6.3.2 Interpretation

Right ear—Pure-tone air and bone conduction threshold testing revealed normal hearing sensitivity at 250 through 8,000 Hz. The SRT revealed a normal ability to receive speech and was in agreement with the PTA. The WRS revealed a normal ability to recognize speech. Immittance testing was not measured due to the surgical history.

Left ear—Pure-tone air and bone conduction threshold testing revealed a moderate and moderately severe conductive hearing loss at 250 and 500 Hz, gradually rising to moderate and mild at 1,000 and 2,000 Hz, sloping to moderate and moderately severe at 3,000 and 4,000 Hz, sloping to profound at 6,000 Hz, and rising to moderately severe at 8,000 Hz. The SRT revealed a moderate loss in the ability to receive speech and was in agreement with the PTA. The WRS revealed a normal ability to recognize speech. Immittance testing was not measured due to the surgical history.

6.3.3 Intervention

An otologic follow-up was scheduled. The audiological recommendations included annual testing to monitor the stability of the hearing loss and an evaluation for left ear amplification and HAT, pending medical clearance.

6.4 Case 4

6.4.1 Case History

A 31-year-old male reported being involved in a car accident 3 months ago. He stated that, since being involved in the car accident, he had experienced difficulty hearing in the left ear. He denied any otalgia, pressure, tinnitus, or dizziness. He stated that all sounds seemed muffled in the left ear, and that he was having trouble localizing sounds. There was no reported history of noise exposure.

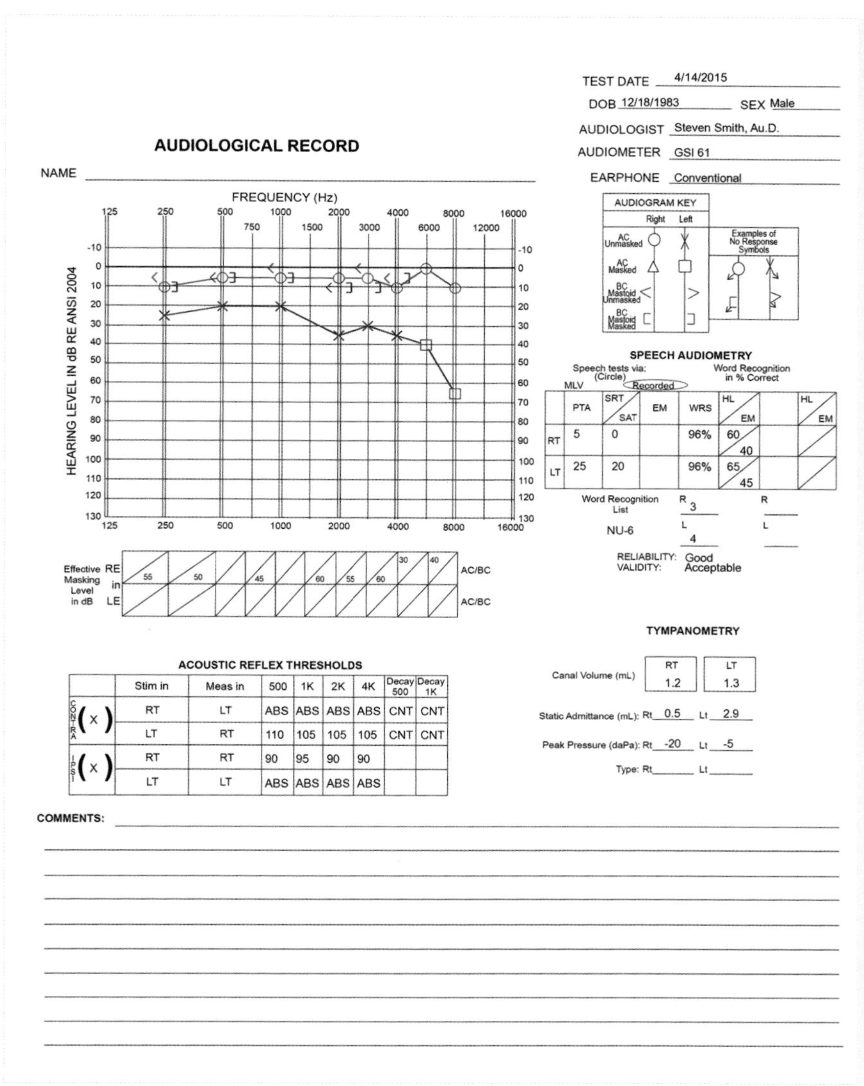

AUDIOLOGICAL RECORD

NAME

TEST DATE 4/14/2015
DOB 12/18/1983 SEX Male
AUDIOLOGIST Steven Smith, Au.D.
AUDIOMETER GSI 61
EARPHONE Conventional

Effective Masking Level in dB

RE in	55	50		45		60	55	60	30	40	AC/BC
LE											AC/BC

ACOUSTIC REFLEX THRESHOLDS

	Stim in	Meas in	500	1K	2K	4K	Decay 500	Decay 1K
CONTRA (X)	RT	LT	ABS	ABS	ABS	ABS	CNT	CNT
	LT	RT	110	105	105	105	CNT	CNT
IPSI (X)	RT	RT	90	95	90	90		
	LT	LT	ABS	ABS	ABS	ABS		

SPEECH AUDIOMETRY

Speech tests via: (Circle) MLV Recorded (circled)

Word Recognition in % Correct

	PTA	SRT / SAT	EM	WRS	HL / EM		HL / EM
RT	5	0		96%	60 / 40		
LT	25	20		96%	65 / 45		

Word Recognition List NU-6: R 3, L 4; R ___, L ___

RELIABILITY: Good
VALIDITY: Acceptable

TYMPANOMETRY

Canal Volume (mL): RT 1.2, LT 1.3

Static Admittance (mL): Rt 0.5 Lt 2.9

Peak Pressure (daPa): Rt -20 Lt -5

Type: Rt ___ Lt ___

COMMENTS:

Fig. 6.4 Audiogram of a patient with hearing loss in the left ear after a car accident. The patient was diagnosed with ossicular discontinuity.

6.4.2 Interpretation

Right ear—Normal hearing from 250 to 8,000 Hz. The SRT was normal in the ability to receive speech and was in agreement with the PTA. The WRS was normal. Immittance testing revealed a normal tympanogram. Acoustic reflex thresholds with stimulation ipsilaterally were normal from 500 to 4,000 Hz and elevated for contralateral stimulation from 500 to 4,000 Hz. Acoustic reflex decay could not be tested due to elevated contralateral acoustic reflex thresholds.

Left ear—Slight conductive hearing loss from 250 to 1,000 Hz, sloping to mild from 2,000 to 6,000 Hz, sloping to moderately severe at 8,000 Hz. The SRT revealed a slight loss in the ability to receive speech and was in agreement with the PTA. The WRS was normal. Immittance testing revealed a hypercompliant tympanogram. The acoustic reflex thresholds with ipsilateral and contralateral stimulation from 500 to 4,000 Hz were absent. Acoustic reflex decay could not be tested due to absent contralateral acoustic reflex thresholds.

6.4.3 Intervention

It was recommended that the patient follow up with an ENT regarding the conductive hearing loss in the left ear. It was determined that the patient had ossicular discontinuity in the left ear. He was provided with the options of surgery to attempt hearing restoration, or amplification for the left ear. He contemplated the options and will follow up when he has determined what he would like to do.

6.5 Case 5

6.5.1 Case History

The patient reported decreased hearing in the right ear for the past few months. The hearing loss did not subside with time, and she developed otalgia. She saw a physician who told her she had an ear infection in the right ear. She was prescribed ear drops, but her symptoms did not subside. She had intermittent tinnitus in the right ear, and that ear occasionally itched. She had a perforation in the right tympanic membrane. She did not report other otologic symptoms or history.

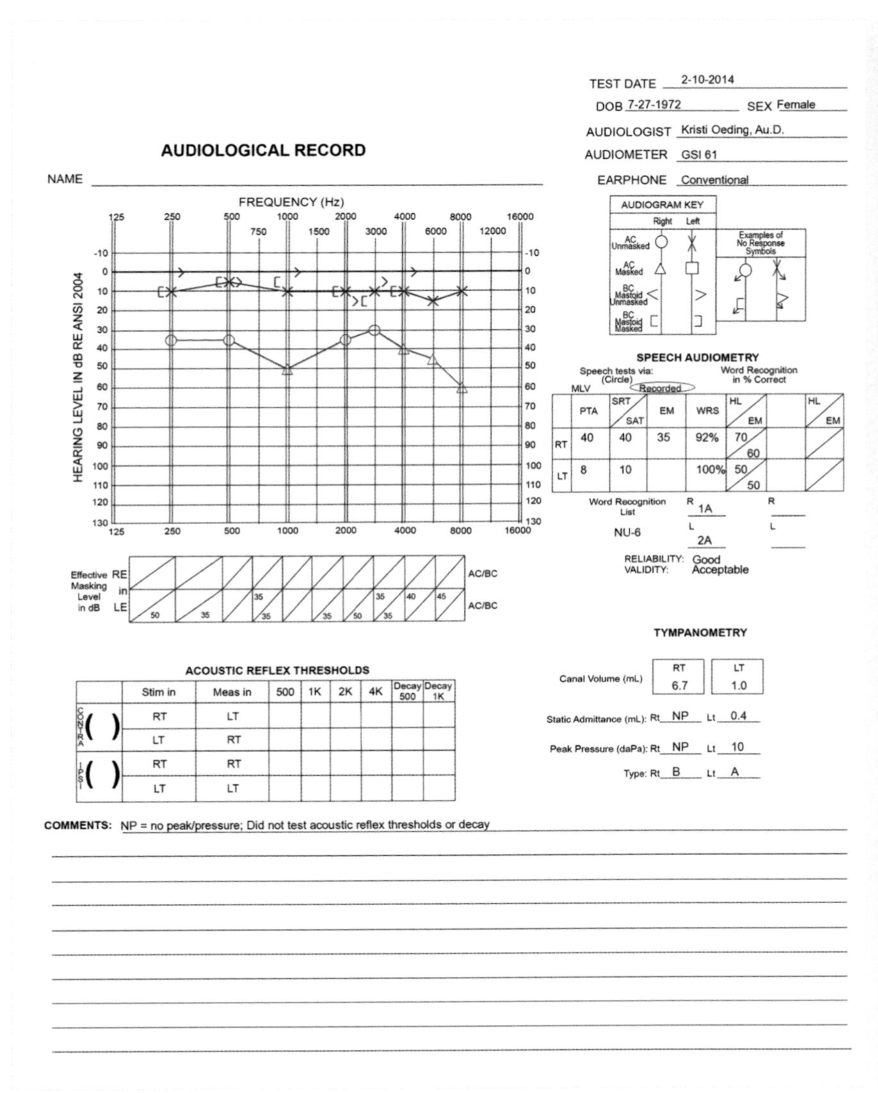

AUDIOLOGICAL RECORD

NAME

TEST DATE 2-10-2014
DOB 7-27-1972 SEX Female
AUDIOLOGIST Kristi Oeding, Au.D.
AUDIOMETER GSI 61
EARPHONE Conventional

SPEECH AUDIOMETRY

Speech tests via: (Circle) MLV Recorded

Word Recognition in % Correct

	PTA	SRT/SAT	EM	WRS	HL/EM	HL/EM
RT	40	40	35	92%	70/60	
LT	8	10		100%	50/50	

Word Recognition List: R 1A, L 2A; NU-6

RELIABILITY: Good
VALIDITY: Acceptable

TYMPANOMETRY

	RT	LT
Canal Volume (mL)	6.7	1.0

Static Admittance (mL): Rt NP Lt 0.4
Peak Pressure (daPa): Rt NP Lt 10
Type: Rt B Lt A

ACOUSTIC REFLEX THRESHOLDS

	Stim in	Meas in	500	1K	2K	4K	Decay 500	Decay 1K
CONTRA	RT	LT						
	LT	RT						
IPSI	RT	RT						
	LT	LT						

COMMENTS: NP = no peak/pressure; Did not test acoustic reflex thresholds or decay

Fig. 6.5 Audiogram of a patient with decreased hearing, otalgia, intermittent tinnitus, and a perforation in the tympanic membrane of the right ear. The patient was diagnosed with a cholesteatoma.

6.5.2 Interpretation

Right ear—Pure-tone thresholds revealed a mild to moderate conductive hearing loss from 250 to 1,000 Hz, rising to a mild conductive hearing loss from 2,000 to 4,000 Hz, and sloping from a moderate to moderately severe hearing loss at 6,000 to 8,000 Hz. The SRT revealed a mild loss in the ability to receive speech and was in agreement with the PTA. The WRS revealed a normal ability to recognize speech. Immittance testing revealed a large ear canal volume and a flat tympanogram. The acoustic reflex thresholds and decay were not measured at this appointment.

Left ear—Pure-tone thresholds were within normal limits from 250 to 8,000 Hz. The SRT revealed a normal ability to receive speech and was in agreement with the PTA. The WRS revealed a normal ability to recognize speech. Immittance testing revealed a normal tympanogram. The acoustic reflex thresholds and decay were not measured at this appointment.

6.5.3 Intervention

A CT scan revealed a cholesteatoma in the middle ear and mastoid. The otologist performed a tympanoplasty, mastoidectomy, and ossicular chain reconstruction.

6.6 Case 6

6.6.1 Case History

A 35-year-old male reported previously diagnosed right-sided otosclerosis. The patient had not had a hearing test completed in more than 2 years, and there was no test available for comparison. He reported increased difficulty understanding speech in noise, and he stated that he was favoring the better-hearing left ear more than in the past. There was no reported history of familial hearing loss or noise exposure. There was no significant health history reported and no history of otosurgery.

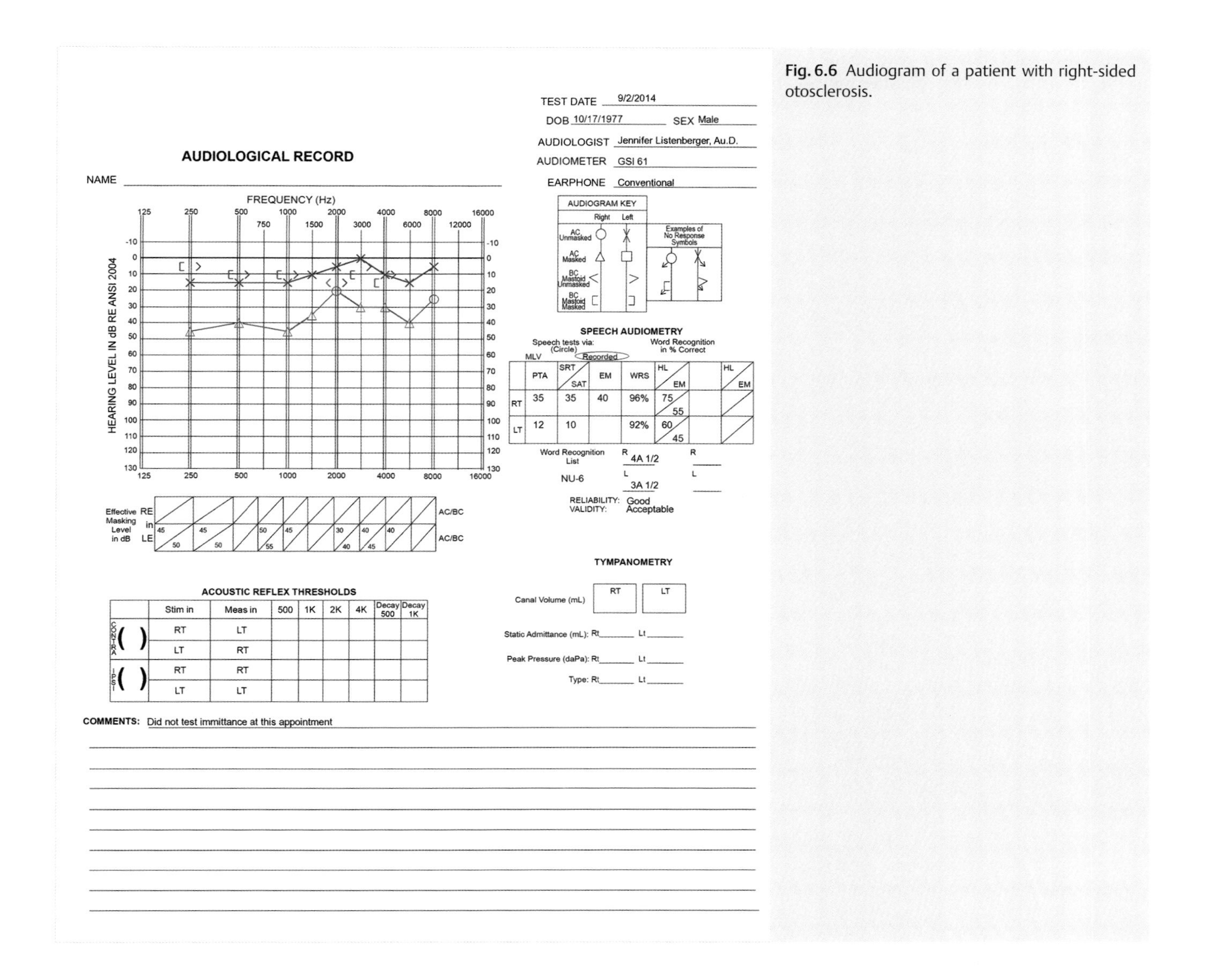

Fig. 6.6 Audiogram of a patient with right-sided otosclerosis.

6.6.2 Interpretation

Right ear—Pure-tone air and bone conduction threshold testing revealed a moderate rising to mild conductive hearing loss from 250 through 1,500 Hz, rising to slight sensorineural hearing loss at 2,000 Hz, then sloping to mild conductive hearing loss at 3,000 through 6,000 Hz, and rising to slight at 8,000 Hz. The SRT revealed a mild loss in the ability to receive speech and was in agreement with the PTA. The WRS indicated a normal ability to recognize speech. Immittance testing was not measured at this appointment.

Left ear—Pure-tone air and bone conduction threshold testing revealed normal hearing sensitivity at 250 through 8,000 Hz. The SRT revealed a normal ability to receive speech and was in agreement with the PTA. The WRS indicated a normal ability to recognize speech. Immittance testing was not measured at this appointment.

6.6.3 Intervention

The patient was scheduled to follow up with an otologist regarding surgical intervention. Annual testing to monitor hearing sensitivity and follow-up with an audiologist regarding amplification, pending medical clearance, were recommended.

6.7 Case 7

6.7.1 Case History

The patient was a 23-year-old female with Treacher Collins syndrome. She stated that she had worn hearing aids when she was a child and had consistently used amplification since that time. She reported that the hearing loss was greater in the lower frequencies and that it was about equal bilaterally. She had tinnitus in both ears, but the tinnitus was not bothersome. She denied dizziness as well as any otalgia or pressure. The appointment was scheduled to start the process of purchasing new hearing aids because her current hearing aids were 5 years old.

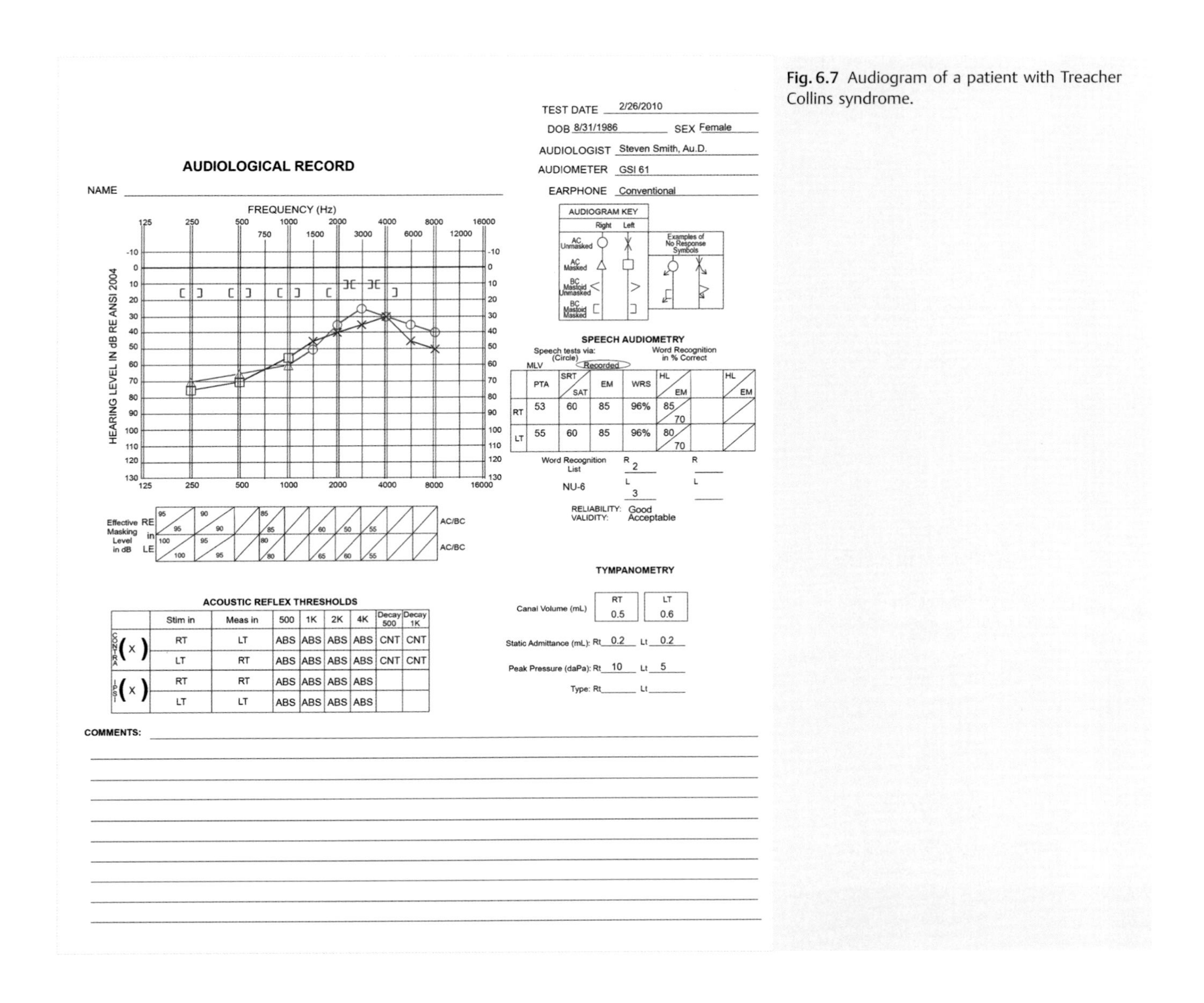

AUDIOLOGICAL RECORD

TEST DATE 2/26/2010
DOB 8/31/1986 SEX Female
AUDIOLOGIST Steven Smith, Au.D.
AUDIOMETER GSI 61
EARPHONE Conventional

NAME

Effective Masking Level in dB

RE	95 / 95	90 / 90		85 / 85		60	50	55			AC/BC
LE	100 / 100	95 / 95		80 / 80		65	60	55			AC/BC

ACOUSTIC REFLEX THRESHOLDS

	Stim in	Meas in	500	1K	2K	4K	Decay 500	Decay 1K
CONTRA (X)	RT	LT	ABS	ABS	ABS	ABS	CNT	CNT
	LT	RT	ABS	ABS	ABS	ABS	CNT	CNT
IPSI (X)	RT	RT	ABS	ABS	ABS	ABS		
	LT	LT	ABS	ABS	ABS	ABS		

COMMENTS:

SPEECH AUDIOMETRY

Speech tests via: (Circle) MLV Recorded — Word Recognition in % Correct

	PTA	SRT / SAT	EM	WRS	HL / EM		HL / EM
RT	53	60	85	96%	85 / 70		
LT	55	60	85	96%	80 / 70		

Word Recognition List NU-6: R 2, L 3

RELIABILITY: Good
VALIDITY: Acceptable

TYMPANOMETRY

Canal Volume (mL): RT 0.5, LT 0.6
Static Admittance (mL): Rt 0.2 Lt 0.2
Peak Pressure (daPa): Rt 10 Lt 5
Type: Rt Lt

Fig. 6.7 Audiogram of a patient with Treacher Collins syndrome.

6.7.2 Interpretation

Right ear—Moderately severe rising to slight conductive hearing loss at 3,000 Hz and sloping to a mild hearing loss. The SRT revealed a moderately severe loss in the ability to receive speech and was in agreement with the PTA. The WRS was normal. Immittance testing revealed a hypocompliant tympanogram. The acoustic reflex thresholds with ipsilateral and contralateral stimulation from 500 to 4,000 Hz were absent. Acoustic reflex decay could not be tested due to absent contralateral acoustic reflex thresholds.

Left ear—Severe rising to mild conductive hearing loss at 4,000 Hz and sloping to a moderate hearing loss. The SRT revealed a moderately severe loss in the ability to receive speech and was in agreement with the PTA. The WRS was normal. Immittance testing revealed a hypocompliant tympanogram. Acoustic reflex thresholds with ipsilateral and contralateral stimulation from 500 to 4,000 Hz were absent. Acoustic reflex decay could not be tested due to absent contralateral acoustic reflex thresholds.

6.7.3 Intervention

The patient was referred to an ENT specialist to obtain medical clearance for hearing aids. She followed up and was fit with bilateral BTE hearing aids with conventional earmolds.

6.8 Case 8

6.8.1 Case History

The patient had left autophony, tinnitus that sounded like static, and an intermittent sensation of pressure and otalgia in the left ear. These symptoms had become greater over the last 2 years. She reported hearing her own voice, chewing, and heartbeat, and a swooshing sound in the left ear. She had a sensation of disorientation and dizziness when she blew her nose or coughed. She did not report other otologic symptoms or history.

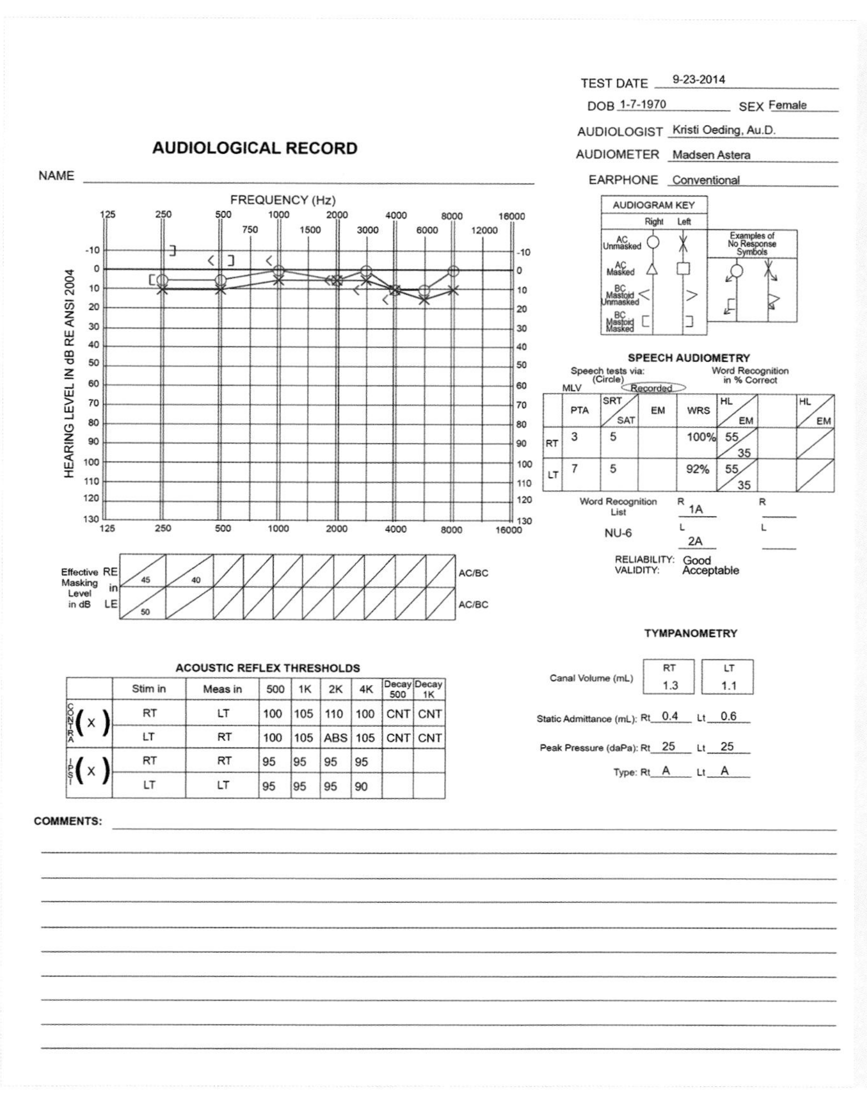

AUDIOLOGICAL RECORD

NAME

TEST DATE 9-23-2014

DOB 1-7-1970 SEX Female

AUDIOLOGIST Kristi Oeding, Au.D.

AUDIOMETER Madsen Astera

EARPHONE Conventional

Effective Masking Level in dB

RE	45, 40	AC/BC
LE	50	AC/BC

SPEECH AUDIOMETRY

Speech tests via: (Circle) MLV Recorded

Word Recognition in % Correct

	PTA	SRT / SAT	EM	WRS	HL / EM		HL / EM
RT	3	5		100%	55 / 35		
LT	7	5		92%	55 / 35		

Word Recognition List NU-6: R 1A, L 2A

RELIABILITY: Good

VALIDITY: Acceptable

ACOUSTIC REFLEX THRESHOLDS

	Stim in	Meas in	500	1K	2K	4K	Decay 500	Decay 1K
CONTRA (X)	RT	LT	100	105	110	100	CNT	CNT
	LT	RT	100	105	ABS	105	CNT	CNT
IPSI (X)	RT	RT	95	95	95	95		
	LT	LT	95	95	95	90		

TYMPANOMETRY

	RT	LT
Canal Volume (mL)	1.3	1.1

Static Admittance (mL): Rt 0.4 Lt 0.6

Peak Pressure (daPa): Rt 25 Lt 25

Type: Rt A Lt A

COMMENTS:

Fig. 6.8 Audiogram of patient with autophony, tinnitus, and intermittent pressure and otalgia in the left ear. The patient was diagnosed with superior semicircular canal dehiscence.

6.8.2 Interpretation

Right ear—Pure-tone thresholds were within normal limits from 250 to 8,000 Hz. The SRT revealed a normal ability to receive speech and was in agreement with the PTA. The WRS revealed a normal ability to recognize speech. Immittance testing was performed and revealed a normal tympanogram. Ipsilateral acoustic reflex thresholds were normal from 500 to 4,000 Hz. Contralateral acoustic reflex thresholds were normal at 500 Hz, elevated at 1,000 and 4,000 Hz, and absent at 2,000 Hz. Acoustic reflex decay could not be tested at 500 Hz due to patient discomfort and at 1,000 Hz due to an elevated contralateral acoustic reflex threshold.

Left ear—Pure-tone thresholds were within normal limits from 250 to 8,000 Hz, except for a conductive component/air–bone gap at 250 and 500 Hz. The SRT revealed a normal ability to receive speech and was in agreement with the PTA. The WRS revealed a normal ability to recognize speech. Immittance testing revealed a normal tympanogram. Ipsilateral acoustic reflex thresholds were normal from 500 to 4,000 Hz. Contralateral acoustic reflex thresholds were normal at 500 and 4,000 Hz and elevated at 1,000 to 2,000 Hz. Acoustic reflex decay could not be tested at 500 Hz due to patient discomfort and at 1,000 Hz due to an elevated contralateral acoustic reflex threshold.

6.8.3 Intervention

A CT scan and VEMP confirmed a left dehiscent superior semicircular canal. If the symptoms worsened, the patient would consider surgery, but currently the symptoms were not affecting her everyday life.

6.9 Case 9

6.9.1 Case History

The patient reported a history of chronic ear infections and multiple surgeries for the left ear as a child and young adult. The last surgery was completed more than 20 years ago. Per the ENT report, the patient had left ear canal soft tissue stenosis. The patient reported having difficulty with cerumen impaction and was seeing an otologist semiannually for cerumen removal. He did have hearing loss in the left ear and had used amplification successfully for many years. He denied any tinnitus, dizziness, or aural pressure or fullness. There was no reported history of familial hearing loss or significant noise exposure. No other significant health history was reported.

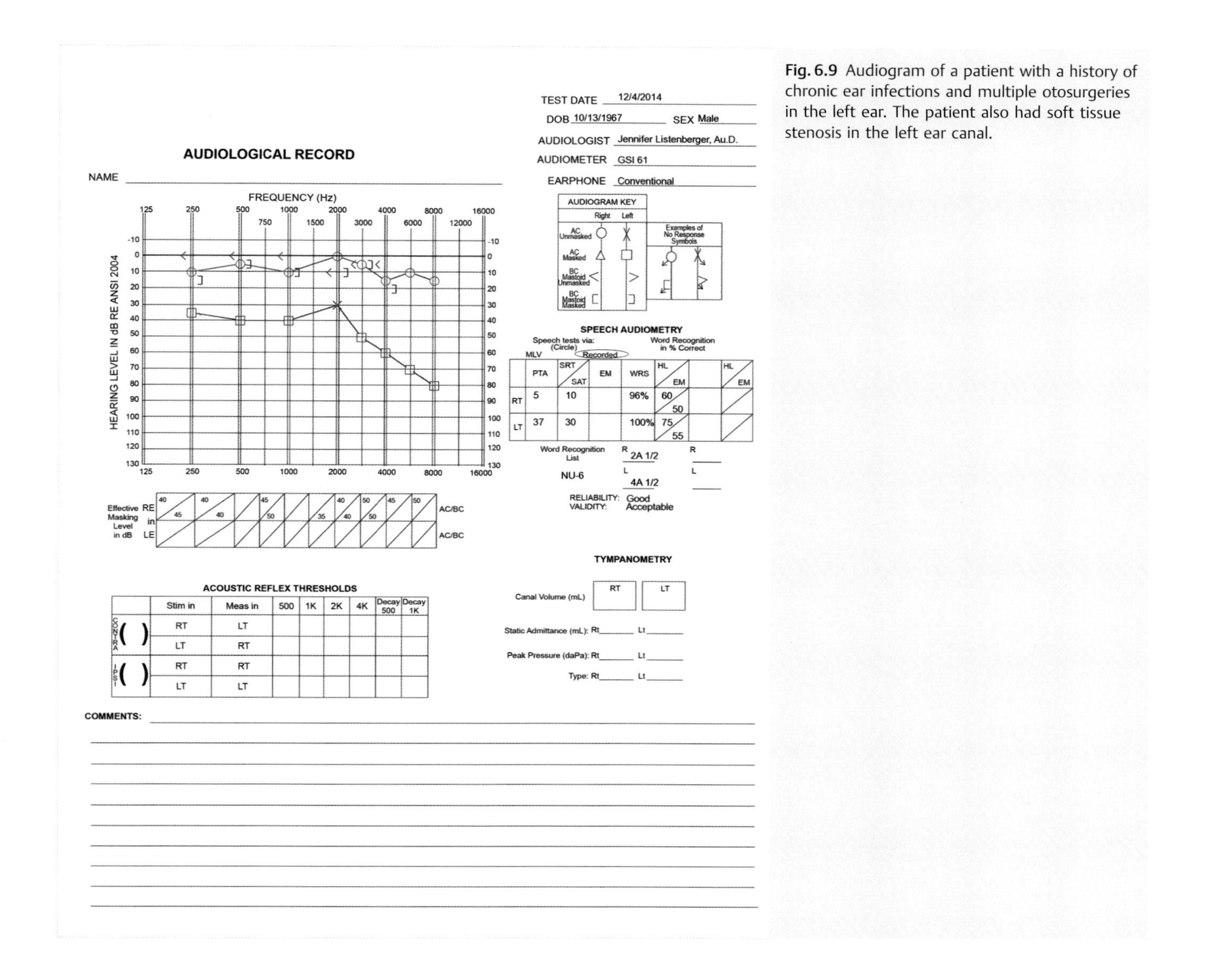

Fig. 6.9 Audiogram of a patient with a history of chronic ear infections and multiple otosurgeries in the left ear. The patient also had soft tissue stenosis in the left ear canal.

6.9.2 Interpretation

Right ear—Pure-tone air and bone conduction threshold testing revealed normal hearing sensitivity at 250 through 8,000 Hz. The SRT revealed a normal ability to receive speech and was in agreement with the PTA. The WRS revealed a normal ability to recognize speech. Immittance testing was not measured due to previous otosurgery.

Left ear—Pure-tone air and bone conduction threshold testing revealed a mild conductive hearing loss at 250 through 2,000 Hz, sloping to moderate to severe mixed hearing loss at 3,000 through 8,000 Hz. The SRT revealed a mild loss in the ability to receive speech and was in agreement with the PTA. The WRS revealed a normal ability to recognize speech. Immittance testing was not measured due to previous otosurgery.

6.9.3 Intervention

The patient was scheduled to follow up with an otologist in 6 months. A hearing test was scheduled for an annual examination to monitor stability of hearing sensitivity. The patient was encouraged to schedule a hearing aid evaluation for new technology.

6.10 Case 10

6.10.1 Case History

The patient was a 41-year-old female who had started to have some otalgia and fullness in her right ear a few days earlier after having difficulties with allergies. This progressed and she now felt she heard very little from the right ear and had a sensation of fullness like she was under water in that ear.

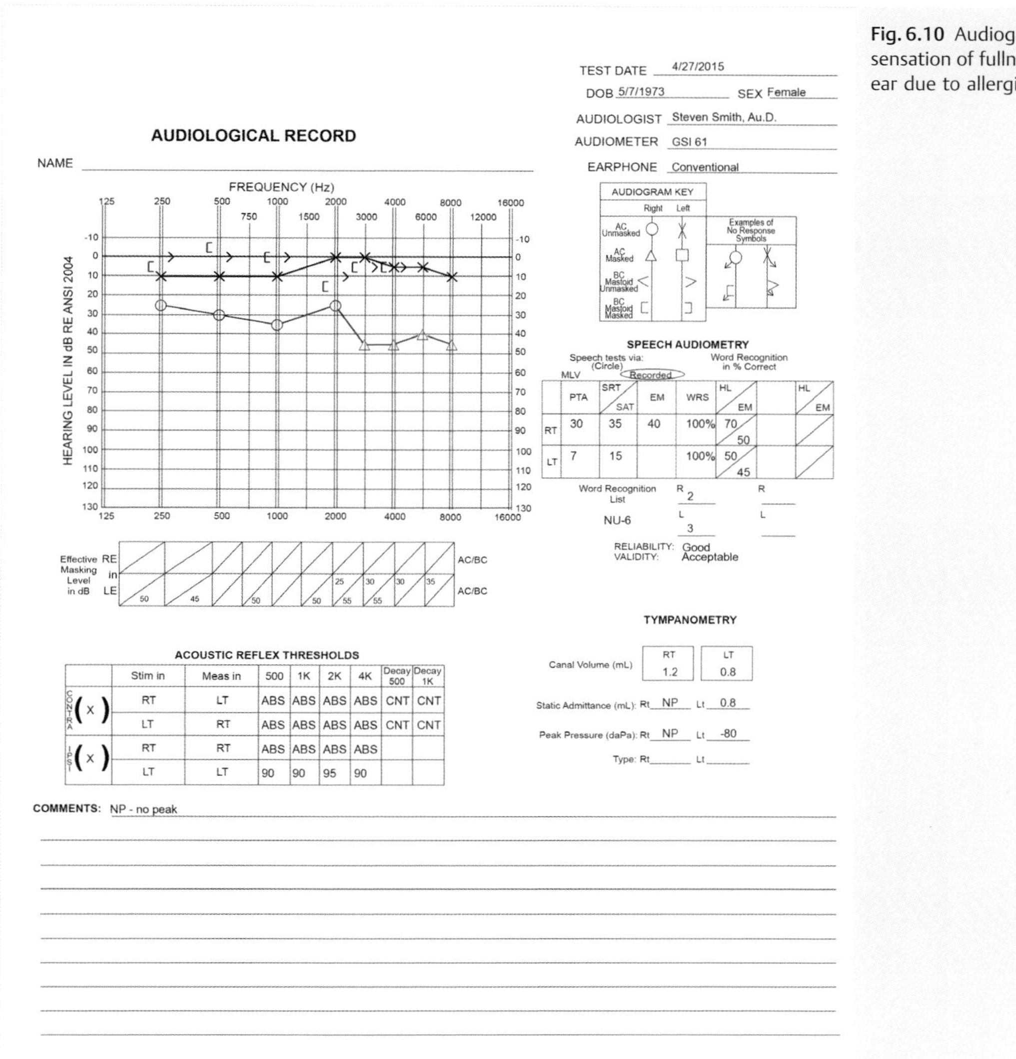

TEST DATE 4/27/2015
DOB 5/7/1973 SEX Female
AUDIOLOGIST Steven Smith, Au.D.
AUDIOMETER GSI 61
EARPHONE Conventional

AUDIOLOGICAL RECORD

NAME

Effective Masking Level in dB

RE in								AC/BC
LE	50	45	50	50	25 / 55	30 / 55	30	35	AC/BC

SPEECH AUDIOMETRY

Speech tests via: (Circle) MLV Recorded

Word Recognition in % Correct

	PTA	SRT / SAT	EM	WRS	HL / EM		HL / EM
RT	30	35	40	100%	70 / 50		
LT	7	15		100%	50 / 45		

Word Recognition List: R 2, L 3 — NU-6

RELIABILITY: Good
VALIDITY: Acceptable

ACOUSTIC REFLEX THRESHOLDS

	Stim in	Meas in	500	1K	2K	4K	Decay 500	Decay 1K
CONTRA (x)	RT	LT	ABS	ABS	ABS	ABS	CNT	CNT
	LT	RT	ABS	ABS	ABS	ABS	CNT	CNT
IPSI (x)	RT	RT	ABS	ABS	ABS	ABS		
	LT	LT	90	90	95	90		

TYMPANOMETRY

	RT	LT
Canal Volume (mL)	1.2	0.8
Static Admittance (mL)	NP	0.8
Peak Pressure (daPa)	NP	-80
Type		

COMMENTS: NP - no peak

Fig. 6.10 Audiogram of a patient with otalgia, a sensation of fullness, and hearing loss in the right ear due to allergies.

6.10.2 Interpretation

Right ear—Slight sloping to a mild conductive hearing loss at 250 through 1,000 Hz, rising to a slight sensorineural hearing loss at 2,000 Hz, sloping to a moderate conductive hearing loss at 3,000 through 8,000 Hz, except for a mild hearing loss at 6,000 Hz. The SRT revealed a mild loss in the ability to receive speech and was in agreement with the PTA. The WRS was normal. Immittance testing revealed a flat tympanogram. The acoustic reflex thresholds with ipsilateral and contralateral stimulation from 500 to 4,000 Hz were absent. Acoustic reflex decay could not be measured due to absent contralateral acoustic reflex thresholds.

Left ear—Normal hearing from 250 to 8,000 Hz. The SRT revealed a normal ability to receive speech and was in agreement with the PTA. The WRS was normal. Immittance testing revealed a normal tympanogram. The acoustic reflexes with ipsilateral stimulation were normal from 500 to 4,000 Hz, and the acoustic reflexes with contralateral stimulation from 500 to 4,000 Hz were absent. Acoustic reflex decay could not be measured due to absent contralateral acoustic reflex thresholds.

6.10.3 Intervention

The patient was referred to an otolaryngologist due to the conductive hearing loss. She was diagnosed with otitis media in the right ear and provided with a nasal spray. She scheduled a 1-month follow-up hearing examination.

6.11 Case 11

6.11.1 Case History

The patient arrived with an interpreter. He reported otalgia in the left ear for several years that had recently increased in intensity. He had a hearing loss in the left ear for several years and had noticed decreased hearing over the past 3 months. He used the right ear to talk on the telephone. He also noted otorrhea and itching in the left ear. The patient was diagnosed with an ear infection in the left ear two weeks earlier, but the symptoms had not subsided with medication. He had a perforation in the left tympanic membrane. He did not report other otologic symptoms or history.

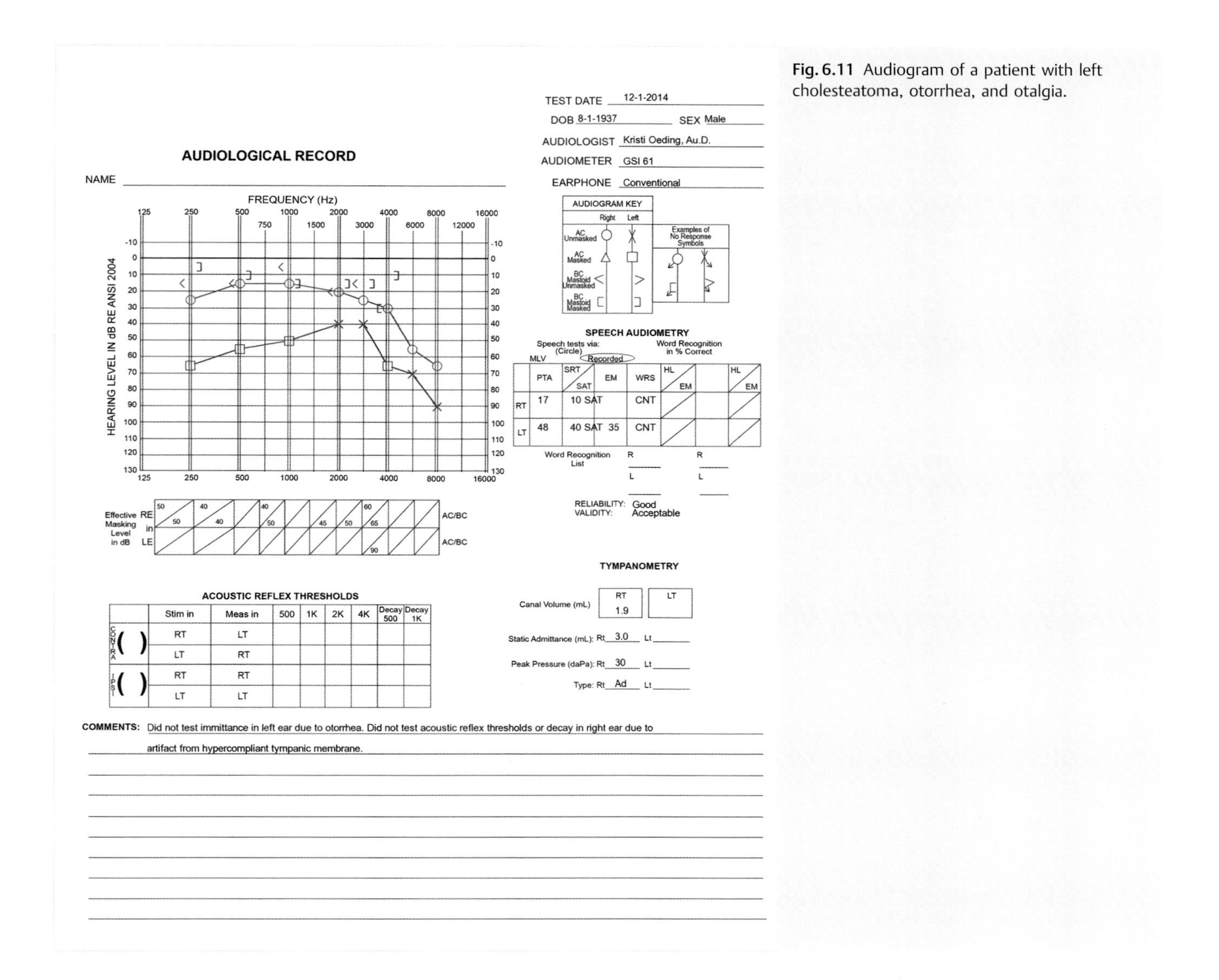

Fig. 6.11 Audiogram of a patient with left cholesteatoma, otorrhea, and otalgia.

6.11.2 Interpretation

Right ear—Pure-tone thresholds were slight sensorineural hearing loss rising to within normal limits from 250–1,000 Hz, sloping from a slight to mild sensorineural hearing loss from 2,000–4,000 Hz, and further sloping to a moderate to moderately severe hearing loss from 6,000–8,000 Hz. SAT revealed a normal ability to detect speech and was in agreement with the PTA. The WRS could not be measured given that English was not the patient's primary language. Immittance testing revealed a hypercompliant tympanogram. Ipsilateral and contralateral acoustic reflex thresholds and decay were not measured due to artifact from a hypercompliant tympanic membrane.

Left ear—Pure-tone thresholds were moderately severe rising to a mild conductive hearing loss from 250 to 3,000 Hz and sloping from a moderately severe to severe conductive hearing loss from 4,000 to 8,000 Hz. The SAT revealed a mild loss in the ability to detect speech and was in agreement with the PTA. The WRS could not be measured because English was not the patient's primary language. Immittance testing was not measured due to otorrhea.

6.11.3 Intervention

A CT scan revealed a cholesteatoma in the left ear. The otologist recommended a tympanoplasty and a mastoidectomy, but the patient was concerned about having surgery. He decided to schedule regular follow-up appointments and to wait and watch the cholesteatoma.

6.12 Case 12

6.12.1 Case History

The patient reported a long-standing history of left-sided eustachian tube dysfunction, chronic serous otitis media, and multiple pressure equalization tubes in the left ear. The last hearing test, completed 3 years ago, revealed a mild conductive hearing loss in the left ear. The patient reported improved hearing after having a tube placed, but hearing in the left ear had deteriorated within the past 3 months. There was no reported history of familial hearing loss or other significant otosurgery. The patient was a competitive dirt bike racer and expressed concerns of high noise levels when racing, but there was no other history of noise exposure.

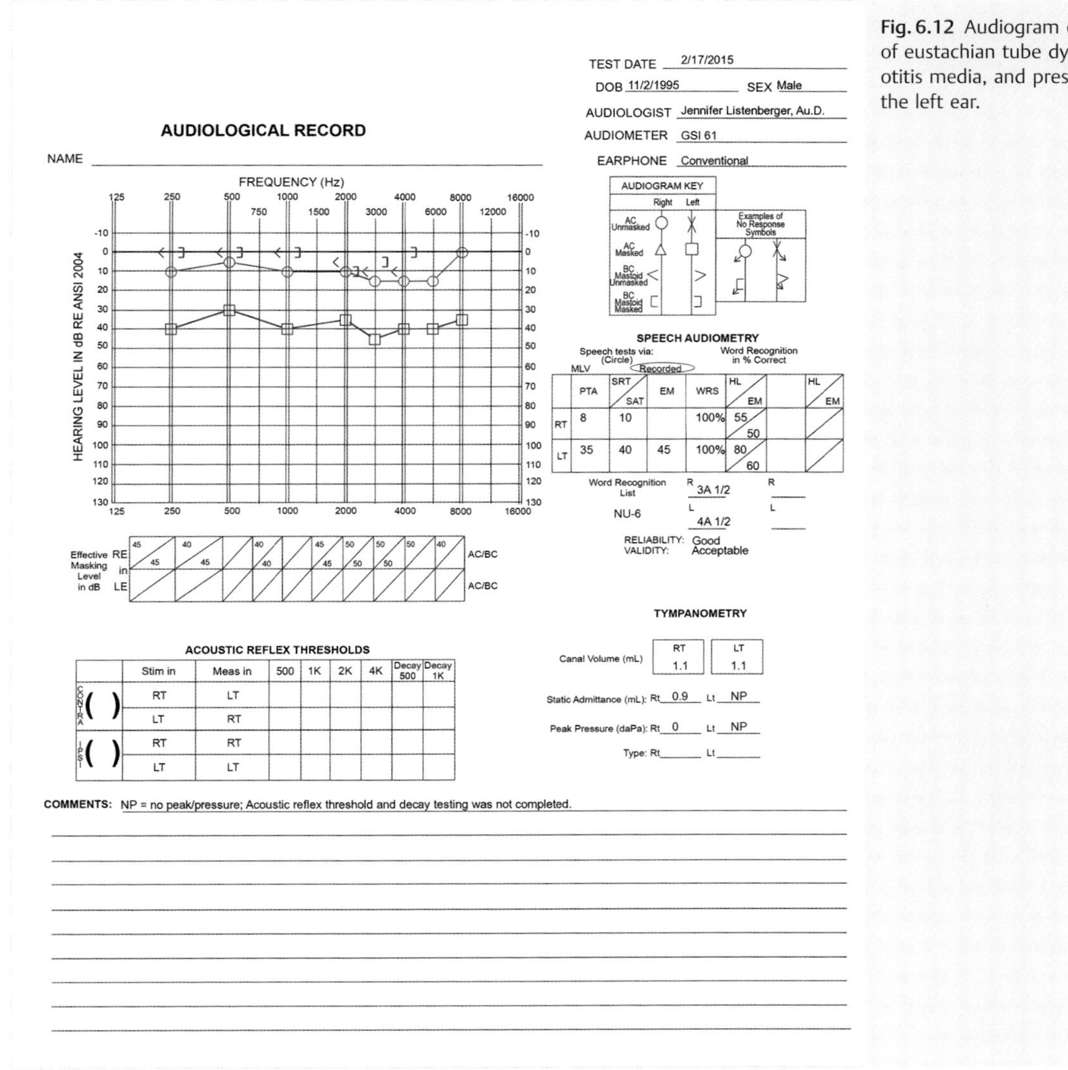

Fig. 6.12 Audiogram of a patient with a history of eustachian tube dysfunction, chronic serous otitis media, and pressure equalization tubes in the left ear.

6.12.2 Interpretation

Right ear—Pure-tone air and bone conduction threshold testing revealed normal hearing sensitivity at 250 through 8,000 Hz. The SRT revealed a normal ability to receive speech and was in agreement with the PTA. The WRS revealed a normal ability to recognize speech. Immittance testing revealed a normal tympanogram. Acoustic reflex threshold and decay testing was not measured.

Left ear—Pure-tone air and bone conduction threshold testing revealed a flat, mild conductive hearing loss at 250 through 8,000 Hz, with a moderate notch at 3,000 Hz. The SRT revealed a mild loss in the ability to receive speech and was in agreement with the PTA. The WRS revealed a normal ability to recognize speech. Immittance testing revealed a flat tympanogram with normal ear canal volume. Acoustic reflex threshold and decay testing was not measured.

6.12.3 Intervention

The patient followed up with an otologist as scheduled. The audiological recommendations were to return for a hearing test after medical management and as needed. Hearing protection was discussed, with an emphasis on custom earplugs for use when riding his dirt bike.

6.13 Case 13

6.13.1 Case History

A 30-year-old female came to the clinic stating she had had a perforated tympanic membrane in the left ear as a child. She underwent surgery for this at that time, but the repair was not successful. She reported that she continues to have hearing loss in the left ear and intermittent otorrhea. She reported otalgia in the left ear. She denied any problem with her hearing in the right ear. She denied dizziness as well as tinnitus.

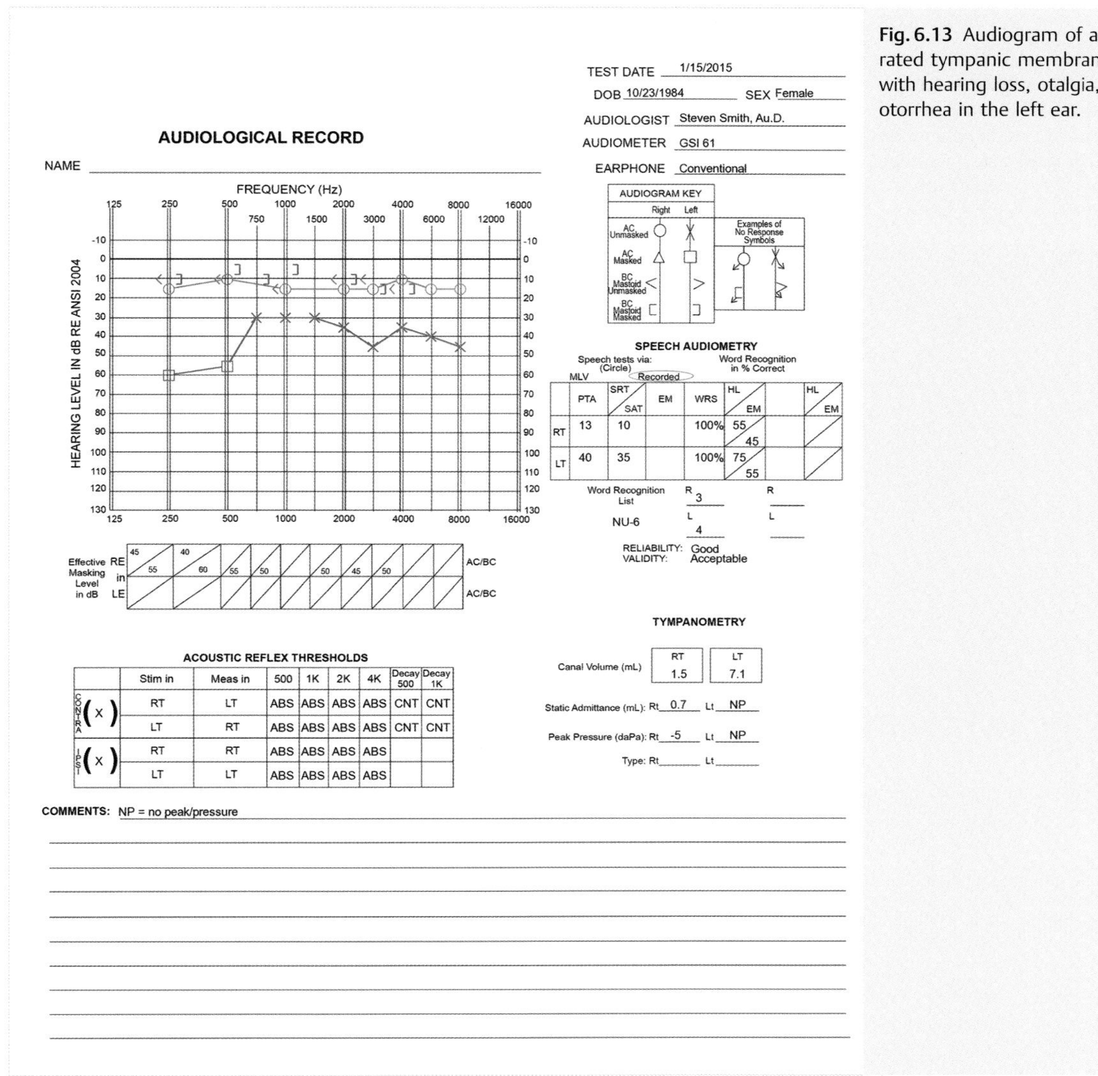

AUDIOLOGICAL RECORD

TEST DATE 1/15/2015
DOB 10/23/1984 SEX Female
AUDIOLOGIST Steven Smith, Au.D.
AUDIOMETER GSI 61
EARPHONE Conventional
NAME

SPEECH AUDIOMETRY

Speech tests via: (Circle) MLV Recorded
Word Recognition in % Correct

	PTA	SRT / SAT	EM	WRS	HL / EM		HL / EM
RT	13	10		100%	55 / 45		
LT	40	35		100%	75 / 55		

Word Recognition List: R 3, L 4
NU-6

RELIABILITY: Good
VALIDITY: Acceptable

Effective Masking Level in dB

	125	250	500	750	1000	1500	2000	3000	4000	6000	8000	
RE in	45 / 55	40 / 60	55	50			50	45	50			AC/BC
LE in												AC/BC

TYMPANOMETRY

	RT	LT
Canal Volume (mL)	1.5	7.1

Static Admittance (mL): Rt 0.7 Lt NP
Peak Pressure (daPa): Rt -5 Lt NP
Type: Rt Lt

ACOUSTIC REFLEX THRESHOLDS

	Stim in	Meas in	500	1K	2K	4K	Decay 500	Decay 1K
CONTRA (x)	RT	LT	ABS	ABS	ABS	ABS	CNT	CNT
	LT	RT	ABS	ABS	ABS	ABS	CNT	CNT
IPSI (x)	RT	RT	ABS	ABS	ABS	ABS		
	LT	LT	ABS	ABS	ABS	ABS		

COMMENTS: NP = no peak/pressure

Fig. 6.13 Audiogram of a patient with a perforated tympanic membrane in the left ear along with hearing loss, otalgia, and intermittent otorrhea in the left ear.

6.13.2 Interpretation

Right ear—Normal hearing from 250 to 8,000 Hz. The SRT was normal in the ability to receive speech and was in agreement with the PTA. The WRS was normal. Immittance testing revealed a normal tympanogram. The acoustic reflex thresholds with ipsilateral and contralateral stimulation from 500 to 4,000 Hz were absent. Acoustic reflex decay could not be measured due to absent contralateral acoustic reflex thresholds.

Left ear—Moderately severe to moderate conductive hearing loss at 250 to 500 Hz, rising to a mild to moderate hearing loss from 750 to 8,000 Hz. The SRT revealed a mild loss in the ability to receive speech and was in agreement with the PTA. The WRS was normal. Immittance testing revealed a flat tympanogram with a large ear canal volume. The acoustic reflex thresholds with ipsilateral and contralateral stimulation from 500 to 4,000 Hz were absent. Acoustic reflex decay could not be measured due to absent contralateral acoustic reflex thresholds.

6.13.3 Intervention

The patient scheduled a consultation with an ENT specialist regarding the perforated tympanic membrane. Imaging studies were ordered to determine the viability of surgical repair. The patient was provided with the option of revision surgery to attempt reconstruction of the tympanic membrane along with ossicular chain reconstruction, or follow-up with amplification. She decided to have surgery, and, if it was not successful, she would consider a hearing aid.

6.14 Case 14

6.14.1 Case History

The patient reported a hearing loss in the left ear. He had a history of recurrent otitis media as a child and had bilateral tympanic membrane perforations. At that time he noted hearing loss bilaterally. He had bilateral tympanoplasties 1 year ago and noted improvement in hearing in the right, but not the left ear. He noted constant, non-bothersome tinnitus in the left ear. He could hear with the left ear, but reported reduced bass for sound. He did not report other otologic symptoms or history.

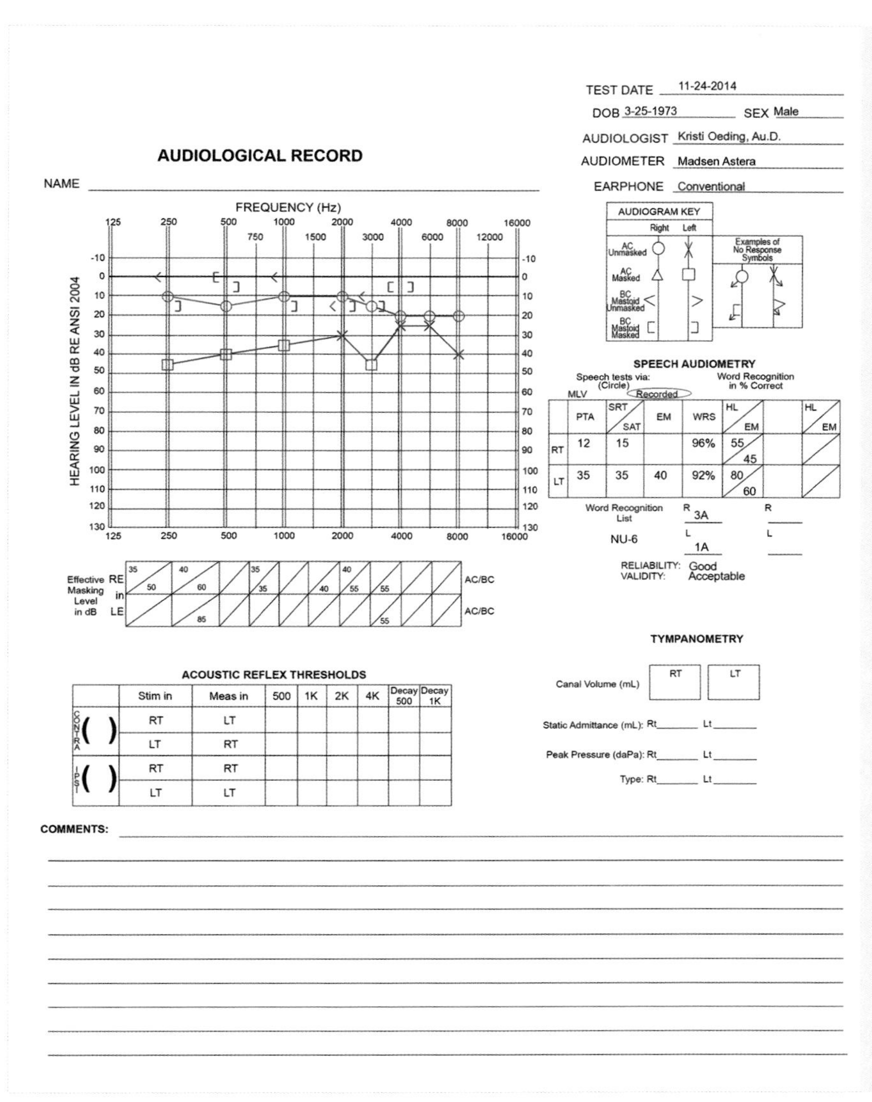

AUDIOLOGICAL RECORD

NAME

TEST DATE 11-24-2014
DOB 3-25-1973 SEX Male
AUDIOLOGIST Kristi Oeding, Au.D.
AUDIOMETER Madsen Astera
EARPHONE Conventional

SPEECH AUDIOMETRY

Speech tests via: (Circle) MLV Recorded

Word Recognition in % Correct

	PTA	SRT/SAT	EM	WRS	HL/EM	HL/EM
RT	12	15		96%	55/45	
LT	35	35	40	92%	80/60	

Word Recognition List NU-6: R 3A, L 1A

RELIABILITY: Good
VALIDITY: Acceptable

TYMPANOMETRY

Canal Volume (mL) RT LT
Static Admittance (mL): Rt___ Lt___
Peak Pressure (daPa): Rt___ Lt___
Type: Rt___ Lt___

ACOUSTIC REFLEX THRESHOLDS

	Stim in	Meas in	500	1K	2K	4K	Decay 500	Decay 1K
CONTRA ( )	RT	LT						
	LT	RT						
IPSI ( )	RT	RT						
	LT	LT						

COMMENTS:

Fig. 6.14 Audiogram of a patient with decreased hearing and constant tinnitus in the left ear and a history of bilateral otitis media and tympanoplasties.

6.14.2 Interpretation

Right ear—Pure-tone thresholds were within normal limits from 250 to 3,000 Hz and sloping to a slight conductive hearing loss from 4,000 to 8,000 Hz. The SRT revealed a normal ability to receive speech and was in agreement with the PTA. The WRS revealed a normal ability to recognize speech. Immittance testing was not performed due to previous otosurgery.

Left ear—Pure-tone thresholds were moderate rising to mild conductive hearing loss from 250 to 2,000 Hz, sloping to a moderate conductive hearing loss at 3,000 Hz, rising to a slight conductive hearing loss at 4,000 to 6,000 Hz, and sloping to a mild hearing loss at 8,000 Hz. The SRT revealed a mild loss in the ability to receive speech and was in agreement with the PTA. The WRS revealed a normal ability to recognize speech. Immittance testing was not performed due to previous otosurgery.

6.14.3 Intervention

The otologist reported both tympanic membranes were still intact, but the left tympanic membrane was slightly retracted. Before determining medical intervention, the patient's records of previous audiograms and otosurgeries were requested to be reviewed. The audiological recommendations included retesting hearing after medical management and a possible hearing aid evaluation for the left ear, depending on the outcome of medical management, HAT, and hearing protection in noise.

6.15 Case 15

6.15.1 Case History

A 53-year-old female arrived with a history of conductive hearing loss in the left ear. The patient had a stapedectomy in the left ear approximately 10 years ago, and the prostheses extruded over time. She reported not noticing any significant improvement in hearing after surgery and no significant changes in hearing over the past 10 years. She reported constant tinnitus in the left that had started immediately after the surgery. The tinnitus was described as a low-level ringing. The patient had used amplification successfully in the left ear for the past 5 years. A hearing test had been completed 3 years ago.

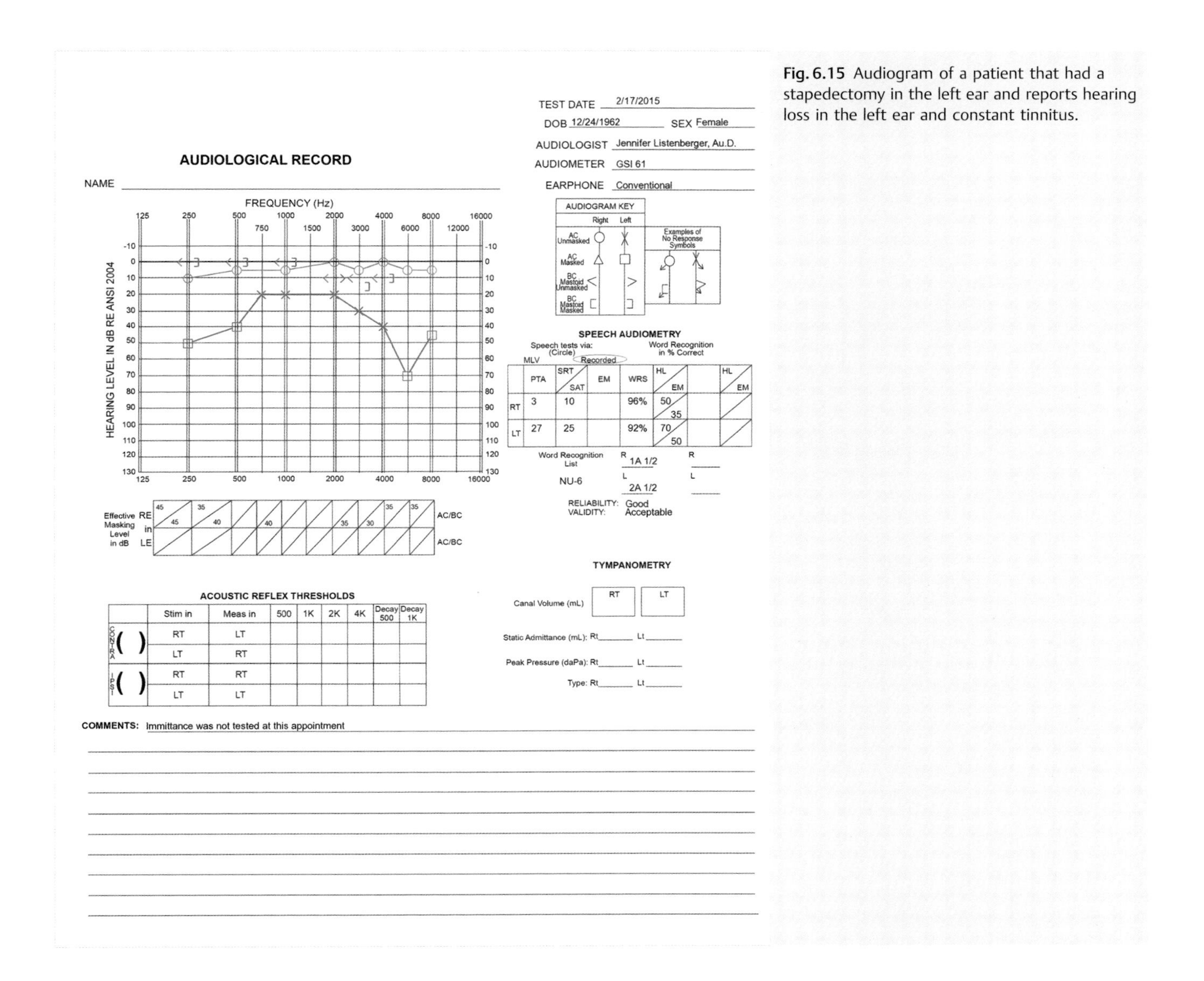

AUDIOLOGICAL RECORD

NAME

TEST DATE 2/17/2015

DOB 12/24/1962 SEX Female

AUDIOLOGIST Jennifer Listenberger, Au.D.

AUDIOMETER GSI 61

EARPHONE Conventional

SPEECH AUDIOMETRY

Speech tests via: (Circle) MLV Recorded

Word Recognition in % Correct

	PTA	SRT / SAT	EM	WRS	HL / EM		HL / EM
RT	3	10		96%	50 / 35		
LT	27	25		92%	70 / 50		

Word Recognition List: NU-6 — R 1A 1/2; L 2A 1/2

RELIABILITY: Good

VALIDITY: Acceptable

TYMPANOMETRY

Canal Volume (mL) RT LT

Static Admittance (mL): Rt___ Lt___

Peak Pressure (daPa): Rt___ Lt___

Type: Rt___ Lt___

ACOUSTIC REFLEX THRESHOLDS

	Stim in	Meas in	500	1K	2K	4K	Decay 500	Decay 1K
CONTRA ( )	RT	LT						
	LT	RT						
IPSI ( )	RT	RT						
	LT	LT						

COMMENTS: Immittance was not tested at this appointment

Fig. 6.15 Audiogram of a patient that had a stapedectomy in the left ear and reports hearing loss in the left ear and constant tinnitus.

6.15.2 Interpretation

Right ear—Pure-tone air and bone conduction threshold testing revealed normal hearing sensitivity at 250 through 8,000 Hz. The SRT revealed a normal ability to receive speech and was in agreement with the PTA. The WRS revealed a normal ability to recognize speech. Immittance testing was not measured at this appointment.

Left ear—Pure-tone air and bone conduction threshold testing revealed a moderate rising to mild conductive hearing loss at 250 and 500 Hz, rising to a slight mixed hearing loss at 750 through 2,000 Hz, sloping to mild to moderately severe at 3,000 through 6,000 Hz, and rising to moderate at 8,000 Hz. The SRT revealed a slight loss in the ability to receive speech and was in agreement with the PTA. The WRS revealed a normal ability to recognize speech. Immittance testing was not measured.

6.15.3 Intervention

The patient followed up with an otologist as scheduled. The audiological recommendations were to return annually for testing to monitor stability of hearing sensitivity, to continue using amplification, and to use hearing protection as needed.

6.16 Case 16

6.16.1 Case History

A 28-year-old male reported that he had fallen a few weeks earlier while in a deer stand about 20 feet off the ground. He landed on his left side, and a branch punctured his left tympanic membrane and the bridge of his nose. He reported that he has had difficulty hearing from his left ear and has been experiencing tinnitus and otalgia in that ear since the fall. His right ear was reportedly normal. He denied any problem with his hearing prior to the accident.

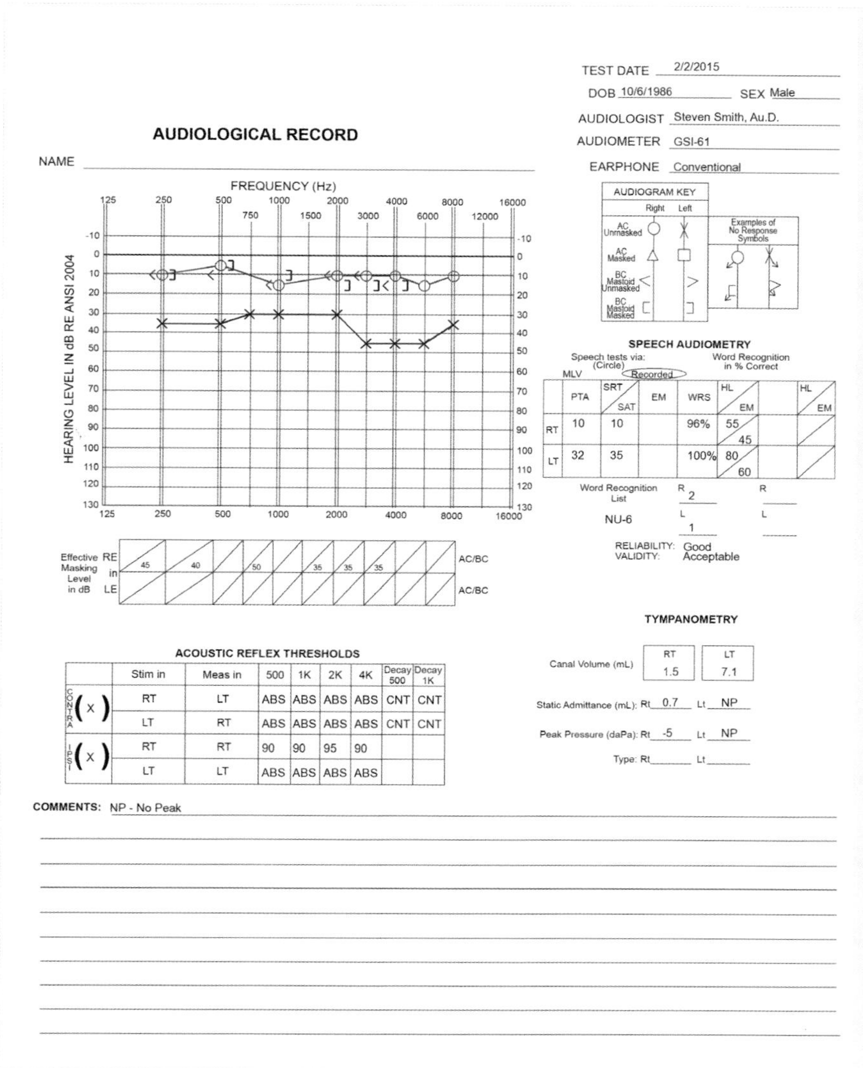

Fig. 6.16 Audiogram of a patient that fell out of a deer stand and sustained a punctured left tympanic membrane causing hearing loss, tinnitus, and otalgia.

6.16.2 Interpretation

Right ear—Normal hearing from 250 to 8,000 Hz. The SRT revealed a normal ability to receive speech and was in agreement with the PTA. The WRS score was normal in the ability to recognize speech. Immittance testing revealed a normal tympanogram. The acoustic reflex thresholds with ipsilateral stimulation were normal between 500 and 4,000 Hz. The acoustic reflex thresholds with contralateral stimulation from 500 to 4,000 Hz were absent. Acoustic reflex decay could not be measured due to absent contralateral acoustic reflex thresholds.

Left ear—Flat mild to moderate conductive hearing loss from 250 to 8,000 Hz. The SRT revealed mild loss in the ability to receive speech and was in agreement with the PTA. The WRS was normal in the ability to recognize speech. Immittance testing revealed a flat tympanogram with a large ear canal volume. The acoustic reflex thresholds with ipsilateral and contralateral stimulation from 500 to 4,000 Hz were absent. Acoustic reflex decay could not be measured due to absent contralateral acoustic reflex thresholds.

6.16.3 Intervention

The patient followed up with an ENT specialist regarding the perforated tympanic membrane. It was determined that the perforation was large, and surgical intervention was recommended. Imaging studies were performed and surgery was scheduled. He will follow up with an audiologist once surgery has been performed to determine if his hearing improves.

6.17 Case 17

6.17.1 Case History

The patient reported a bilateral hearing loss for the last 2 weeks. There was a sensation of fullness/fluid bilaterally. She noted tinnitus bilaterally that started 2 weeks ago. She had seasonal allergies and reported that she currently had symptoms of allergies. She did not report other otologic symptoms or history.

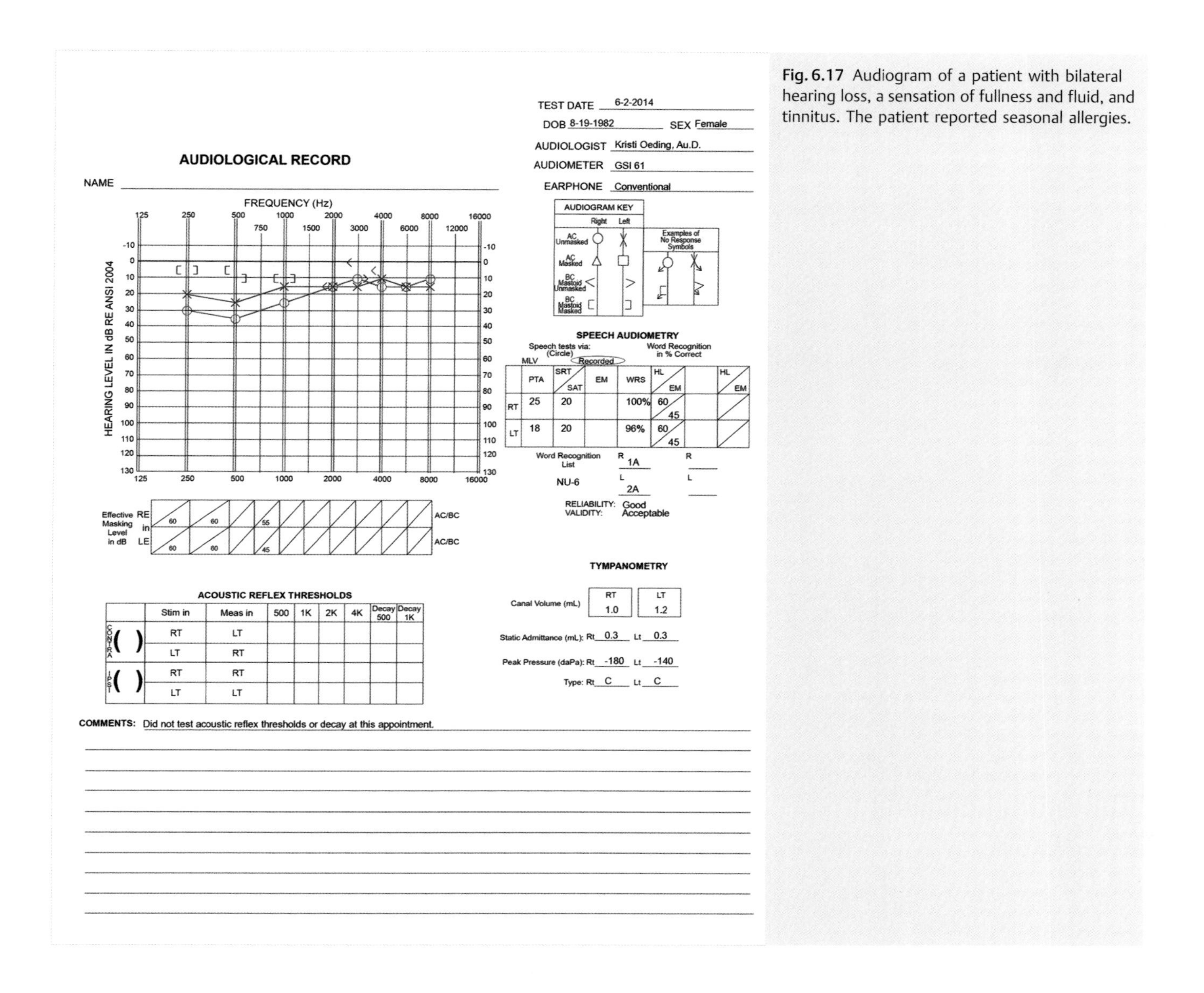

AUDIOLOGICAL RECORD

NAME

TEST DATE 6-2-2014

DOB 8-19-1982 SEX Female

AUDIOLOGIST Kristi Oeding, Au.D.

AUDIOMETER GSI 61

EARPHONE Conventional

SPEECH AUDIOMETRY

Speech tests via: (Circle) MLV Recorded

Word Recognition in % Correct

	PTA	SRT / SAT	EM	WRS	HL / EM		HL / EM
RT	25	20		100%	60 / 45		
LT	18	20		96%	60 / 45		

Word Recognition List: NU-6 — R 1A, L 2A; R ___, L ___

RELIABILITY: Good
VALIDITY: Acceptable

Effective Masking Level in dB

RE	60	60	55									AC/BC
LE	60	60	45									AC/BC

ACOUSTIC REFLEX THRESHOLDS

	Stim in	Meas in	500	1K	2K	4K	Decay 500	Decay 1K
CONTRA ( )	RT	LT						
	LT	RT						
IPSI ( )	RT	RT						
	LT	LT						

TYMPANOMETRY

	RT	LT
Canal Volume (mL)	1.0	1.2
Static Admittance (mL)	0.3	0.3
Peak Pressure (daPa)	-180	-140
Type	C	C

COMMENTS: Did not test acoustic reflex thresholds or decay at this appointment.

Fig. 6.17 Audiogram of a patient with bilateral hearing loss, a sensation of fullness and fluid, and tinnitus. The patient reported seasonal allergies.

6.17.2 Interpretation

Right ear—Pure-tone thresholds were mild rising to slight conductive hearing loss from 250 to 1,000 Hz and rising to normal hearing sensitivity from 2,000 to 8,000 Hz. The SRT revealed a slight loss in the ability to receive speech and was in agreement with the PTA. The WRS revealed a normal ability to recognize speech. Immittance testing was performed and revealed excessive negative pressure on the tympanogram. The acoustic reflex thresholds and decay were not measured at this appointment.

Left ear—Pure-tone thresholds were slight conductive hearing loss from 250 to 500 Hz and rising to normal hearing sensitivity from 1,000 to 8,000 Hz. The SRT revealed a slight loss in the ability to receive speech and was in agreement with the PTA. The WRS revealed a normal ability to recognize speech. Immittance testing was measured and revealed excessive negative pressure on the tympanogram. The acoustic reflex thresholds and decay were not tested at this appointment.

6.17.3 Intervention

The otologist noted fluid behind both tympanic membranes. The patient was provided with an Otovent. The audiological recommendations included retesting hearing post medical management and in 1 year and use of hearing protection in noise.

6.18 Case 18

6.18.1 Case History

A 22-year-old male reported a lifelong history of ear infections and ear problems, including a cholesteatoma. He has had multiple otosurgeries throughout the years bilaterally. His last surgery was completed in the right ear approximately 1 year ago for a revision canal wall down mastoidectomy with an ossicular chain reconstruction with total ossicular replacement. A tympanostomy tube was placed in the reconstructed right middle ear. There was a long-standing history of a large, left-sided tympanic membrane perforation.

This young male attempted to use amplification in the right ear 3 years ago, but did not perceive a significant benefit. The hearing aid no longer fit the reconstructed ear. The hearing in the right ear was poorer than the hearing in the left. He believed he had some difficulty hearing, but felt he had adjusted to the hearing loss because he had it for so long. His greatest concern was maintaining the hearing he had, as he did report going to places with high noise levels.

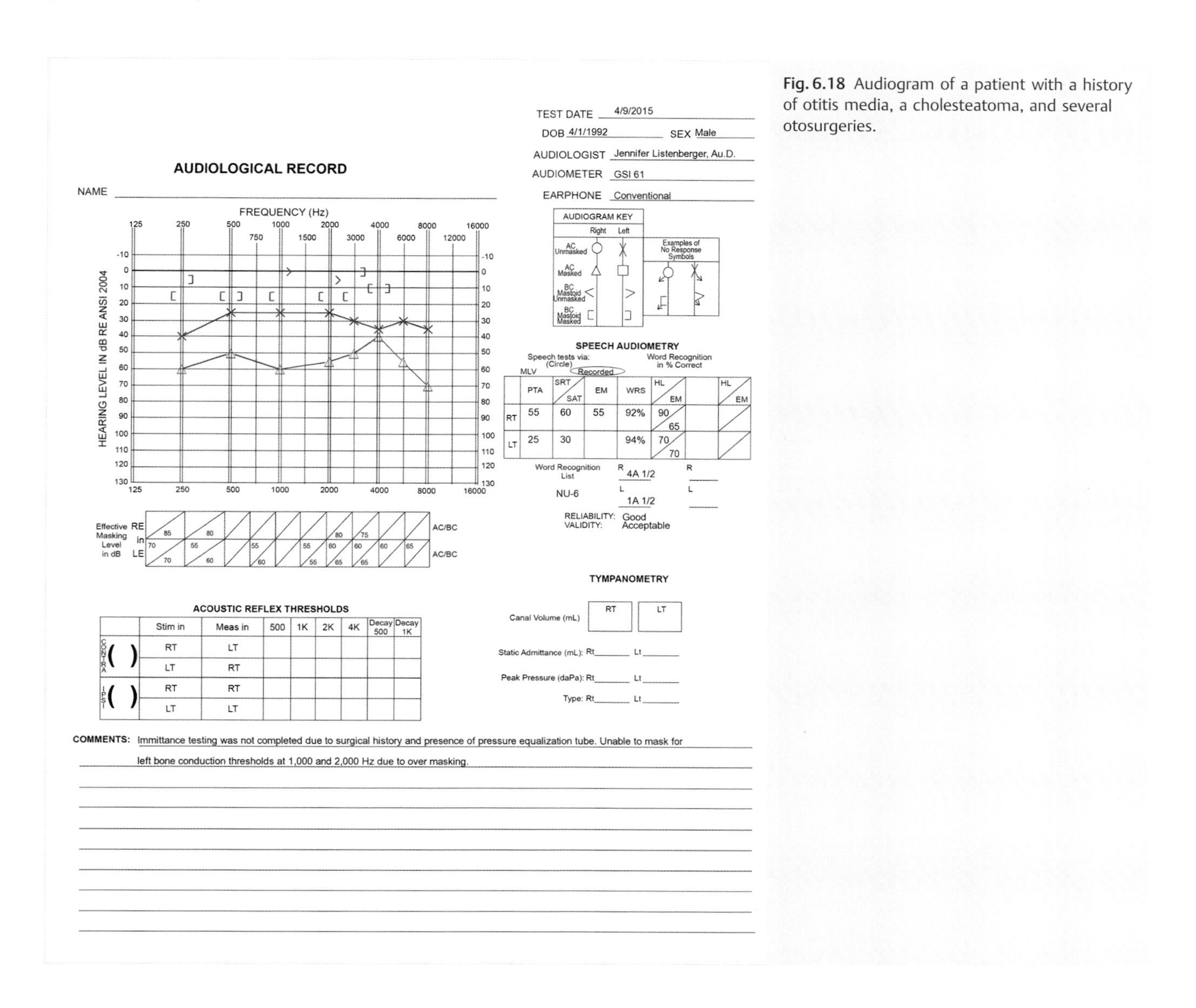

Fig. 6.18 Audiogram of a patient with a history of otitis media, a cholesteatoma, and several otosurgeries.

6.18.2 Interpretation

Right ear—Pure-tone air and bone conduction threshold testing revealed a moderately severe to mild conductive hearing loss at 250 through 4,000 Hz, sloping to moderate to moderately severe at 6,000 through 8,000 Hz. The SRT revealed a moderately severe loss in the ability to receive speech and was in agreement with the PTA. The WRS revealed a normal ability to recognize speech. Immittance testing was not measured due to a significant surgical history.

Left ear—Pure-tone air and bone conduction threshold testing revealed a mild conductive hearing loss at 250 Hz, rising to a slight mixed hearing loss at 500 through 2,000 Hz, and sloping to a mild conductive hearing loss at 3,000 through 8,000 Hz. The SRT revealed a mild loss in the ability to receive speech and was in agreement with the PTA. The WRS revealed a normal ability to recognize speech. Immittance testing was not measured due to the large tympanic membrane perforation and surgical history.

6.18.3 Intervention

The patient followed up with an otologist as scheduled. The audiological recommendations were to return annually for a hearing test to monitor the stability of hearing and to be evaluated for use of amplification and HAT, and to wear hearing protection when exposed to high levels of noise.

6.19 Case 19

6.19.1 Case History

The patient reported that she had had multiple surgeries on her left ear and multiple ear infections in the left ear over the last few years. She reported that she used a hearing aid in the left ear and was unable to wear it much of the time due to otorrhea. She reported that her right ear was hearing well and did not have problems.

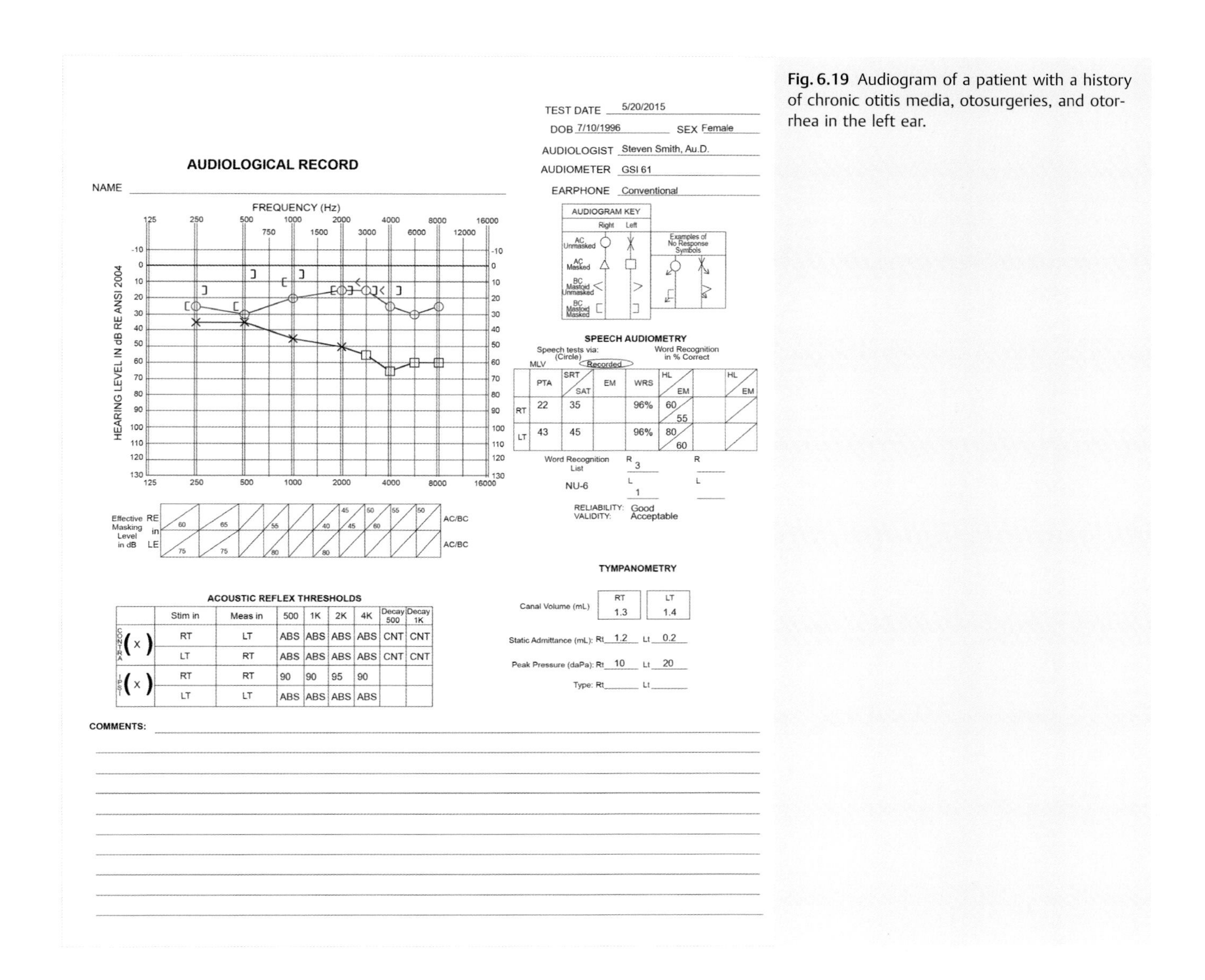

AUDIOLOGICAL RECORD

NAME

TEST DATE 5/20/2015
DOB 7/10/1996 SEX Female
AUDIOLOGIST Steven Smith, Au.D.
AUDIOMETER GSI 61
EARPHONE Conventional

SPEECH AUDIOMETRY

Speech tests via: (Circle) MLV Recorded

Word Recognition in % Correct

	PTA	SRT / SAT	EM	WRS	HL / EM		HL / EM
RT	22	35		96%	60 / 55		
LT	43	45		96%	80 / 60		

Word Recognition List NU-6: R 3, L 1; R ___, L ___

RELIABILITY: Good
VALIDITY: Acceptable

TYMPANOMETRY

	RT	LT
Canal Volume (mL)	1.3	1.4

Static Admittance (mL): Rt 1.2 Lt 0.2

Peak Pressure (daPa): Rt 10 Lt 20

Type: Rt ___ Lt ___

ACOUSTIC REFLEX THRESHOLDS

	Stim in	Meas in	500	1K	2K	4K	Decay 500	Decay 1K
CONTRA	RT	LT	ABS	ABS	ABS	ABS	CNT	CNT
	LT	RT	ABS	ABS	ABS	ABS	CNT	CNT
IPSI	RT	RT	90	90	95	90		
	LT	LT	ABS	ABS	ABS	ABS		

COMMENTS:

Fig. 6.19 Audiogram of a patient with a history of chronic otitis media, otosurgeries, and otorrhea in the left ear.

6.19.2 Interpretation

Right ear—Slight and mild sensorineural hearing loss from 250 to 500 Hz, rising to a slight sensorineural hearing loss at 1,000 Hz to normal hearing sensitivity at 2,000 to 3,000 Hz, and sloping to slight at 4,000 to 8,000 Hz, with a mild notch at 6,000 Hz. The SRT revealed a mild loss in the ability to receive speech and was relatively in agreement with the PTA. The WRS revealed a normal ability to recognize speech. Immittance testing revealed a normal tympanogram. Acoustic reflex thresholds with ipsilateral stimulation were normal from 500 to 4,000 Hz and absent for contralateral stimulation. Acoustic reflex decay could not be measured due to absent contralateral acoustic reflex thresholds.

Left ear—Mild gradually sloping to a moderately severe conductive hearing loss at 250 to 8,000 Hz. The SRT revealed a moderate loss in the ability to receive speech and was in agreement with the PTA. The WRS revealed a normal ability to recognize speech. Immittance testing revealed a hypocompliant tympanogram. The acoustic reflex thresholds were absent with ipsilateral and contralateral stimulation from 500 to 4,000 Hz. Acoustic reflex decay could not be measured due to absent contralateral acoustic reflex thresholds.

6.19.3 Intervention

The patient was referred to an ENT specialist for follow-up regarding the otorrhea. This was treated; however, it was determined that the hearing aid may be contributing to the persistence of the infection, and she was counseled regarding the possible use of a BAHA. She was considering it and may follow through with surgery for the BAHA.

6.20 Case 20

6.20.1 Case History

The patient reported that he flew last week and, when the plane was descending, heard a popping sound in the right ear and had otalgia. Since this incident, hearing had been muffled in the right ear, and he noted intermittent tinnitus in the right ear. He did not have any symptoms in the left ear. He had a family history of hearing loss, with his parents acquiring hearing loss later in life. He did not report other otologic symptoms or history.

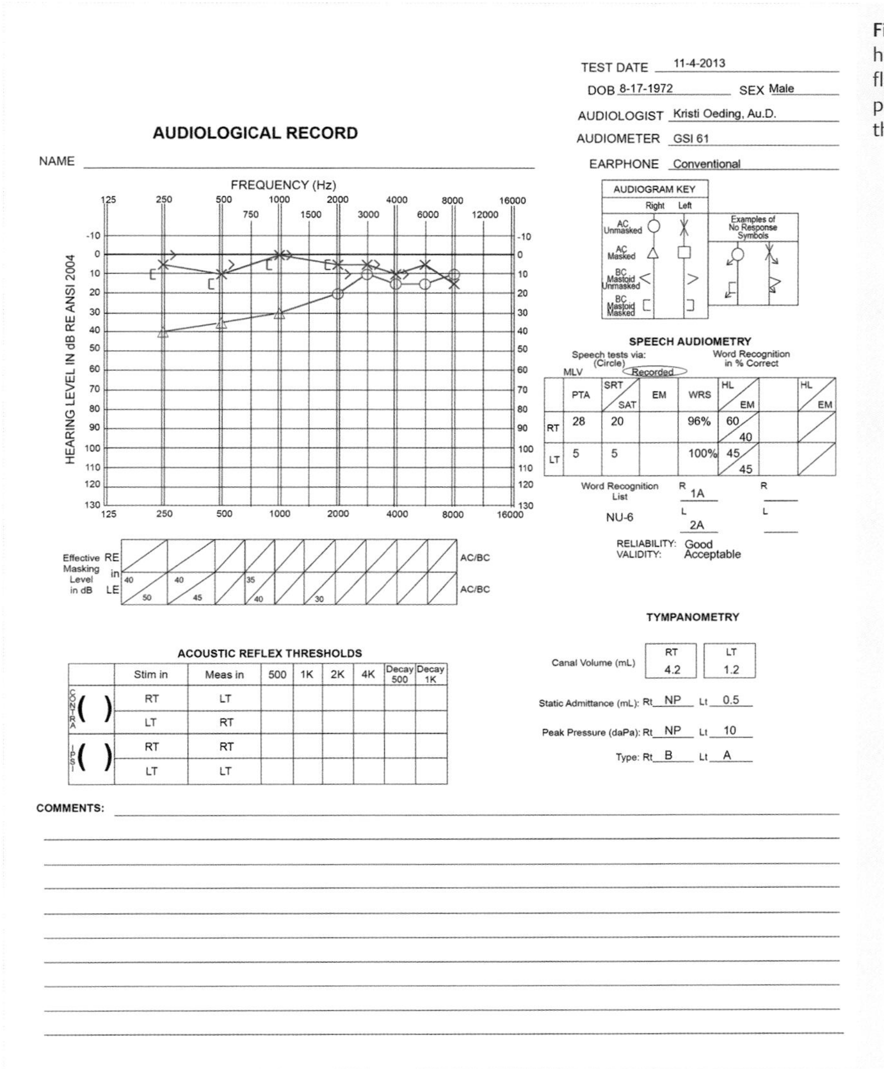

AUDIOLOGICAL RECORD

NAME

TEST DATE 11-4-2013

DOB 8-17-1972 SEX Male

AUDIOLOGIST Kristi Oeding, Au.D.

AUDIOMETER GSI 61

EARPHONE Conventional

Effective Masking Level in dB

	250	500	1000	2000	
RE in					AC/BC
LE	40 / 50	40 / 45	35 / 40	30	AC/BC

SPEECH AUDIOMETRY

Speech tests via: (Circle) MLV Recorded

Word Recognition in % Correct

	PTA	SRT / SAT	EM	WRS	HL / EM		HL / EM
RT	28	20		96%	60 / 40		
LT	5	5		100%	45 / 45		

Word Recognition List NU-6: R 1A, L 2A; R ___, L ___

RELIABILITY: Good

VALIDITY: Acceptable

TYMPANOMETRY

	RT	LT
Canal Volume (mL)	4.2	1.2

Static Admittance (mL): Rt NP Lt 0.5

Peak Pressure (daPa): Rt NP Lt 10

Type: Rt B Lt A

ACOUSTIC REFLEX THRESHOLDS

	Stim in	Meas in	500	1K	2K	4K	Decay 500	Decay 1K
CONTRA ( )	RT	LT						
	LT	RT						
IPSI ( )	RT	RT						
	LT	LT						

COMMENTS:

Fig. 6.20 Audiogram of a patient with decreased hearing and tinnitus in the right ear following a flight. When the airplane was descending, the patient heard a popping sound and had otalgia in the right ear.

6.20.2 Interpretation

Right ear—Pure-tone thresholds were mild, rising to a slight conductive hearing loss from 250 to 2,000 Hz and rising to normal hearing sensitivity from 3,000 to 8,000 Hz. The SRT revealed a slight loss in the ability to receive speech and was in agreement with the PTA. The WRS revealed a normal ability to recognize speech. Immittance testing revealed a flat tympanogram with a large ear canal volume. Acoustic reflex thresholds and decay were not measured at this appointment.

Left ear—Pure-tone thresholds were normal hearing sensitivity from 250 to 8,000 Hz. The SRT revealed a normal ability to receive speech and was in agreement with the PTA. The WRS revealed a normal ability to recognize speech. Immittance testing revealed a normal tympanogram. Acoustic reflex thresholds and decay were not measured at this appointment.

6.20.3 Intervention

The otologist noted a small perforation in the right tympanic membrane. If the perforation did not heal, a tympanoplasty would be performed. The audiological recommendations included retesting hearing post-medical management and in 1 year and use of hearing protection in noise.

6.21 Case 21

6.21.1 Case History

A 41-year-old female reported a long-standing history of hearing loss bilaterally, multiple otosurgeries, chronic ear infections, and a cholesteatoma, with her last ear infection occurring a few months ago in the right ear. She reported a significant deterioration in her hearing bilaterally over the past few years. She reported her last surgery in her left ear was 2 years ago. She reported having multiple hearing tests, but none were available for comparison at this time. There was a report of constant bilateral tinnitus that sometimes interfered with her ability to fall asleep, but usually music was helpful. There was some familial hearing loss, but mostly in older family members. There was no significant history of noise exposure or ototoxic treatments. Per chart review of previous records, otosurgeries included canal wall down tympanomastoidectomies and ossiculoplasty.

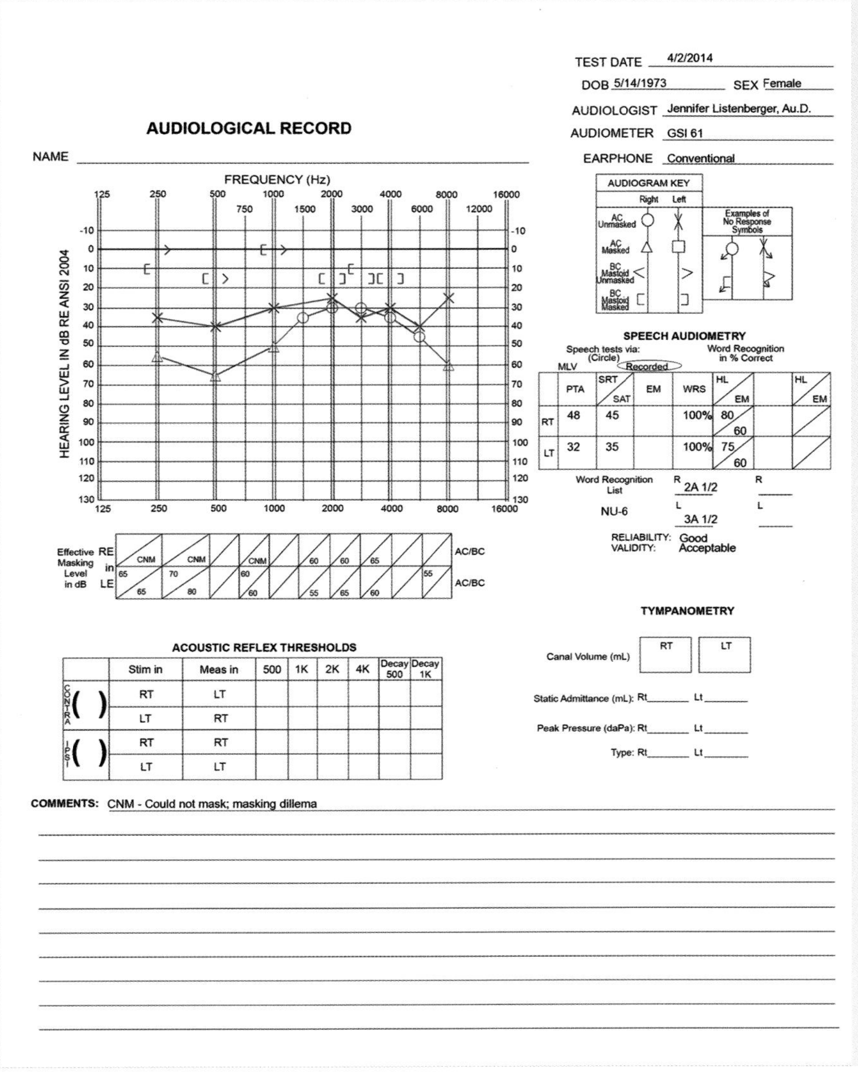

Fig. 6.21 Audiogram of a patient with decreased hearing bilaterally along with a history of multiple otosurgeries and chronic otitis media bilaterally, and a cholesteatoma in the right ear.

6.21.2 Interpretation

Right ear—Pure-tone air and bone conduction threshold testing revealed a moderate to moderately severe conductive hearing loss at 250 through 500 Hz, rising to moderate to mild at 1,000 through 4,000 Hz, and sloping to moderate to moderately severe at 6,000 through 8,000 Hz. The SRT revealed a moderate loss in the ability to receive speech and was in agreement with the PTA. The WRS revealed a normal ability to recognize speech. Immittance testing was not measured due to surgical history.

Left ear—Pure-tone air and bone conduction threshold testing revealed a mild, predominantly conductive hearing loss at 250 through 6,000 Hz, except for a slight sensorineural hearing loss at 2,000 Hz and 8,000 Hz. The SRT revealed a mild loss in the ability to receive speech and was in agreement with the PTA. The WRS revealed a normal ability to recognize speech. Immittance testing was not measured due to her surgical history.

6.21.3 Intervention

The patient continued the scheduled follow-ups with the otologist. The audiological recommendations included returning for a hearing test after medical management and annually to monitor the stability of hearing, returning for a hearing aid evaluation, use of HAT, and use of hearing protection in noise.

6.22 Case 22

6.22.1 Case History

The patient reported a decrease in her hearing in the right ear that started many years ago and has progressed to the point where she does not feel she can hear from the right side. She stated she has tinnitus in the right ear and has recently had some dizziness as well. She denied otalgia as well as fullness in her ears. She reported that the left ear hears well.

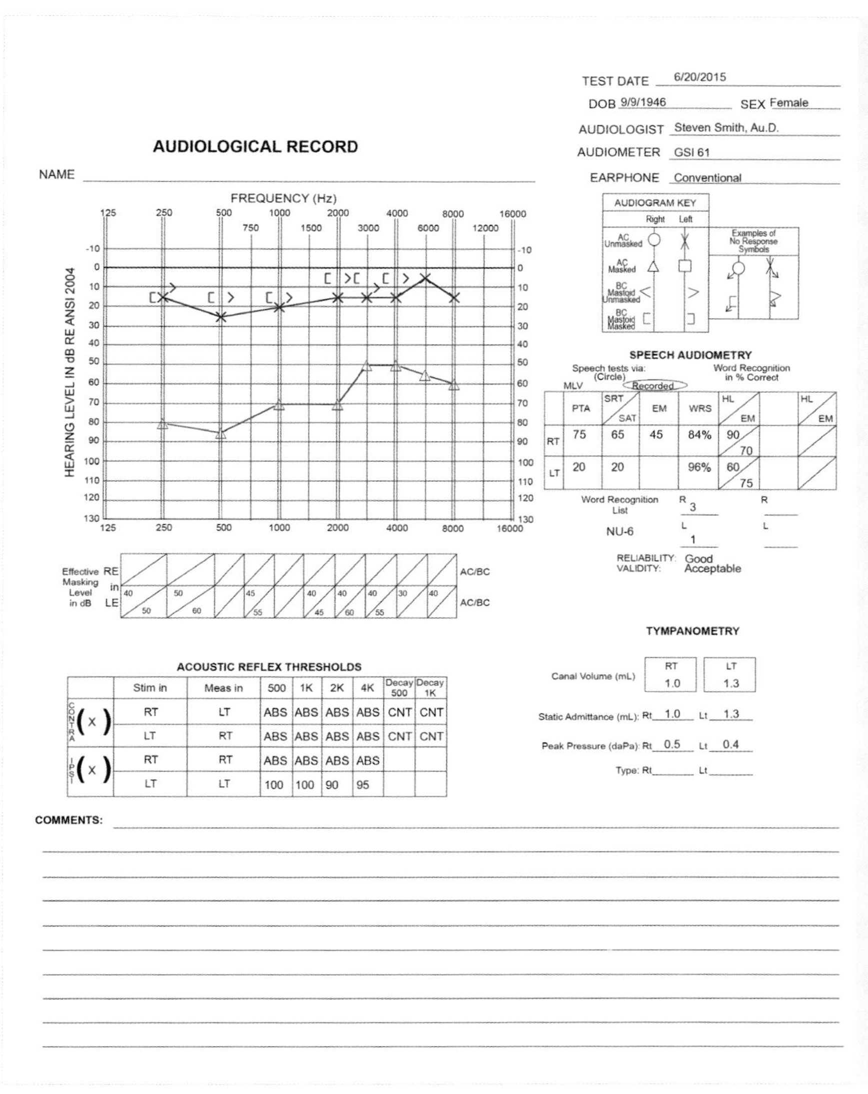

AUDIOLOGICAL RECORD

NAME

TEST DATE 6/20/2015

DOB 9/9/1946 SEX Female

AUDIOLOGIST Steven Smith, Au.D.

AUDIOMETER GSI 61

EARPHONE Conventional

Effective Masking Level in dB

	250	500	750	1000	1500	2000	3000	4000	6000	8000	
RE in LE	40 / 50	50 / 60		45 / 55		40 / 45	40 / 60	40 / 55	30	40	AC/BC

SPEECH AUDIOMETRY

Speech tests via: (Circle) MLV Recorded

Word Recognition in % Correct

	PTA	SRT / SAT	EM	WRS	HL / EM	HL / EM
RT	75	65	45	84%	90 / 70	
LT	20	20		96%	60 / 75	

Word Recognition List: R 3, L 1

NU-6

RELIABILITY: Good

VALIDITY: Acceptable

TYMPANOMETRY

	RT	LT
Canal Volume (mL)	1.0	1.3

Static Admittance (mL): Rt 1.0 Lt 1.3

Peak Pressure (daPa): Rt 0.5 Lt 0.4

Type: Rt ____ Lt ____

ACOUSTIC REFLEX THRESHOLDS

	Stim in	Meas in	500	1K	2K	4K	Decay 500	Decay 1K
CONTRA (x)	RT	LT	ABS	ABS	ABS	ABS	CNT	CNT
	LT	RT	ABS	ABS	ABS	ABS	CNT	CNT
IPSI (x)	RT	RT	ABS	ABS	ABS	ABS		
	LT	LT	100	100	90	95		

COMMENTS:

Fig. 6.22 Audiogram of a patient with decreased hearing and tinnitus in the right ear along with a recent onset of dizziness. The patient was diagnosed with otosclerosis.

6.22.2 Interpretation

Right ear—Severe rising to a moderately severe conductive hearing loss at 250 to 2,000 Hz, rising to moderate at 3,000 to 6,000 Hz, and sloping to moderately severe at 8,000. The SRT revealed a moderately severe loss in the ability to receive speech and was in agreement with the PTA. The WRS revealed a slight difficulty in the ability to recognize speech. Immittance testing revealed a normal tympanogram. The acoustic reflexes were absent from 500 to 4,000 Hz to ipsilateral and contralateral stimulation. Acoustic reflex decay could not be measured due to absent contralateral acoustic reflex thresholds.

Left ear—Normal hearing sensitivity at 250 Hz, sloping to a slight sensorineural hearing loss at 500 through 1,000 Hz, rising to normal hearing sensitivity at 2,000 to 8,000 Hz. The SRT revealed a slight loss in the ability to receive speech and was in agreement with the PTA. The WRS revealed a normal ability to recognize speech. Immittance testing revealed a normal tympanogram. The acoustic reflexes with ipsilateral stimulation were normal from 500 to 4,000 Hz and absent for contralateral stimulation. Acoustic reflex decay could not be measured due to absent contralateral acoustic reflex thresholds.

6.22.3 Intervention

The patient was referred to an ENT specialist, and she was eventually diagnosed with otosclerosis in the right ear. She was advised by the ENT specialist regarding surgical intervention and amplification. The patient was undecided and will schedule an appointment when she decides whether or not she wants to pursue amplification or surgery.

6.23 Case 23

6.23.1 Case History

The patient reported decreased hearing in the left ear for the past 10 weeks. The decreased hearing started after 6 weeks of radiation for cancer of the left tonsil. She had constant humming tinnitus in the left ear, and her voice echoed in that ear. She did not have hearing loss or otologic symptoms in the right ear. She also noted some imbalance. She had a family history of hearing loss, with her mother having hearing loss later in life. She did not report other otologic symptoms or history.

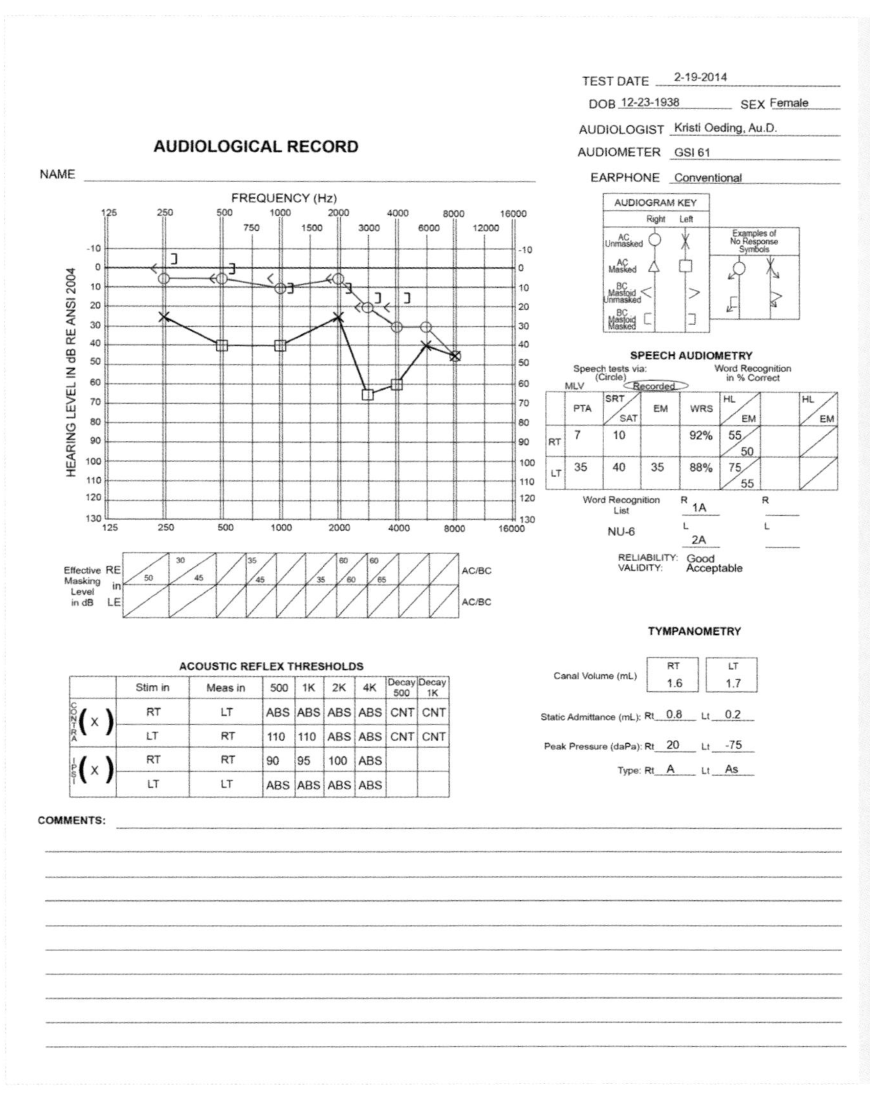

AUDIOLOGICAL RECORD

NAME

TEST DATE 2-19-2014
DOB 12-23-1938 SEX Female
AUDIOLOGIST Kristi Oeding, Au.D.
AUDIOMETER GSI 61
EARPHONE Conventional

SPEECH AUDIOMETRY

Speech tests via: (Circle) MLV Recorded

Word Recognition in % Correct

	PTA	SRT / SAT	EM	WRS	HL / EM
RT	7	10		92%	55 / 50
LT	35	40	35	88%	75 / 55

Word Recognition List: R 1A; L 2A

NU-6

RELIABILITY: Good
VALIDITY: Acceptable

ACOUSTIC REFLEX THRESHOLDS

	Stim in	Meas in	500	1K	2K	4K	Decay 500	Decay 1K
CONTRA (X)	RT	LT	ABS	ABS	ABS	ABS	CNT	CNT
	LT	RT	110	110	ABS	ABS	CNT	CNT
IPSI (X)	RT	RT	90	95	100	ABS		
	LT	LT	ABS	ABS	ABS	ABS		

TYMPANOMETRY

	RT	LT
Canal Volume (mL)	1.6	1.7

Static Admittance (mL): Rt 0.8 Lt 0.2

Peak Pressure (daPa): Rt 20 Lt -75

Type: Rt A Lt As

COMMENTS:

Fig. 6.23 Audiogram of a patient with decreased hearing in the left ear following radiation treatment for cancer of the left tonsil. The patient also reported constant tinnitus and her voice echoed in the left ear.

6.23.2 Interpretation

Right ear—Pure-tone thresholds revealed normal hearing sensitivity from 250 to 2,000 Hz and sloping from a slight to moderate sensorineural hearing loss from 3,000 to 8,000 Hz. The SRT revealed a normal ability to receive speech and was in agreement with the PTA. The WRS revealed a normal ability to recognize speech. Immittance testing revealed a normal tympanogram. Ipsilateral acoustic reflex thresholds were within normal limits from 500 to 2,000 Hz and absent at 4,000 Hz, and contralateral reflex thresholds were elevated at 500 to 1,000 Hz and absent at 2,000 to 4,000 Hz. Acoustic reflex decay could not be measured due to elevated contralateral acoustic reflex thresholds.

Left ear—Pure-tone thresholds revealed a slight sloping to mild conductive hearing loss from 250 to 1,000 Hz, rising to slight at 2,000 Hz, sloping to moderately severe at 3,000 to 4,000 Hz, and rising to mild to moderate hearing loss at 6,000 to 8,000 Hz. The SRT revealed a mild loss in the ability to receive speech and was in agreement with the PTA. The WRS revealed a slight difficulty in the ability to recognize speech. Immittance testing revealed a hypocompliant tympanogram. The ipsilateral and contralateral acoustic reflex thresholds were absent at 500 to 4,000 Hz. Acoustic reflex decay could not be measured due to absent contralateral acoustic reflex thresholds.

6.23.3 Intervention

The otologist noted otitis media with effusion in the left ear. The patient was going to try an Otovent before a pressure equalization tube. The audiological recommendations included a hearing test after medical management, annual testing to monitor hearing sensitivity due to radiation therapy, possible use of HAT, and use of hearing protection in noise.

6.24 Case 24

6.24.1 Case History

The patient was diagnosed with lichen planus approximately 8 years ago, but it started to affect her ears only 2 years ago. She reported a history of otosclerosis and a stapedectomy in the left ear in 1993 and in the right ear in 2004. She stated her hearing was essentially normal after the surgeries but then started to deteriorate approximately 2 years ago. She reported hearing better with the right ear and said that the hearing had recently deteriorated quickly, but had been relatively stable for the past 2 years. The patient reported some improvement when taking an injected anti-inflammatory medication, but she stopped taking the medication for a month. Since she had stopped taking the medication, her hearing had deteriorated, and no noticeable improvements were reported after she had taken the medication again for 1 month. Physician notes stated there was excessive tympanic membrane scarring bilaterally. The patient reported hearing tests had been completed over the past few years, but they were not available for comparison.

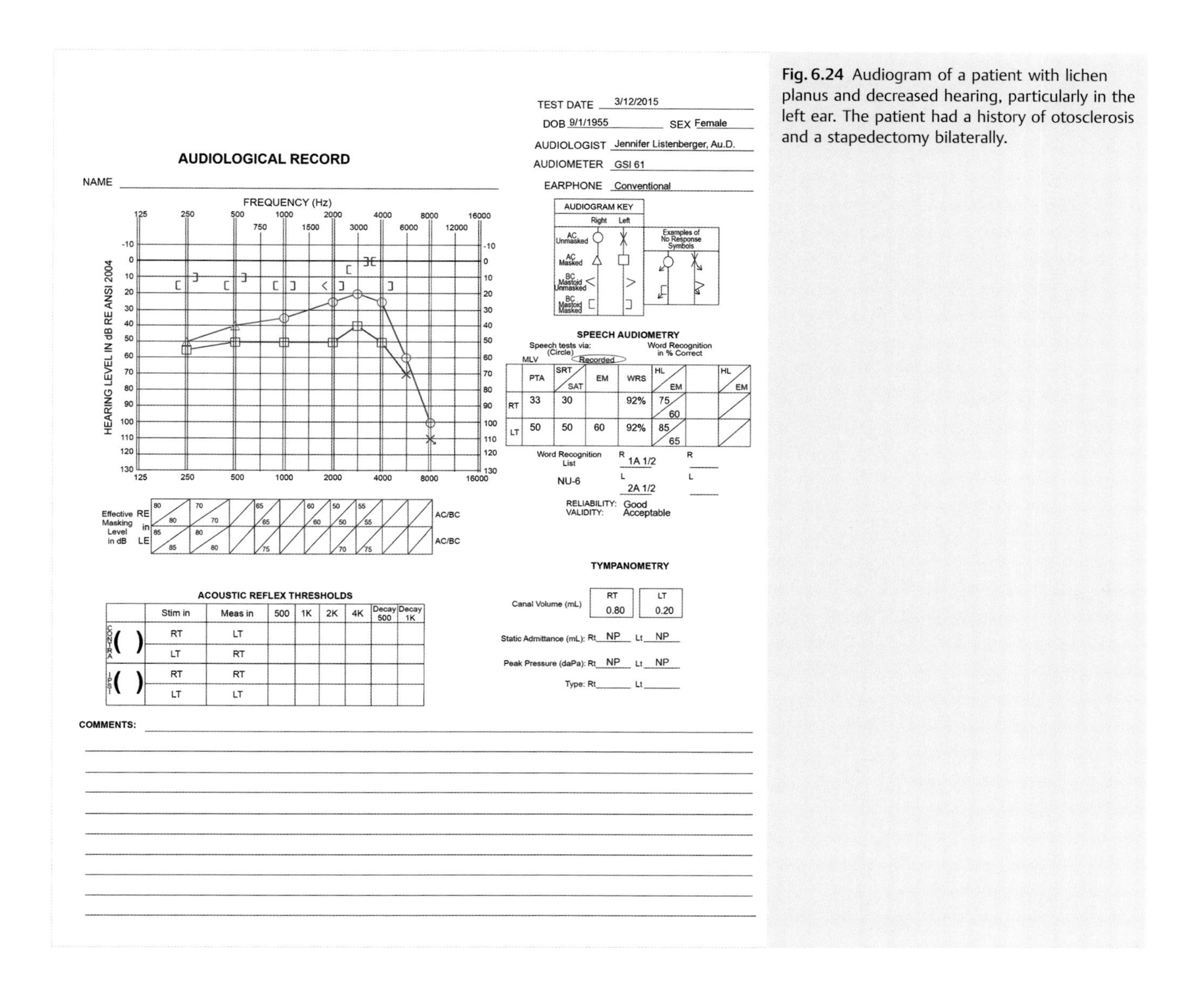

Fig. 6.24 Audiogram of a patient with lichen planus and decreased hearing, particularly in the left ear. The patient had a history of otosclerosis and a stapedectomy bilaterally.

6.24.2 Interpretation

Right ear—Pure-tone air and bone conduction threshold testing revealed a moderate rising to mild conductive hearing loss at 250 through 1,000 Hz, rising to a slight mixed hearing loss at 2,000 through 4,000 Hz, and steeply sloping to moderately severe to profound at 6,000 and 8,000 Hz. The SRT revealed a mild loss in the ability to receive speech and was in agreement with the PTA. The WRS revealed a normal ability to recognize speech. Immittance testing revealed a flat tympanogram with normal ear canal volume. Acoustic reflex threshold and decay testing were not measured at this appointment.

Left ear—Pure-tone air and bone conduction threshold testing revealed a moderate conductive hearing loss at 250 through 4,000 Hz, except for a rise to mild at 3,000 Hz, then sloping to moderately severe to profound at 6,000 and 8,000 Hz. There was no measurable response within the equipment limits at 8,000 Hz. The SRT revealed a moderate loss in the ability to receive speech and was in agreement with the PTA. The WRS revealed a normal ability to recognize speech. Immittance testing revealed a flat tympanogram with a small ear canal volume. Acoustic reflex threshold and decay testing were not measured at this appointment.

6.24.3 Intervention

The patient will follow up with the otologist as scheduled. The audiological recommendations were to return for a hearing test to monitor stability of auditory sensitivity and to schedule a hearing aid evaluation to discuss amplification and HAT.

6.25 Case 25

6.25.1 Case History

The patient reported a sudden onset of hearing loss and tinnitus in the right ear immediately following a fall and head trauma approximately 2 weeks prior to the hearing test. The patient's parents were present and provided a detailed history. The patient suffered a skull fracture through the right temporal bone and a concussion. The patient reported that he had hearing in the right ear, but sound was muffled and seemed far away. There was no reported improvement in symptoms over the past 2 weeks. There was no history of hearing loss or tinnitus prior to the head trauma.

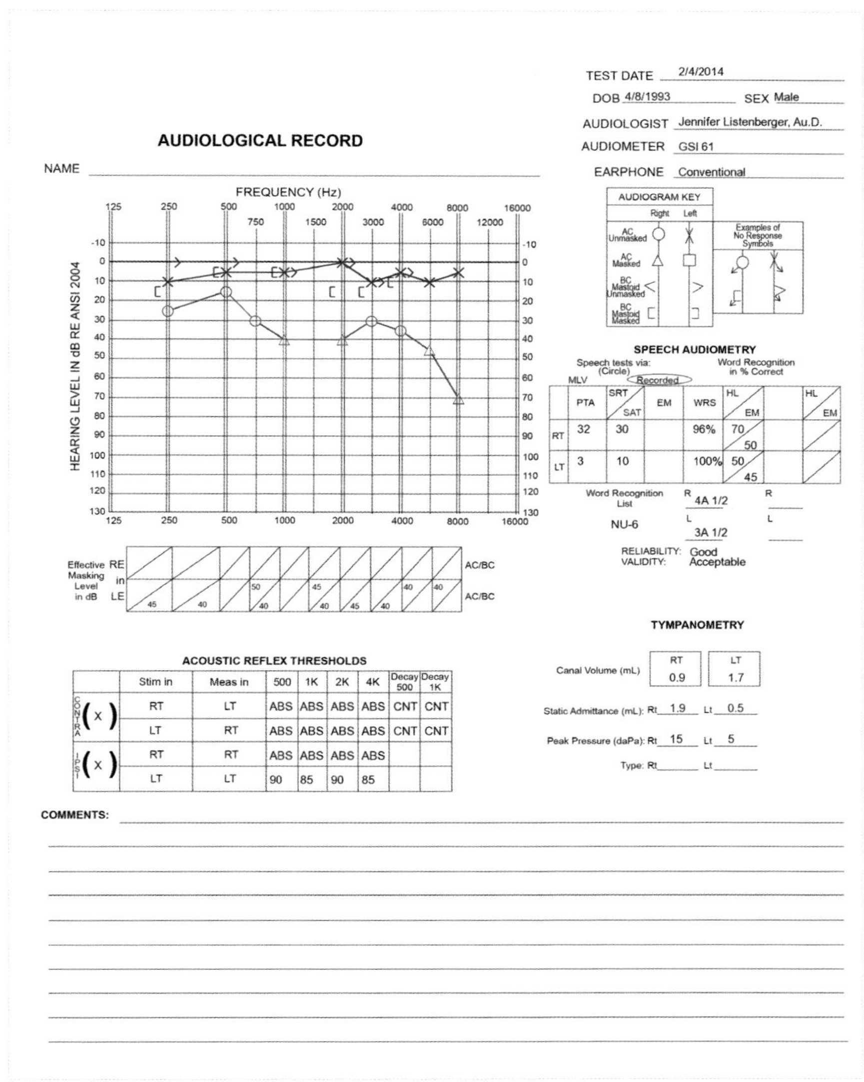

AUDIOLOGICAL RECORD

NAME

TEST DATE 2/4/2014
DOB 4/8/1993 SEX Male
AUDIOLOGIST Jennifer Listenberger, Au.D.
AUDIOMETER GSI 61
EARPHONE Conventional

SPEECH AUDIOMETRY

Speech tests via: (Circle) MLV Recorded — Word Recognition in % Correct

	PTA	SRT/SAT	EM	WRS	HL/EM		HL/EM
RT	32	30		96%	70/50		
LT	3	10		100%	50/45		

Word Recognition List: R 4A 1/2; L 3A 1/2
NU-6

RELIABILITY: Good
VALIDITY: Acceptable

Effective Masking Level in dB (AC/BC): LE 45, 40, 40, 40, 45, 40; RE 50, 45, 40, 40

ACOUSTIC REFLEX THRESHOLDS

	Stim in	Meas in	500	1K	2K	4K	Decay 500	Decay 1K
CONTRA (x)	RT	LT	ABS	ABS	ABS	ABS	CNT	CNT
	LT	RT	ABS	ABS	ABS	ABS	CNT	CNT
IPSI (x)	RT	RT	ABS	ABS	ABS	ABS		
	LT	LT	90	85	90	85		

TYMPANOMETRY

	RT	LT
Canal Volume (mL)	0.9	1.7
Static Admittance (mL)	1.9	0.5
Peak Pressure (daPa)	15	5
Type		

COMMENTS:

Fig. 6.25 Audiogram of a patient with a sudden onset of hearing loss and tinnitus in the right ear following a fall and head trauma. The patient suffered a skull fracture through the right temporal bone and a concussion.

6.25.2 Interpretation

Right ear—Pure-tone air and bone conduction threshold testing revealed a slight sensorineural hearing loss at 250 Hz, rising to normal at 500 Hz, sloping to mild conductive hearing loss at 750 through 4,000 Hz, and sloping to moderate to moderately severe at 6,000 through 8,000 Hz. The SRT revealed a mild loss in the ability to receive speech and was in agreement with the PTA. The WRS revealed a normal ability to recognize speech. Immittance testing revealed a hypercompliant tympanogram. The acoustic reflex thresholds were absent for ipsilateral and contralateral stimulation at 500 through 4,000 Hz. Acoustic reflex decay could not be measured due to absent contralateral acoustic reflex thresholds.

Left ear—Pure-tone air and bone conduction threshold testing revealed normal hearing sensitivity at 250 through 8,000 Hz. The SRT revealed a normal ability to receive speech and was in agreement with the PTA. The WRS revealed a normal ability to recognize speech. Immittance testing revealed a normal tympanogram. The acoustic reflex thresholds were within normal limits for ipsilateral stimulation and absent for contralateral stimulation at 500 through 4,000 Hz. Acoustic reflex decay could not be measured due to absent contralateral acoustic reflex thresholds.

6.25.3 Intervention

The patient will follow up with the otologist as scheduled. The audiological recommendations were to return for a hearing test after medical management and as needed and to use hearing protection in noise.

6.26 Case 26

6.26.1 Case History

The patient reported a slight decrease in hearing over the last few years. He had intermittent tinnitus and a slight sensation of fullness in the left ear. He also reported a family history of hearing loss, with his mother acquiring hearing loss in her early forties. He did not report other otologic symptoms or history.

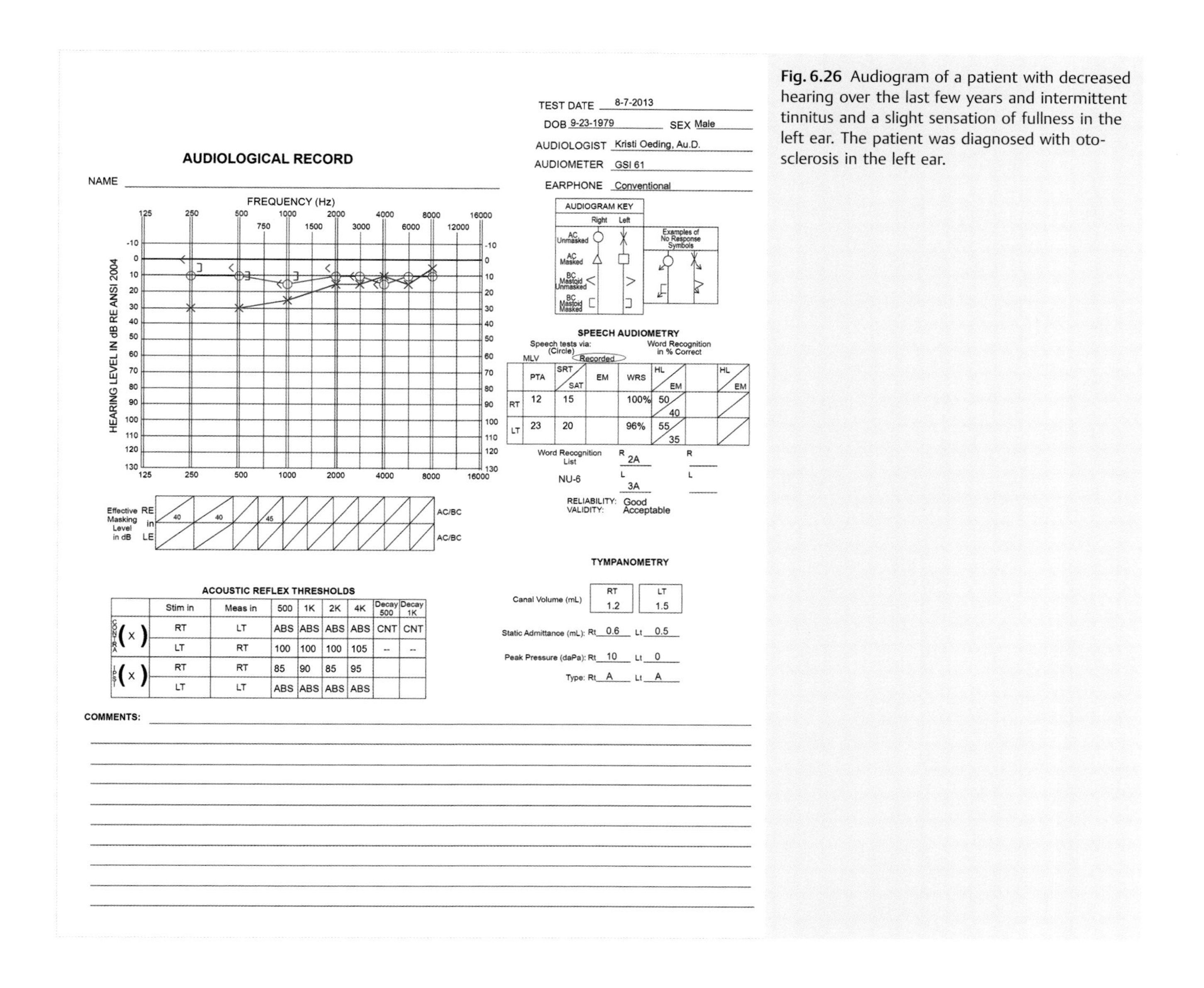

AUDIOLOGICAL RECORD

NAME

TEST DATE 8-7-2013
DOB 9-23-1979 SEX Male
AUDIOLOGIST Kristi Oeding, Au.D.
AUDIOMETER GSI 61
EARPHONE Conventional

SPEECH AUDIOMETRY

Speech tests via: (Circle) MLV Recorded

Word Recognition in % Correct

	PTA	SRT / SAT	EM	WRS	HL / EM		HL / EM
RT	12	15		100%	50 / 40		
LT	23	20		96%	55 / 35		

Word Recognition List NU-6: R 2A; L 3A

RELIABILITY: Good
VALIDITY: Acceptable

TYMPANOMETRY

	RT	LT
Canal Volume (mL)	1.2	1.5
Static Admittance (mL)	0.6	0.5
Peak Pressure (daPa)	10	0
Type	A	A

ACOUSTIC REFLEX THRESHOLDS

	Stim in	Meas in	500	1K	2K	4K	Decay 500	Decay 1K
CONTRA (X)	RT	LT	ABS	ABS	ABS	ABS	CNT	CNT
	LT	RT	100	100	100	105	--	--
IPSI (X)	RT	RT	85	90	85	95		
	LT	LT	ABS	ABS	ABS	ABS		

COMMENTS:

Fig. 6.26 Audiogram of a patient with decreased hearing over the last few years and intermittent tinnitus and a slight sensation of fullness in the left ear. The patient was diagnosed with otosclerosis in the left ear.

6.26.2 Interpretation

Right ear—Pure-tone thresholds were within normal limits from 250 to 8,000 Hz. The SRT revealed a normal ability to receive speech and was in agreement with the PTA. The WRS revealed a normal ability to recognize speech. Immittance testing revealed a normal tympanogram. The ipsilateral acoustic reflex thresholds were normal from 500 to 4,000 Hz. The contralateral acoustic reflex thresholds were normal from 500 to 2,000 Hz and elevated at 4,000 Hz. Acoustic reflex decay was negative at 500 and 1,000 Hz.

Left ear—Pure-tone thresholds revealed a mild rising to slight conductive hearing loss from 250 to 1,000 Hz and rising to normal hearing sensitivity from 2,000 to 8,000 Hz. The SRT revealed a slight loss in the ability to receive speech and was in agreement with the PTA. The WRS revealed a normal ability to recognize speech. Immittance testing revealed a normal tympanogram. The ipsilateral and contralateral acoustic reflex thresholds were absent from 500 to 4,000 Hz. Acoustic reflex decay could not be measured due to absent contralateral acoustic reflex thresholds at 500 and 1,000 Hz.

6.26.3 Intervention

The otologist ordered a CT scan, which revealed otosclerosis in the left ear. The progression of otosclerosis will be monitored, and surgery may be an option in the future. The audiological recommendations included annual hearing tests and hearing protection in noise.

6.27 Case 27

6.27.1 Case History

A 23-year-old male returned to the office for follow-up testing to monitor sensitivity of hearing due to a long-standing history of bilateral conductive hearing loss. The patient presented with a significant history of ear pathology and otosurgery with a tympanic membrane perforation in the left ear and a cholesteatoma and ossicular chain reconstruction in the right ear. The last hearing test was completed in June 2014. The patient reported he was fitted with amplification for the right ear approximately two years prior to testing, but he never consistently used the hearing aid and the hearing aid no longer fit due to aural reconstruction.

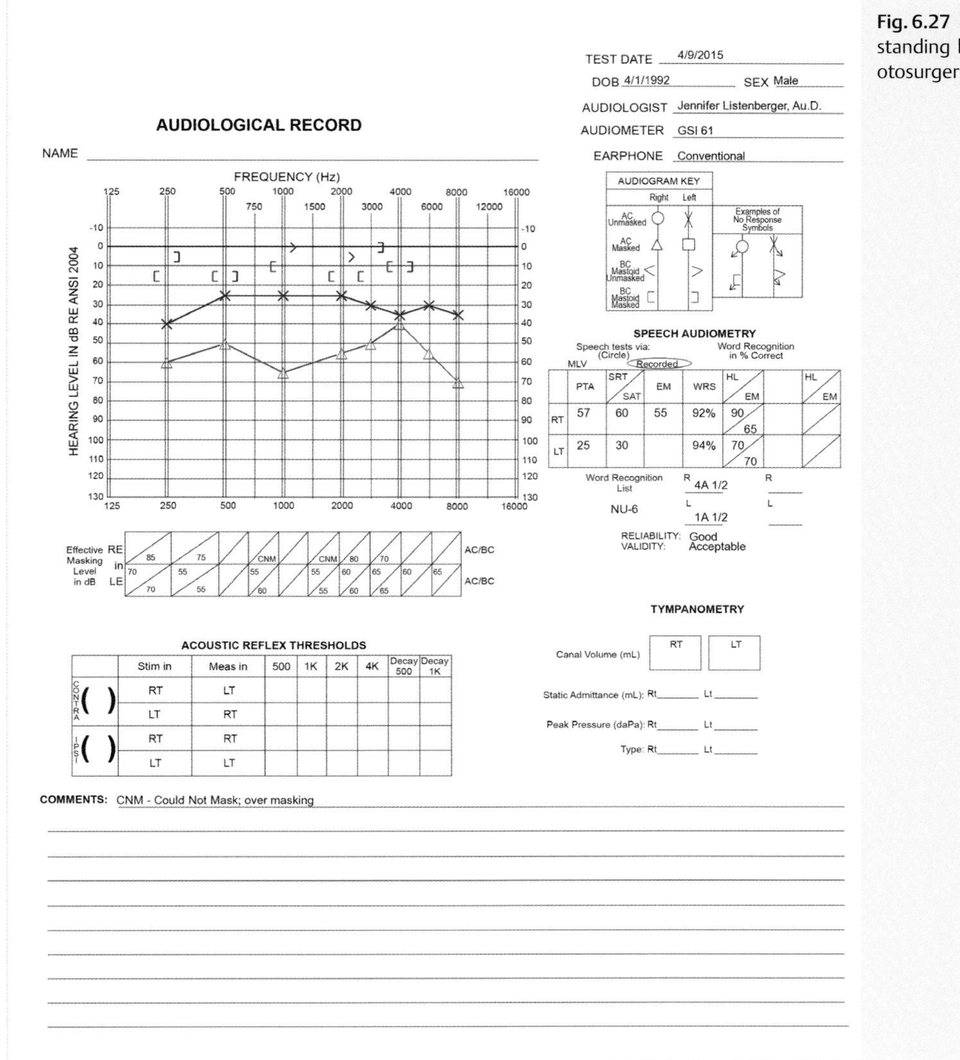

AUDIOLOGICAL RECORD

NAME

TEST DATE 4/9/2015

DOB 4/1/1992 SEX Male

AUDIOLOGIST Jennifer Listenberger, Au.D.

AUDIOMETER GSI 61

EARPHONE Conventional

Effective Masking Level in dB

RE in: 85, 75, CNM, CNM, 80, 70 (AC/BC)

LE in: 70, 55, 55, 55, 65, 60, 65 / 70, 55, 60, 55, 60, 65 (AC/BC)

SPEECH AUDIOMETRY

Speech tests via: (Circle) MLV Recorded

Word Recognition in % Correct

	PTA	SRT/SAT	EM	WRS	HL/EM	HL/EM
RT	57	60	55	92%	90/65	
LT	25	30		94%	70/70	

Word Recognition List NU-6: R 4A 1/2; L 1A 1/2

RELIABILITY: Good

VALIDITY: Acceptable

ACOUSTIC REFLEX THRESHOLDS

	Stim in	Meas in	500	1K	2K	4K	Decay 500	Decay 1K
CONTRA ( )	RT	LT						
	LT	RT						
IPSI ( )	RT	RT						
	LT	LT						

TYMPANOMETRY

Canal Volume (mL) RT LT

Static Admittance (mL): Rt____ Lt____

Peak Pressure (daPa): Rt____ Lt____

Type: Rt____ Lt____

COMMENTS: CNM - Could Not Mask; over masking

Fig. 6.27 Audiogram of a patient with a long-standing history of hearing loss and a history of otosurgery bilaterally.

6.27.2 Interpretation

Right ear—Pure-tone air and bone conduction threshold testing revealed an essentially flat moderate and moderately severe conductive hearing loss at 250 through 8,000 Hz, with a rise to mild at 4,000 Hz. The SRT revealed moderately severe loss in the ability to receive speech and was in agreement with the PTA. The WRS revealed a normal ability to recognize speech. Immittance testing was not measured due to the surgical history.

Left ear—Pure-tone air and bone conduction threshold testing revealed a flat slight and mild predominantly conductive hearing loss at 250 through 8,000 Hz, except for sensorineural hearing loss at 500 Hz. The SRT revealed a mild loss in the ability to receive speech and was in agreement with the PTA. The WRS revealed a normal ability to recognize speech. Immittance testing was not measured due to the surgical history.

6.27.3 Intervention

The test results were reviewed and the thresholds and WRS did not change from the test completed 1 year earlier. The patient was encouraged to follow up with his physician as recommended. The audiological recommendations included annual testing to monitor hearing sensitivity, hearing aid evaluation to discuss amplification and HAT, and hearing protection in noise.

6.28 Case 28

6.28.1 Case History

A 26-year-old female with a long-standing history of unilateral conductive hearing loss was seen for follow-up testing to monitor her hearing sensitivity. The patient had a history of cholesteatoma and had multiple surgeries for the left ear starting when she was 2 years old. The last surgery was a mastoidectomy with an ossicular chain reconstruction approximately 11 years ago in 2004. The patient denied tinnitus or dizziness. She wore a hearing aid in the left ear.

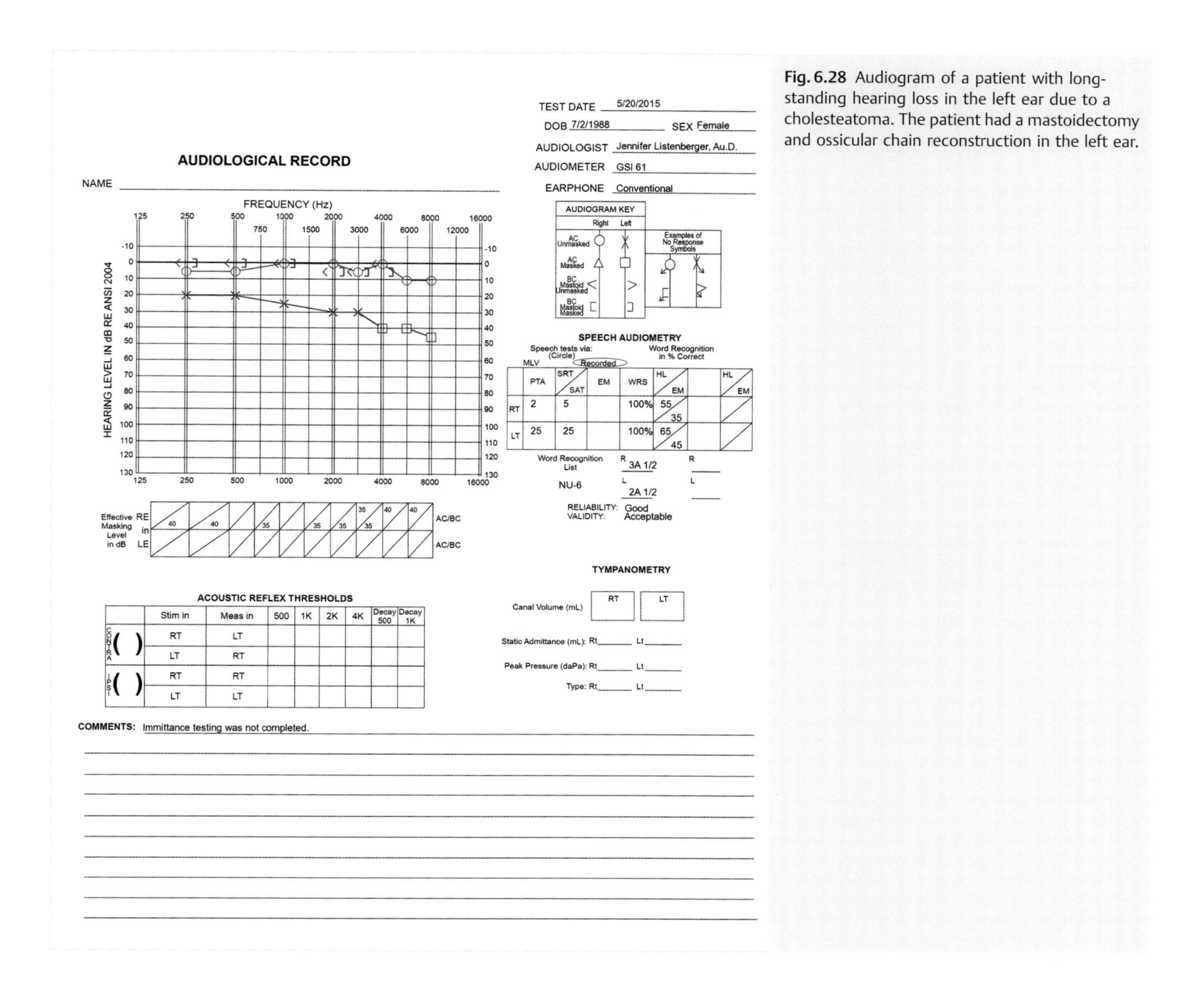

AUDIOLOGICAL RECORD

NAME

TEST DATE 5/20/2015
DOB 7/2/1988 SEX Female
AUDIOLOGIST Jennifer Listenberger, Au.D.
AUDIOMETER GSI 61
EARPHONE Conventional

Effective Masking Level in dB

	250	500	750	1000	1500	2000	3000	4000	6000	8000	
RE in	40	40		35		35	35 / 35	35	40	40	AC/BC
LE											AC/BC

SPEECH AUDIOMETRY

Speech tests via: (Circle) MLV Recorded

Word Recognition in % Correct

	PTA	SRT / SAT	EM	WRS	HL / EM		HL / EM
RT	2	5		100%	55 / 35		
LT	25	25		100%	65 / 45		

Word Recognition List NU-6: R 3A 1/2; L 2A 1/2

RELIABILITY: Good
VALIDITY: Acceptable

ACOUSTIC REFLEX THRESHOLDS

	Stim in	Meas in	500	1K	2K	4K	Decay 500	Decay 1K
CONTRA ( )	RT	LT						
	LT	RT						
IPSI ( )	RT	RT						
	LT	LT						

TYMPANOMETRY

Canal Volume (mL) RT LT
Static Admittance (mL): Rt____ Lt____
Peak Pressure (daPa): Rt____ Lt____
Type: Rt____ Lt____

COMMENTS: Immittance testing was not completed.

Fig. 6.28 Audiogram of a patient with long-standing hearing loss in the left ear due to a cholesteatoma. The patient had a mastoidectomy and ossicular chain reconstruction in the left ear.

6.28.2 Interpretation

Right ear—Pure-tone air and bone conduction threshold testing revealed normal hearing sensitivity at 250 through 8,000 Hz. The SRT revealed a normal ability to receive speech and was in agreement with the PTA. The WRS revealed a normal ability to recognize speech. Immittance testing was not measured at this appointment.

Left ear—Pure-tone air and bone conduction threshold testing revealed a slight sloping to mild conductive hearing loss at 250 through 6,000 Hz, sloping to moderate at 8,000 Hz. The SRT revealed a slight loss in the ability to receive speech and was in agreement with the PTA. The WRS revealed a normal ability to recognize speech. Immittance testing was not measured at this appointment.

6.28.3 Intervention

The patient will follow up with the otologist as scheduled. The audiological recommendations were to return for a hearing test annually to monitor hearing sensitivity, to use hearing protection in noise, and to continue use of amplification.

6.29 Case 29

6.29.1 Case History

The patient reported that he was mowing the lawn and a branch punctured his right tympanic membrane. He had otalgia, hearing loss, and tinnitus in the right ear since the incident. He had a history of ear infections bilaterally as a child. He did not report other otologic symptoms or history.

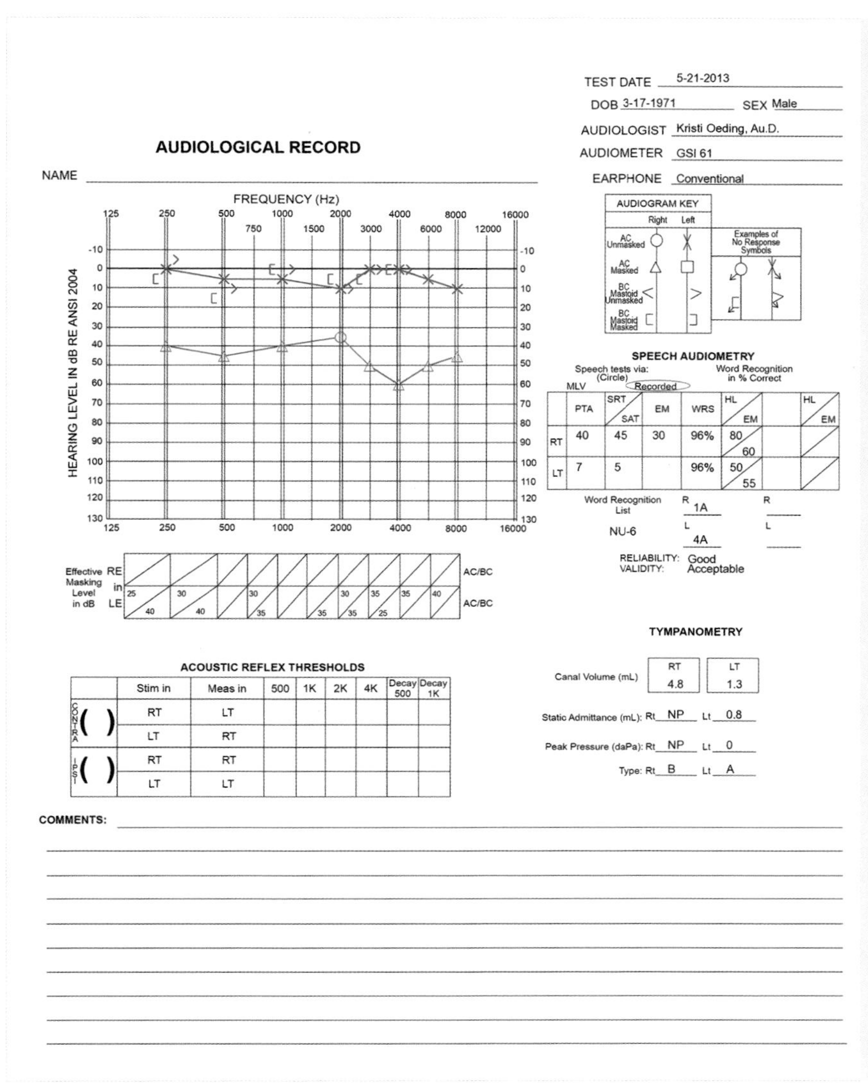

AUDIOLOGICAL RECORD

NAME

TEST DATE 5-21-2013

DOB 3-17-1971 SEX Male

AUDIOLOGIST Kristi Oeding, Au.D.

AUDIOMETER GSI 61

EARPHONE Conventional

FREQUENCY (Hz)

HEARING LEVEL IN dB RE ANSI 2004

AUDIOGRAM KEY

	Right	Left
AC Unmasked	O	X
AC Masked	△	□
BC Mastoid Unmasked	<	>
BC Mastoid Masked	[	]

Examples of No Response Symbols

Effective Masking Level in dB

	125	250	500	750	1000	1500	2000	3000	4000	6000	8000
RE AC/BC											
LE AC/BC	25 / 40	30 / 40	30 / 35			30 / 35	35 / 35	35 / 25	40		

SPEECH AUDIOMETRY

Speech tests via: (Circle) MLV Recorded

Word Recognition in % Correct

	PTA	SRT/SAT	EM	WRS	HL/EM		HL/EM
RT	40	45	30	96%	80 / 60		
LT	7	5		96%	50 / 55		

Word Recognition List NU-6: R 1A, L 4A

RELIABILITY: Good

VALIDITY: Acceptable

TYMPANOMETRY

	RT	LT
Canal Volume (mL)	4.8	1.3
Static Admittance (mL)	NP	0.8
Peak Pressure (daPa)	NP	0
Type	B	A

ACOUSTIC REFLEX THRESHOLDS

	Stim in	Meas in	500	1K	2K	4K	Decay 500	Decay 1K
CONTRA ( )	RT	LT						
	LT	RT						
IPSI ( )	RT	RT						
	LT	LT						

COMMENTS:

Fig. 6.29 Audiogram of a patient with a punctured right tympanic membrane from a branch when he was mowing the lawn. The patient reported otalgia, hearing loss, and tinnitus in the right ear.

6.29.2 Interpretation

Right ear—Pure-tone thresholds revealed a mild conductive hearing loss from 250 to 2,000 Hz, except for a moderate conductive hearing loss at 500 Hz, sloping to a moderate to moderately severe conductive hearing loss from 3,000 to 4,000 Hz, and rising to moderate from 6,000 to 8,000 Hz. The SRT revealed a moderate loss in the ability to receive speech and was in agreement with the PTA. The WRS revealed a normal ability to recognize speech. Immittance testing was performed and revealed a flat tympanogram with a large ear canal volume. Acoustic reflex thresholds and decay were not measured at this appointment.

Left ear—Pure-tone thresholds were within normal limits from 250 to 8,000 Hz. The SRT revealed a normal ability to receive speech and was in agreement with the PTA. The WRS revealed a normal ability to recognize speech. Immittance testing was performed and revealed a normal tympanogram. The acoustic reflex thresholds and decay were not measured at this appointment.

6.29.3 Intervention

The otologist ordered a CT scan, and ossicular discontinuity was noted. The otologist planned to perform a tympanoplasty and ossicular chain reconstruction. The audiological recommendations included retesting his hearing after surgery and annually as well as use of hearing protection in noise.

6.30 Case 30

6.30.1 Case History

The patient returned for testing due to decreased hearing in the right ear. He has a long-standing history of bilateral conductive hearing loss due to chronic otitis media with effusion and eustachian tube dysfunction. He had a history of multiple surgeries for tympanic membrane reconstruction. A hearing test was completed 1 year ago when pressure equalization tubes were placed bilaterally. The right tube had extruded. The patient also reported aural pressure in the right ear.

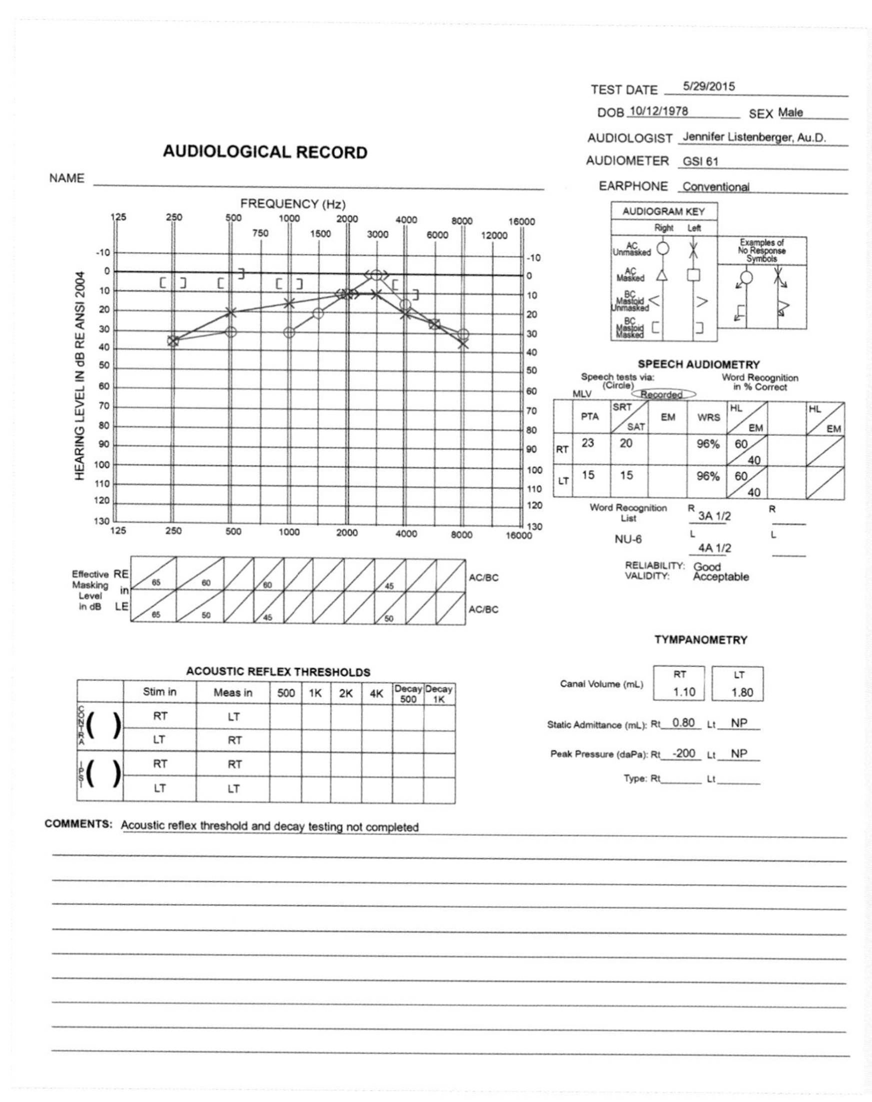

AUDIOLOGICAL RECORD

NAME

TEST DATE 5/29/2015
DOB 10/12/1978 SEX Male
AUDIOLOGIST Jennifer Listenberger, Au.D.
AUDIOMETER GSI 61
EARPHONE Conventional

SPEECH AUDIOMETRY

Speech tests via: (Circle) MLV Recorded

	PTA	SRT/SAT	EM	WRS	HL/EM
RT	23	20		96%	60/40
LT	15	15		96%	60/40

Word Recognition List NU-6: R 3A 1/2; L 4A 1/2

RELIABILITY: Good
VALIDITY: Acceptable

Effective Masking Level in dB: RE 65, 60, 60, 45; LE 65, 50, 45, 50

TYMPANOMETRY

Canal Volume (mL): RT 1.10; LT 1.80
Static Admittance (mL): Rt 0.80 Lt NP
Peak Pressure (daPa): Rt -200 Lt NP
Type: Rt ___ Lt ___

ACOUSTIC REFLEX THRESHOLDS

	Stim in	Meas in	500	1K	2K	4K	Decay 500	Decay 1K
CONTRA	RT	LT						
	LT	RT						
IPSI	RT	RT						
	LT	LT						

COMMENTS: Acoustic reflex threshold and decay testing not completed

Fig. 6.30 Audiogram of a patient with decreased hearing in the right ear and a history of bilateral chronic otitis media and eustachian tube dysfunction. The patient has had multiple tympanoplasties and has had pressure equalization tubes.

6.30.2 Interpretation

Right ear—Pure-tone air and bone conduction threshold testing revealed a mild conductive hearing loss at 250 through 1,000 Hz, rising to slight at 1,500 Hz, rising to normal hearing sensitivity at 2,000 through 4,000 Hz, then sloping to slight to mild at 6,000 and 8,000 Hz. The SRT revealed a slight loss in the ability to receive speech and was in agreement with the PTA. The WRS revealed a normal ability to recognize speech. Immittance testing revealed a tympanogram with excessive negative pressure. Acoustic reflex threshold and decay testing was not measured at this appointment.

Left ear—Pure-tone air and bone conduction threshold testing revealed a mild rising to slight conductive hearing loss at 250 through 500 Hz, rising to normal hearing sensitivity at 1,000 through 3,000 Hz, then sloping to a slight sloping to mild sensorineural hearing loss at 4,000 through 8,000 Hz. The SRT revealed a normal ability to receive speech and was in agreement with the PTA. The WRS revealed a normal ability to recognize speech. Immittance testing revealed a flat tympanogram with a normal ear canal volume. Acoustic reflex threshold and decay testing was not measured at this appointment.

6.30.3 Intervention

The patient will return for medical follow-up per recommendation of the ENT specialist. The audiological recommendations were to return for a hearing test after medical management and annually to monitor hearing sensitivity, to return to discuss amplification and use of HAT, and to use hearing protection in noise.

7 Mixed Hearing Loss Cases

7.1 Case 1

7.1.1 Case History

The patient reported that 20 years ago he had a cyst in his left ear that caused an infection. The cyst was removed and the infection was cleared. This resulted in hearing loss in the left ear. Surgery was attempted to repair the middle ear and restore hearing, but this was unsuccessful. He reported that he has used a hearing aid in the left ear occasionally since that time. The patient stated that he started to have decreased hearing in his right ear approximately 3 years ago. He stated that he frequently has fluid in his middle ear causing hearing loss. He had multiple tubes placed in each ear and stated that they eventually fell out. He currently had a tube placed in the right ear. He reported pain and pressure at times in the right ear. He had intermittent tinnitus bilaterally. He denied dizziness or loud noise exposure as well as a family history of hearing loss.

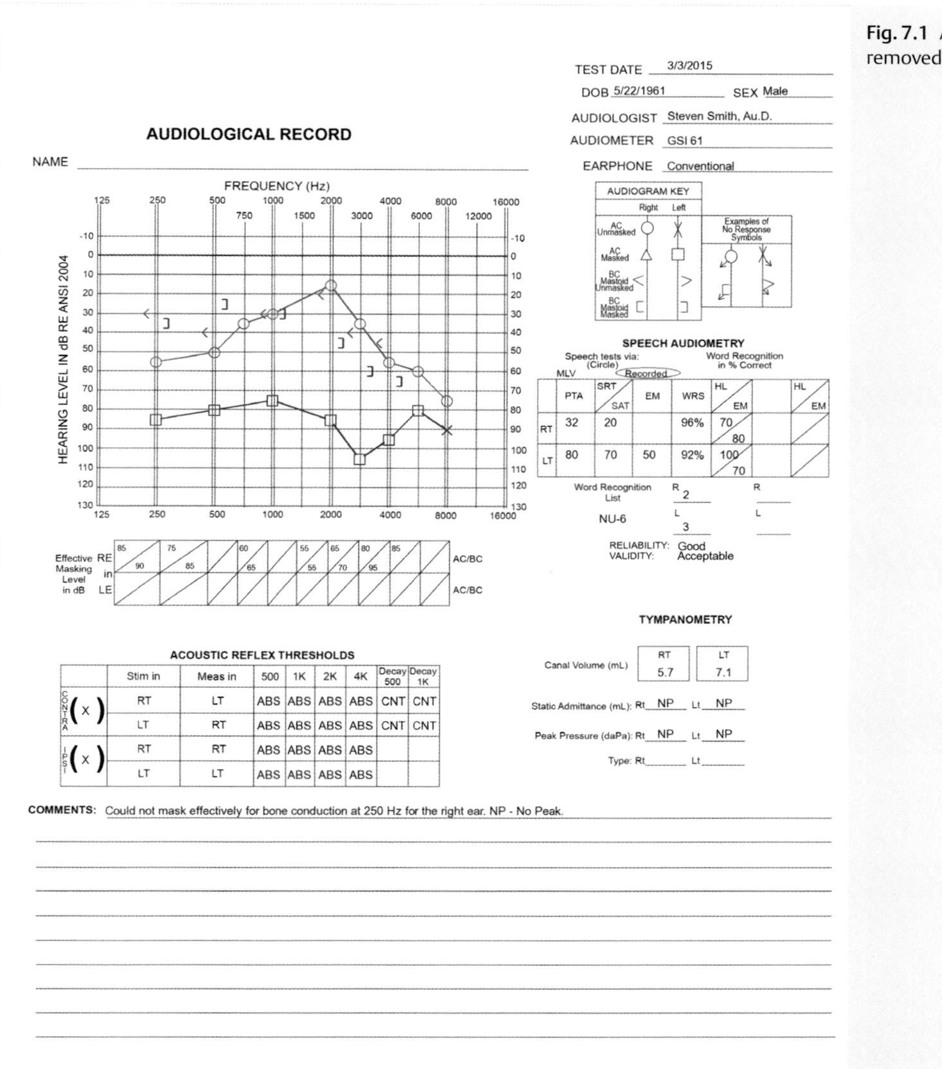

TEST DATE 3/3/2015

DOB 5/22/1961 SEX Male

AUDIOLOGIST Steven Smith, Au.D.

AUDIOMETER GSI 61

EARPHONE Conventional

AUDIOLOGICAL RECORD

NAME

Effective Masking Level in dB

RE in	85/90	75/85		60/65		55/55	65/70	80/95	85/		AC/BC
LE											AC/BC

SPEECH AUDIOMETRY

Speech tests via: (Circle) MLV (Recorded) — Word Recognition in % Correct

	PTA	SRT/SAT	EM	WRS	HL/EM		HL/EM
RT	32	20		96%	70/80		
LT	80	70	50	92%	100/70		

Word Recognition List: NU-6 — R 2, L 3; R ___, L ___

RELIABILITY: Good
VALIDITY: Acceptable

TYMPANOMETRY

	RT	LT
Canal Volume (mL)	5.7	7.1

Static Admittance (mL): Rt NP Lt NP

Peak Pressure (daPa): Rt NP Lt NP

Type: Rt ___ Lt ___

ACOUSTIC REFLEX THRESHOLDS

	Stim in	Meas in	500	1K	2K	4K	Decay 500	Decay 1K
CONTRA (x)	RT	LT	ABS	ABS	ABS	ABS	CNT	CNT
	LT	RT	ABS	ABS	ABS	ABS	CNT	CNT
IPSI (x)	RT	RT	ABS	ABS	ABS	ABS		
	LT	LT	ABS	ABS	ABS	ABS		

COMMENTS: Could not mask effectively for bone conduction at 250 Hz for the right ear. NP - No Peak.

Fig. 7.1 Audiogram of a patient who had a cyst removed from the left ear.

7.1.2 Interpretation

Right ear—Moderate mixed hearing loss, gradually rising to normal hearing sensitivity at 2,000 Hz, then sloping to severe sensorineural hearing loss. The SRT revealed a slight loss in the ability to receive speech and was relatively in agreement with the PTA. The WRS was normal. Immittance testing revealed a flat tympanogram with a large ear canal volume. The acoustic reflex thresholds with ipsilateral and contralateral stimulation from 500 to 4,000 Hz were absent. Acoustic reflex decay could not be measured.

Left ear—Severe mixed hearing loss with a profound mixed hearing loss notch at 3,000 and 4,000 Hz. The SRT revealed a moderately severe loss in the ability to receive speech and was in agreement with the PTA. The WRS was normal. Immittance testing revealed a flat tympanogram with a large ear canal volume. The acoustic reflex thresholds with ipsilateral and contralateral stimulation from 500 to 4,000 Hz were absent. Acoustic reflex decay could not be measured.

7.1.3 Intervention

The patient was referred to an ENT specialist for treatment of the ear infection in the right ear and for follow-up on the left ear. He was encouraged to continue use of a hearing aid for the left ear and to follow up for a hearing aid evaluation for the right ear pending medical clearance.

7.2 Case 2

7.2.1 Case History

The patient reported bilateral hearing loss due to otosclerosis for several years. She had otosurgery in her left ear. She wore an ITC hearing aid in the left ear that had an omnidirectional microphone and was intermittent. She had worn a hearing aid for 10 years. She also reported bilateral tinnitus for several years. She had a family history of hearing loss through her father and grandfather. She had a history of noise exposure from hunting. She did not report other otologic symptoms or history.

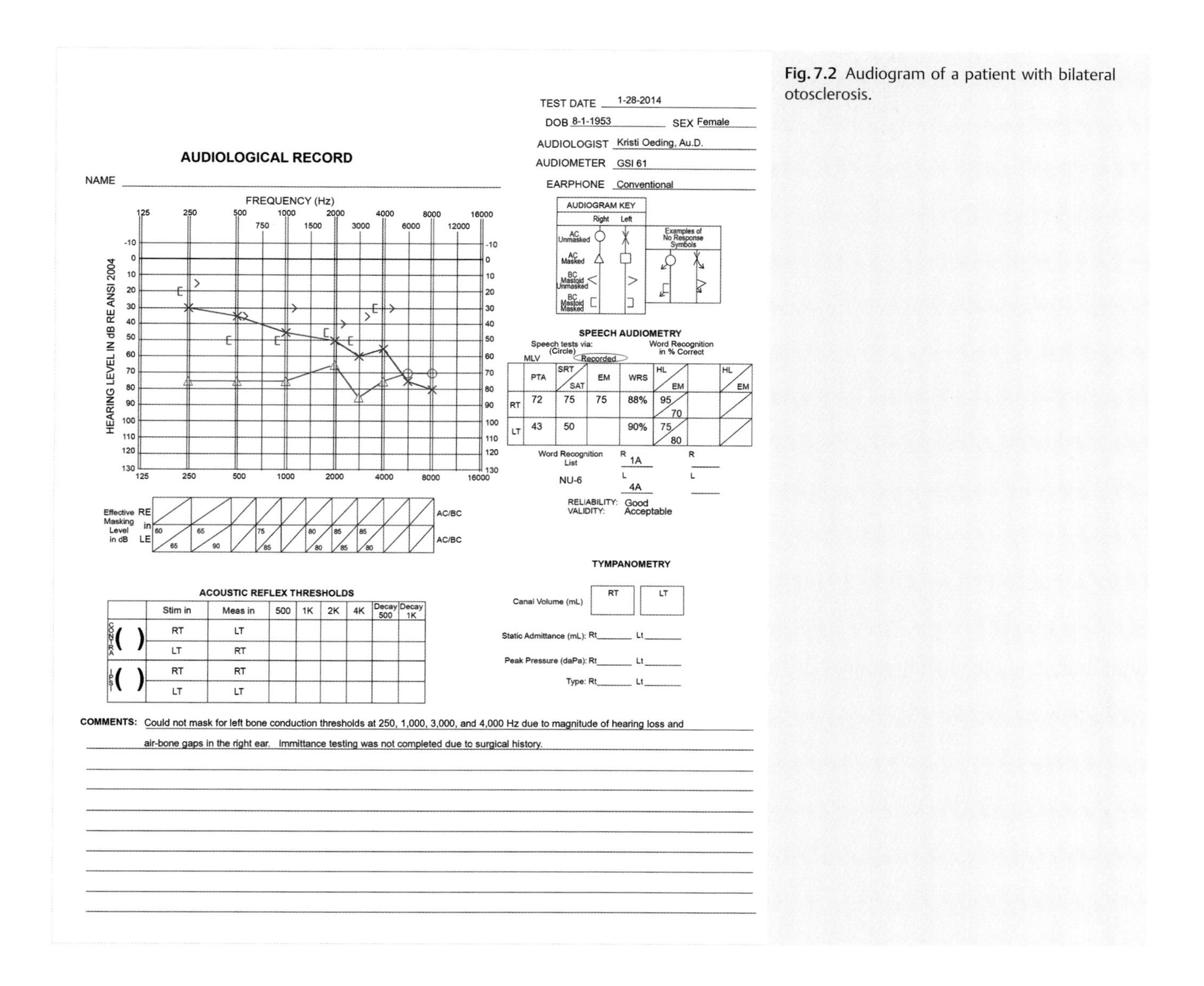

AUDIOLOGICAL RECORD

NAME

TEST DATE 1-28-2014

DOB 8-1-1953 SEX Female

AUDIOLOGIST Kristi Oeding, Au.D.

AUDIOMETER GSI 61

EARPHONE Conventional

SPEECH AUDIOMETRY

Speech tests via: (Circle) MLV Recorded

Word Recognition in % Correct

	PTA	SRT/SAT	EM	WRS	HL/EM	HL/EM
RT	72	75	75	88%	95/70	
LT	43	50		90%	75/80	

Word Recognition List: R 1A, L 4A

NU-6

RELIABILITY: Good

VALIDITY: Acceptable

TYMPANOMETRY

Canal Volume (mL) RT LT

Static Admittance (mL): Rt_____ Lt_____

Peak Pressure (daPa): Rt_____ Lt_____

Type: Rt_____ Lt_____

Effective Masking Level in dB: RE in 60, 65, 75, 80, 85, 85; LE 65, 90, 85, 80, 85, 80

ACOUSTIC REFLEX THRESHOLDS

	Stim in	Meas in	500	1K	2K	4K	Decay 500	Decay 1K
CONTRA ( )	RT	LT						
	LT	RT						
IPSI ( )	RT	RT						
	LT	LT						

COMMENTS: Could not mask for left bone conduction thresholds at 250, 1,000, 3,000, and 4,000 Hz due to magnitude of hearing loss and air-bone gaps in the right ear. Immittance testing was not completed due to surgical history.

Fig. 7.2 Audiogram of a patient with bilateral otosclerosis.

7.2.2 Interpretation

Right ear—Pure-tone thresholds revealed a severe mixed hearing loss from 250 to 1,000 Hz, rising to moderately severe at 2,000 Hz, sloping to severe from 3,000 to 4,000 Hz, and rising to moderately severe from 6,000 to 8,000 Hz. The SRT revealed a severe loss in the ability to receive speech and was in agreement with the PTA. The WRS revealed a slight difficulty in the ability to recognize speech. Immittance testing was not measured due to the previous otosurgery.

Left ear—Pure-tone thresholds revealed a mild to moderately severe mixed hearing loss from 250 to 3,000 Hz, rising to moderate at 4,000 Hz, and sloping to severe from 6,000 to 8,000 Hz. The SRT revealed a moderate loss in the ability to receive speech and was in agreement with the PTA. The WRS revealed a normal ability to recognize speech. Immittance testing was not measured due to the previous otosurgery.

7.2.3 Intervention

The otologist recommended a hearing aid trial before considering otosurgery. Other audiological recommendations included an annual hearing test, HAT, and hearing protection in noise. She was fit with binaural BTE hearing aids and perceived significant benefit from her hearing aids.

7.3 Case 3

7.3.1 Case History

The patient reported a long-standing history of hearing loss with a sudden hearing loss occurring in the right ear over 20 years ago and a gradual deterioration in hearing in the left ear. The patient's last hearing examination was completed in 2005 and revealed a mixed hearing loss in the left ear and a profound sensorineural hearing loss in the right with no measurable thresholds within the limits of the audiometer. He had used amplification for the left ear and had noticed his hearing aid was not providing as much benefit as in the past. The patient denied tinnitus, dizziness, or aural pressure or fullness. There was no significant history of otosurgery, ear pathology, familial hearing loss, or noise exposure.

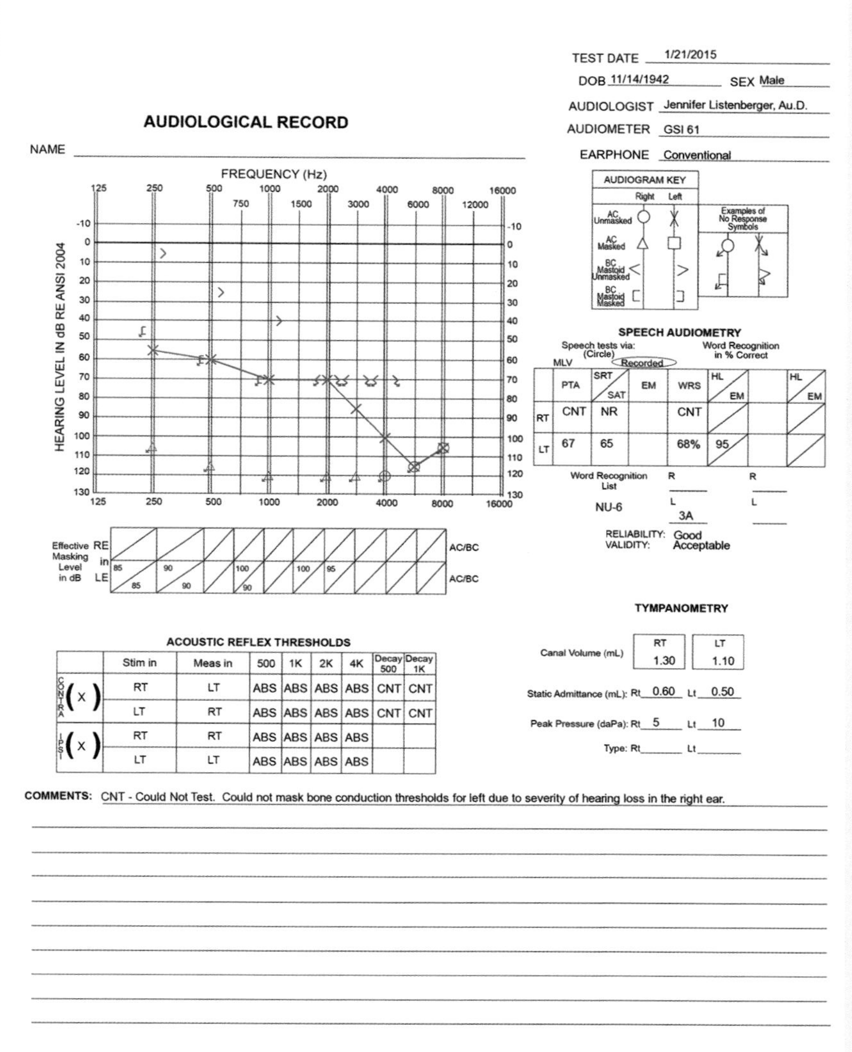

AUDIOLOGICAL RECORD

NAME ____

TEST DATE 1/21/2015
DOB 11/14/1942 SEX Male
AUDIOLOGIST Jennifer Listenberger, Au.D.
AUDIOMETER GSI 61
EARPHONE Conventional

FREQUENCY (Hz): 125, 250, 500, 750, 1000, 1500, 2000, 3000, 4000, 6000, 8000, 12000, 16000

HEARING LEVEL IN dB RE ANSI 2004: -10, 0, 10, 20, 30, 40, 50, 60, 70, 80, 90, 100, 110, 120, 130

AUDIOGRAM KEY: Right, Left; AC Unmasked; AC Masked; BC Mastoid Unmasked; BC Mastoid Masked; Examples of No Response Symbols

Effective Masking Level in dB: RE; LE — 85, 85, 90, 90, 100, 90, 100, 95 — AC/BC

SPEECH AUDIOMETRY

Speech tests via: (Circle) MLV Recorded

Word Recognition in % Correct

	PTA	SRT / SAT	EM	WRS	HL / EM		HL / EM
RT	CNT	NR		CNT			
LT	67	65		68%	95		

Word Recognition List: NU-6; R ____; L 3A

RELIABILITY: Good
VALIDITY: Acceptable

TYMPANOMETRY

	RT	LT
Canal Volume (mL)	1.30	1.10

Static Admittance (mL): Rt 0.60 Lt 0.50
Peak Pressure (daPa): Rt 5 Lt 10
Type: Rt ____ Lt ____

ACOUSTIC REFLEX THRESHOLDS

	Stim in	Meas in	500	1K	2K	4K	Decay 500	Decay 1K
CONTRA (x)	RT	LT	ABS	ABS	ABS	ABS	CNT	CNT
	LT	RT	ABS	ABS	ABS	ABS	CNT	CNT
IPSI (x)	RT	RT	ABS	ABS	ABS	ABS		
	LT	LT	ABS	ABS	ABS	ABS		

COMMENTS: CNT - Could Not Test. Could not mask bone conduction thresholds for left due to severity of hearing loss in the right ear.

Fig. 7.3 Audiogram showing a sudden hearing loss in the right ear and a gradual hearing loss in the left ear.

7.3.2 Interpretation

Right ear—Pure-tone air and bone conduction thresholds revealed a profound sensorineural hearing loss with no measurable response for pure-tone air or bone conduction thresholds within the limits of the audiometer. The SRT and SAT revealed no measurable response within the limits of the audiometer. WRS testing could not be completed due to the severity of the hearing thresholds. Immittance testing revealed a normal tympanogram and absent acoustic reflex thresholds from 500 to 4,000 Hz for ipsilateral and contralateral stimulation. Acoustic reflex decay could not be measured.

Left ear—Pure-tone air and bone conduction thresholds revealed a moderate sloping to moderately severe mixed hearing loss at 500 to 2,000 Hz, sloping to severe at 3,000 Hz, and sloping to profound at 4,000 to 8,000 Hz. The SRT revealed a moderately severe loss in the ability to receive speech and was in agreement with the PTA. The WRS revealed a moderate difficulty in the ability to recognize speech. Immittance testing revealed a normal tympanogram and absent acoustic reflex thresholds from 500 to 4,000 Hz for ipsilateral and contralateral stimulation. Acoustic reflex decay could not be measured.

7.3.3 Intervention

The otologic consultation concluded that there was possible otosclerosis for the left ear, but surgical intervention was not recommended and the patient was medically cleared for new amplification. The audiological recommendations were to complete an annual hearing test to monitor progression of hearing loss and to return for an evaluation for new hearing aid technology options, including left BICROS and HAT.

7.4 Case 4

7.4.1 Case History

A 29-year-old female stated that she had a cholesteatoma removed from her left ear many years ago. Reportedly, her ear continued to have otorrhea after this was removed, and it was determined that the cholesteatoma had caused a cerebrospinal fluid leak. This was repaired as well and, since that time, she has had hearing difficulties in her left ear. She recently began to note that her hearing in the left ear began to decrease further. She expressed concerns that the cholesteatoma may have returned. She reported some current drainage in her left ear along with some pain and tinnitus. She believed that she heard well in her right ear.

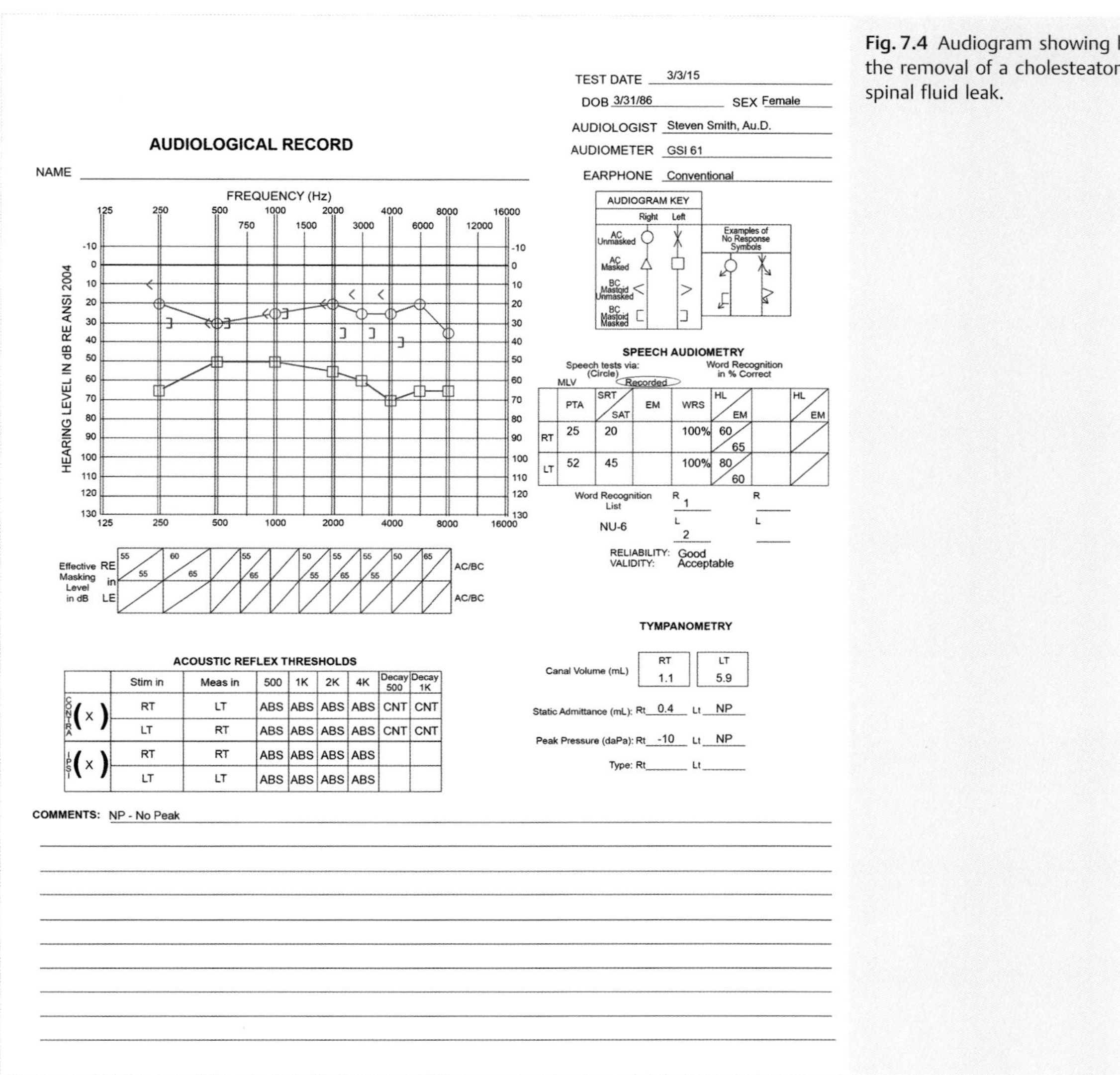

AUDIOLOGICAL RECORD

NAME

TEST DATE 3/3/15
DOB 3/31/86 SEX Female
AUDIOLOGIST Steven Smith, Au.D.
AUDIOMETER GSI 61
EARPHONE Conventional

SPEECH AUDIOMETRY

Speech tests via: MLV (Circle) Recorded
Word Recognition in % Correct

	PTA	SRT / SAT	EM	WRS	HL / EM		HL / EM
RT	25	20		100%	60 / 65		
LT	52	45		100%	80 / 60		

Word Recognition List: R 1, L 2
NU-6

RELIABILITY: Good
VALIDITY: Acceptable

Effective Masking Level in dB RE (AC/BC): 55, 55, 60, 65, 55, 65, 50, 55, 55, 65, 55, 55, 50, 65

TYMPANOMETRY

	RT	LT
Canal Volume (mL)	1.1	5.9

Static Admittance (mL): Rt 0.4 Lt NP
Peak Pressure (daPa): Rt -10 Lt NP
Type: Rt ____ Lt ____

ACOUSTIC REFLEX THRESHOLDS

	Stim in	Meas in	500	1K	2K	4K	Decay 500	Decay 1K
CONTRA	RT	LT	ABS	ABS	ABS	ABS	CNT	CNT
CONTRA	LT	RT	ABS	ABS	ABS	ABS	CNT	CNT
IPSI	RT	RT	ABS	ABS	ABS	ABS		
IPSI	LT	LT	ABS	ABS	ABS	ABS		

COMMENTS: NP - No Peak

Fig. 7.4 Audiogram showing hearing loss after the removal of a cholesteatoma and a cerebrospinal fluid leak.

7.4.2 Interpretation

Right ear—Flat slight to mild sensorineural hearing loss from 250 through 8,000 Hz. The SRT revealed a slight loss in the ability to receive speech and was in agreement with the PTA. The WRS was normal. Immittance testing revealed a normal tympanogram. The acoustic reflex thresholds with ipsilateral and contralateral stimulation were absent from 500 to 4,000 Hz. Acoustic reflex decay could not be measured.

Left ear—Moderately severe rising to moderate mixed hearing loss at 250 through 2,000 Hz, sloping to moderately severe at 3,000 to 8,000 Hz. The SRT revealed a moderate loss in the ability to receive speech and was in agreement with the PTA. The WRS was normal. Immittance testing revealed a flat tympanogram with a large ear canal volume. The acoustic reflex thresholds with ipsilateral and contralateral stimulation from 500 to 4,000 Hz were absent. Acoustic reflex decay could not be measured.

7.4.3 Intervention

The patient followed up with an ENT physician, and an MRI was ordered to determine the presence of a cholesteatoma or to determine the possibility of a new cerebrospinal fluid leak.

7.5 Case 5

7.5.1 Case History

The patient reported bilateral progressive hearing loss for the last 25 years, with the right ear being poorer than the left ear. He had intermittent bilateral ringing tinnitus and a "motor noise" in the left ear along with a constant hum. The patient also had intermittent bilateral ringing tinnitus. He had intermittent bilateral otalgia and a sensation of pressure. Loud, sudden, high-frequency sounds were bothersome and at times painful to his ears. Such sounds included a cup hitting a table, a soda can opening, or someone sneezing. The sensitivity had increased over the last 2 years. He attributed this to having had a shotgun fired near his ears about 2 years ago without hearing protection. His left ear was more sensitive, and he usually wore an earplug, rather than his hearing aid, in the left ear. He often turned the right hearing aid off in anticipation of loud sounds. He had severe episodes of dizziness 10 years ago, but now he only occasionally experienced dizziness when he bent over. He had a history of ear infections over the past 7 years and had several sets of pressure equalization tubes. He had a family history of hearing loss because his father had hearing loss, likely due to noise exposure. He had a history of occupational noise exposure from working as a carpenter for over 30 years. He had worn binaural BTE hearing aids for about 15 years. He did not report other otologic symptoms or history.

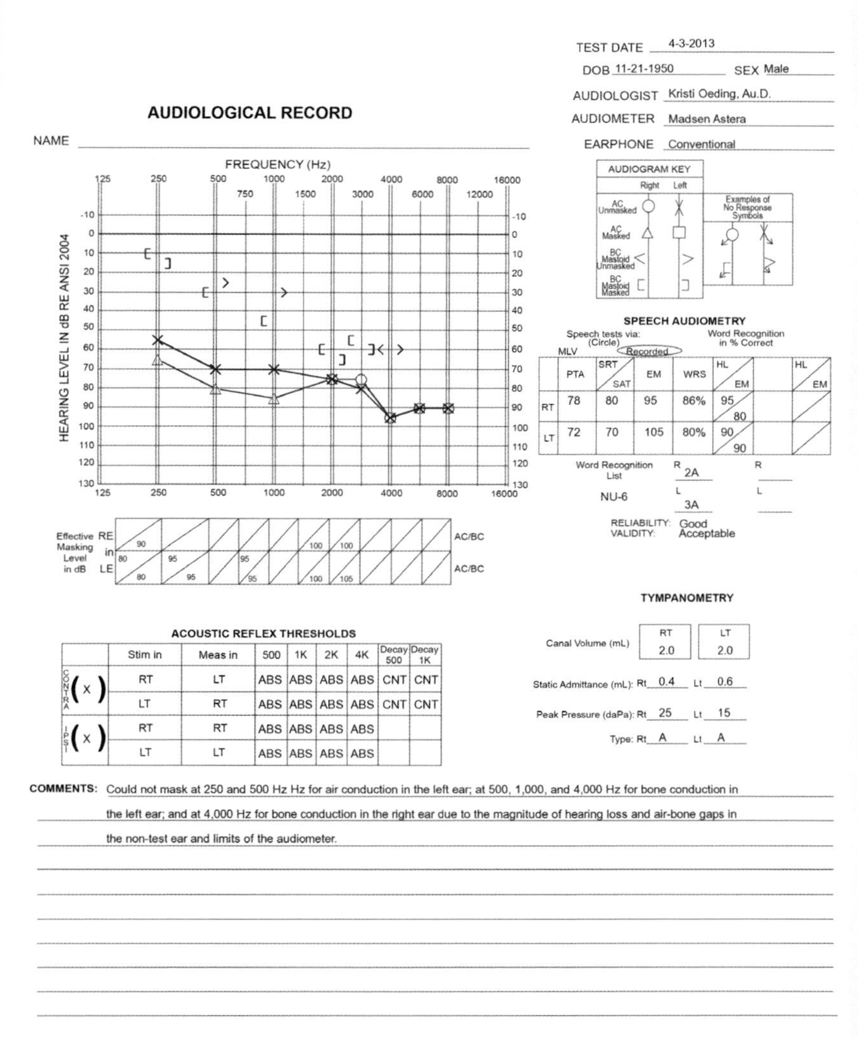

AUDIOLOGICAL RECORD

NAME

TEST DATE 4-3-2013

DOB 11-21-1950 SEX Male

AUDIOLOGIST Kristi Oeding, Au.D.

AUDIOMETER Madsen Astera

EARPHONE Conventional

SPEECH AUDIOMETRY

Speech tests via: (Circle) MLV Recorded

Word Recognition in % Correct

	PTA	SRT / SAT	EM	WRS	HL / EM	HL / EM
RT	78	80	95	86%	95 / 80	
LT	72	70	105	80%	90 / 90	

Word Recognition List NU-6: R 2A, L 3A

RELIABILITY: Good

VALIDITY: Acceptable

TYMPANOMETRY

	RT	LT
Canal Volume (mL)	2.0	2.0

Static Admittance (mL): Rt 0.4 Lt 0.6

Peak Pressure (daPa): Rt 25 Lt 15

Type: Rt A Lt A

Effective Masking Level in dB (AC/BC): RE 90, 80, 95, 95, 100, 100; LE 80, 95, 95, 100, 105

ACOUSTIC REFLEX THRESHOLDS

	Stim in	Meas in	500	1K	2K	4K	Decay 500	Decay 1K
CONTRA	RT	LT	ABS	ABS	ABS	ABS	CNT	CNT
	LT	RT	ABS	ABS	ABS	ABS	CNT	CNT
IPSI	RT	RT	ABS	ABS	ABS	ABS		
	LT	LT	ABS	ABS	ABS	ABS		

COMMENTS: Could not mask at 250 and 500 Hz Hz for air conduction in the left ear; at 500, 1,000, and 4,000 Hz for bone conduction in the left ear; and at 4,000 Hz for bone conduction in the right ear due to the magnitude of hearing loss and air-bone gaps in the non-test ear and limits of the audiometer.

Fig. 7.5 Audiogram of a patient with gradual hearing loss over years with increasing tinnitus and hyperacusis/recruitment.

7.5.2 Interpretation

Right ear—Pure-tone thresholds revealed a moderately severe to severe mixed hearing loss from 250 to 3,000 Hz, sloping to a profound mixed hearing loss at 4,000 Hz, and rising to a severe hearing loss from 6,000 to 8,000 Hz. The SRT revealed a severe loss in the ability to receive speech and was in agreement with the PTA. The WRS revealed a slight difficulty in the ability to recognize speech. Immittance testing revealed a normal tympanogram, and the ipsilateral and contralateral acoustic reflex thresholds were absent from 500 to 4,000 Hz. Acoustic reflex decay could not be measured.

Left ear—Pure-tone thresholds revealed a moderate to moderately severe mixed hearing loss from 250 to 1,000 Hz, sloping to a severe to profound mixed hearing loss from 2,000 to 4,000 Hz, and rising to a severe hearing loss from 6,000 to 8,000 Hz. The SRT revealed a moderately severe loss in the ability to receive speech and was in agreement with the PTA. The WRS revealed a slight difficulty in the ability to recognize speech. Immittance testing revealed a normal tympanogram, and the ipsilateral and contralateral acoustic reflex thresholds were absent from 500 to 4,000 Hz.

7.5.3 Intervention

The otologist diagnosed the patient with left external otitis and attributed the hearing loss to noise exposure and otosclerosis of the oval window and labyrinth. The otologist ordered a CT scan and prescribed Ciprodex ear drops (Alcon) for the external otitis. The patient was also diagnosed with hyperacusis, although it may also have been recruitment due to the degree of hearing loss. The CT scan confirmed otosclerosis bilaterally. The audiological recommendations included a hyperacusis evaluation, hearing aid evaluation, and HAT evaluation, and use of hearing protection in noise. The patient was fit with new hearing aids with an algorithm that suppressed impulse sounds, and he did well with the hearing aids.

7.6 Case 6

7.6.1 Case History

The patient had a long-standing history of hearing loss bilaterally and used amplification. The last audiometric examination from 3 years ago revealed a primarily sensorineural hearing loss with mixed thresholds present at 250 to 1,000 Hz, with air–bone gaps of 10 to 15 dB HL. The patient had noticed a significant increase in difficulty with hearing soft speech in his work environment, even with the use of amplification. There was some familial history of hearing loss in that two of the patient's five siblings had hearing loss. There was no reported history of ear pathology, otosurgery, or noise exposure. The patient denied any tinnitus or dizziness.

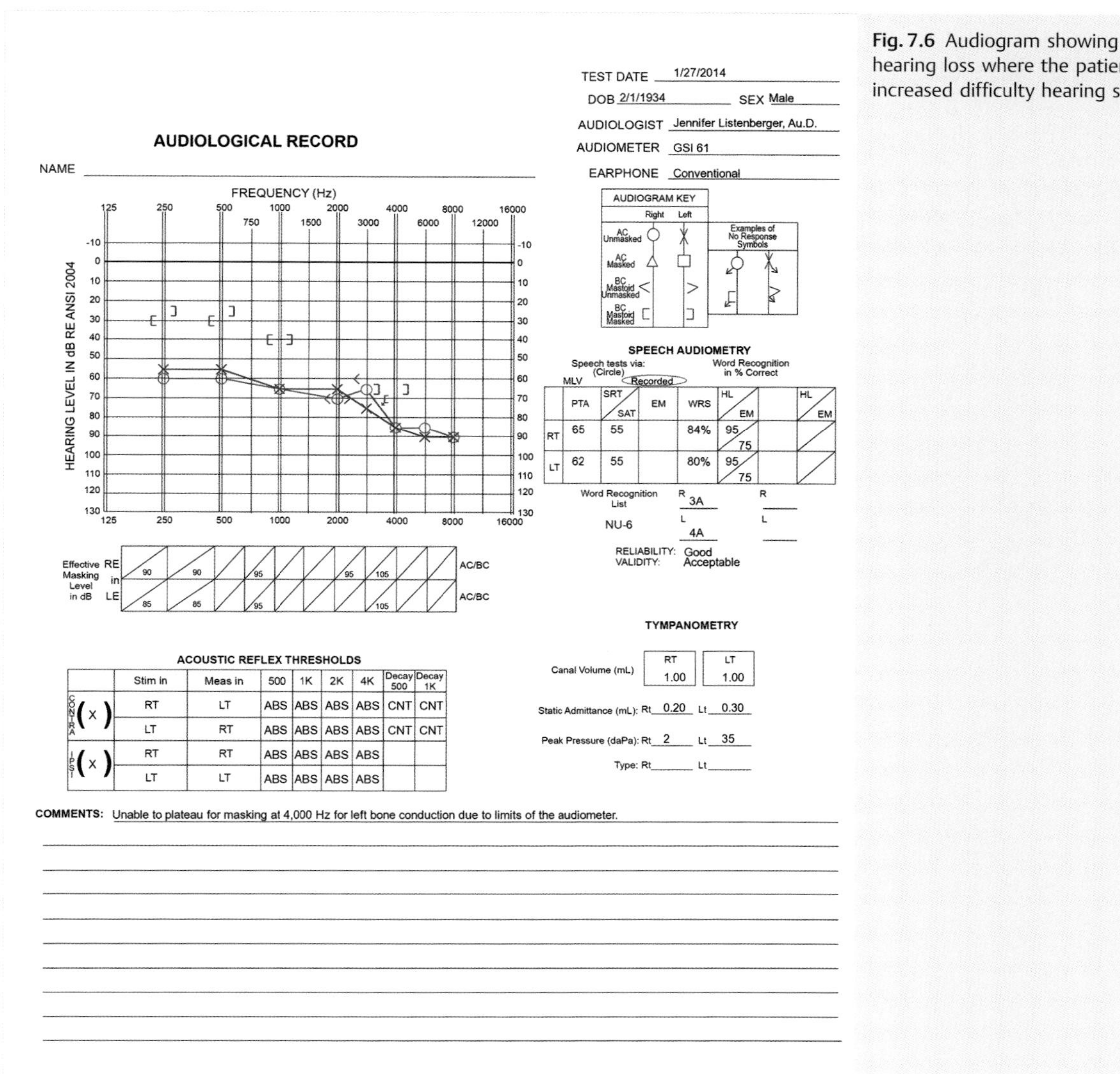

AUDIOLOGICAL RECORD

NAME

TEST DATE 1/27/2014
DOB 2/1/1934 SEX Male
AUDIOLOGIST Jennifer Listenberger, Au.D.
AUDIOMETER GSI 61
EARPHONE Conventional

Effective Masking Level in dB
RE: 90 90 95 95 105 AC/BC
LE: 85 85 95 105 AC/BC

SPEECH AUDIOMETRY

Speech tests via: (Circle) MLV Recorded
Word Recognition in % Correct

	PTA	SRT/SAT	EM	WRS	HL/EM		HL/EM
RT	65	55		84%	95/75		
LT	62	55		80%	95/75		

Word Recognition List NU-6: R 3A, L 4A

RELIABILITY: Good
VALIDITY: Acceptable

ACOUSTIC REFLEX THRESHOLDS

	Stim in	Meas in	500	1K	2K	4K	Decay 500	Decay 1K
CONTRA (X)	RT	LT	ABS	ABS	ABS	ABS	CNT	CNT
	LT	RT	ABS	ABS	ABS	ABS	CNT	CNT
IPSI (X)	RT	RT	ABS	ABS	ABS	ABS		
	LT	LT	ABS	ABS	ABS	ABS		

TYMPANOMETRY

	RT	LT
Canal Volume (mL)	1.00	1.00

Static Admittance (mL): Rt 0.20 Lt 0.30
Peak Pressure (daPa): Rt 2 Lt 35
Type: Rt____ Lt____

COMMENTS: Unable to plateau for masking at 4,000 Hz for left bone conduction due to limits of the audiometer.

Fig. 7.6 Audiogram showing a long-standing hearing loss where the patient had noticed increased difficulty hearing softer sounds.

7.6.2 Interpretation

Right ear—Pure-tone air and bone conduction thresholds revealed a moderately severe hearing loss at 250 to 3,000 Hz and sloping to severe at 4,000 to 8,000 Hz, with a mixed hearing loss at 250 to 1,000 Hz with air–bone gaps of 25 to 30 dB HL and a sensorineural hearing loss at 2,000 to 4,000 Hz. The SRT revealed a moderate loss in the ability to receive speech and was in agreement with the PTA. The WRS revealed a slight difficulty in the ability to recognize speech. Immittance testing revealed a hypocompliant tympanogram and absent acoustic reflex thresholds from 500 to 4,000 Hz to ipsilateral and contralateral stimulation. Acoustic reflex decay could not be measured.

Left ear—Pure-tone air and bone conduction thresholds revealed moderate gradually sloping to moderately severe hearing loss at 250 to 2,000 Hz and sloping to severe at 3,000 to 8,000 Hz, with a mixed hearing loss at 250 to 1,000 and 4,000 Hz with air–bone gaps of 20 to 30 dB HL and a sensorineural hearing loss at 2,000 to 3,000 Hz. The SRT revealed a moderate loss in the ability to receive speech and was in agreement with the PTA. The WRS revealed a slight difficulty in the ability to recognize speech. Immittance testing revealed a normal tympanogram and absent acoustic reflex thresholds from 500 to 4,000 Hz to ipsilateral and contralateral stimulation. Acoustic reflex decay could not be measured.

7.6.3 Intervention

The patient was referred to an ENT specialist due to progression of the conductive hearing loss. Per the ENT specialist's report, the patient was diagnosed with bilateral otosclerosis, and surgical options were discussed. The patient was not interested in surgery at that time. The audiological recommendations were to continue use of amplification, follow up for an evaluation for new technology and style of hearing aids, complete an evaluation for HAT, follow up annually for hearing testing to monitor progression of the hearing loss, and to follow up with an ENT specialist as recommended.

7.7 Case 7

7.7.1 Case History

The patient was a 74-year-old male who had cancer in his neck on the right side. He had surgery to remove the tumor and received radiation therapy to the right side of his head and neck. He reported that his hearing declined bilaterally since treatment, with the right ear having poorer hearing than the left ear. He reported a perforated tympanic membrane in the right ear that may be due to ear infections and the after-effects of radiation. He reported intermittent drainage from the right ear. He stated that he has trouble hearing in most situations, especially in noise. He denied any otalgia. The patient expressed interest in hearing aids to help him improve his hearing.

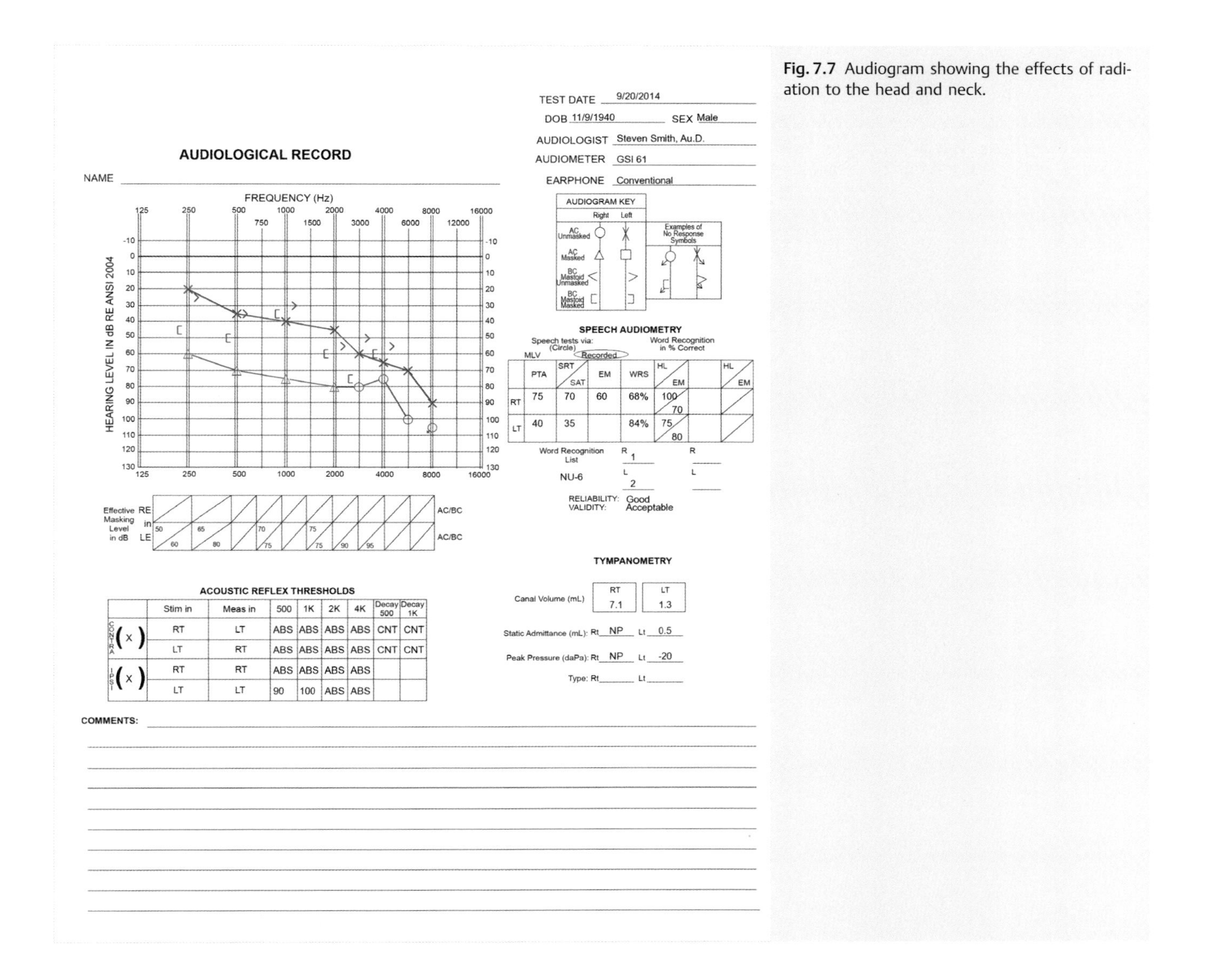

AUDIOLOGICAL RECORD

NAME

TEST DATE 9/20/2014

DOB 11/9/1940 SEX Male

AUDIOLOGIST Steven Smith, Au.D.

AUDIOMETER GSI 61

EARPHONE Conventional

Effective Masking Level in dB

RE in										AC/BC
LE	50 / 60	65 / 80	70 / 75	75 / 75	90	95				AC/BC

SPEECH AUDIOMETRY

Speech tests via: (Circle) MLV Recorded

Word Recognition in % Correct

	PTA	SRT / SAT	EM	WRS	HL / EM	HL / EM
RT	75	70	60	68%	100 / 70	
LT	40	35		84%	75 / 80	

Word Recognition List: R 1, L 2; R ___, L ___

NU-6

RELIABILITY: Good

VALIDITY: Acceptable

ACOUSTIC REFLEX THRESHOLDS

	Stim in	Meas in	500	1K	2K	4K	Decay 500	Decay 1K
CONTRA (x)	RT	LT	ABS	ABS	ABS	ABS	CNT	CNT
	LT	RT	ABS	ABS	ABS	ABS	CNT	CNT
IPSI (x)	RT	RT	ABS	ABS	ABS	ABS		
	LT	LT	90	100	ABS	ABS		

TYMPANOMETRY

	RT	LT
Canal Volume (mL)	7.1	1.3

Static Admittance (mL): Rt NP Lt 0.5

Peak Pressure (daPa): Rt NP Lt -20

Type: Rt ___ Lt ___

COMMENTS:

Fig. 7.7 Audiogram showing the effects of radiation to the head and neck.

7.7.2 Interpretation

Right ear—Moderately severe sloping to a severe mixed hearing loss at 250 to 4,000 Hz, sloping to profound with no measurable response within the limits of the audiometer at 8,000 Hz. The SRT revealed a moderately severe loss in the ability to receive speech and was in agreement with the PTA. The WRS revealed moderate difficulty in the ability to recognize speech. Immittance testing revealed a flat tympanogram with a large ear canal volume. The acoustic reflex thresholds with ipsilateral and contralateral stimulation from 500 to 4,000 Hz were absent. Acoustic reflex decay could not be measured.

Left ear—Slight sloping to moderate sensorineural hearing loss at 250 through 2,000 Hz, sloping to moderately severe to severe at 3,000 to 8,000 Hz. The SRT revealed mild difficulty in the ability to receive speech and was in agreement with the PTA. The WRS revealed a slight difficulty in the ability to recognize speech. Immittance testing revealed a normal tympanogram. The acoustic reflex thresholds with ipsilateral stimulation from 500 to 2,000 Hz were within normal limits and were absent from 2,000 to 4,000 Hz. Contralateral stimulation revealed absent acoustic reflex thresholds from 500 to 4,000 Hz. Acoustic reflex decay could not be measured.

7.7.3 Intervention

The patient was referred to an ENT specialist for treatment of the recurring ear infection in the right ear and the perforated tympanic membrane. A hearing test after treatment was recommended along with a hearing aid evaluation pending medical clearance.

7.8 Case 8

7.8.1 Case History

The patient reported decreased hearing in the left ear since her last hearing test about 1 year ago. She had a history of a sudden sensorineural hearing loss in the right ear that did not improve with intratympanic dexamethasone injections. She reported a history of chronic otitis media and eustachian tube dysfunction bilaterally. She had a history of bilateral PE tubes. She still had a tube in the left ear. She stated she had constant bilateral ringing tinnitus. She did not report other otologic symptoms or history.

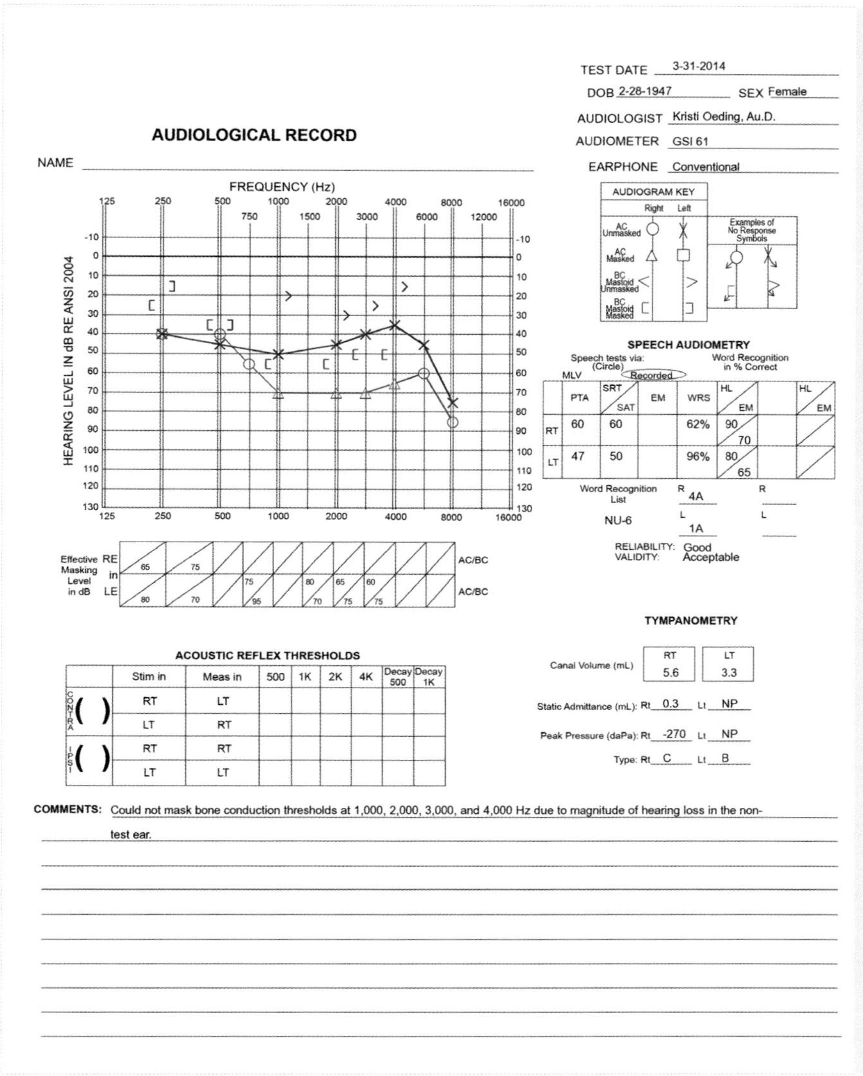

Fig. 7.8 Audiogram of a patient with a sudden sensorineural hearing loss in the right ear who also had bilateral otitis media.

7.8.2 Interpretation

Right ear—Pure-tone thresholds revealed a mild mixed hearing loss from 250 to 500 Hz, sloping to a moderate to moderately severe mixed hearing loss from 750 to 6,000 Hz, and sloping to a severe hearing loss at 8,000 Hz. The SRT revealed a moderately severe loss in the ability to receive speech and was in agreement with the PTA. The WRS revealed moderate difficulty in the ability to recognize speech. Immittance testing revealed excessive negative pressure and a large ear canal volume on the tympanogram. The ipsilateral and contralateral acoustic reflex thresholds and reflex decay were not measured at this appointment.

Left ear—Pure-tone thresholds revealed a mild to moderate mixed hearing loss from 250 to 2,000 Hz, rising to a mild mixed hearing loss from 3,000 to 4,000 Hz, and sloping to a moderate to severe hearing loss from 6,000 to 8,000 Hz. The SRT revealed a moderate loss in the ability to receive speech and was in agreement with the PTA. The WRS revealed a normal ability to recognize speech. Immittance testing revealed a flat tympanogram with a large ear canal volume. The ipsilateral and contralateral acoustic reflex thresholds and reflex decay were not measured at this appointment.

7.8.3 Intervention

The otologist noted that there was still a perforation in the left tympanic membrane from the previous PE tube placement. Bilateral eustachian tube dysfunction was noted. The otologist recommended keeping her ears dry and having a hearing aid evaluation. Other audiological recommendations included an annual hearing test, HAT, and hearing protection in noise.

7.9 Case 9

7.9.1 Case History

A 57-year-old female arrived with a reported history of bilateral otosclerosis. A stapedectomy and revision were completed for each ear, with the last surgery being completed on the left ear approximately 4 years ago. The patient's father had hearing loss but no reported history of otosurgery. There was no significant history of noise exposure. The last hearing test was completed 4 years ago after surgery for the left ear, but the hearing test results were not available for comparison. The patient reported a significant improvement in hearing bilaterally after the revision was completed. There were no significant communication difficulties reported at that time. The patient did report constant tinnitus in the right ear that was described as a steady buzzing and ringing. There was a report of dizziness that was described as being off balance with head movement.

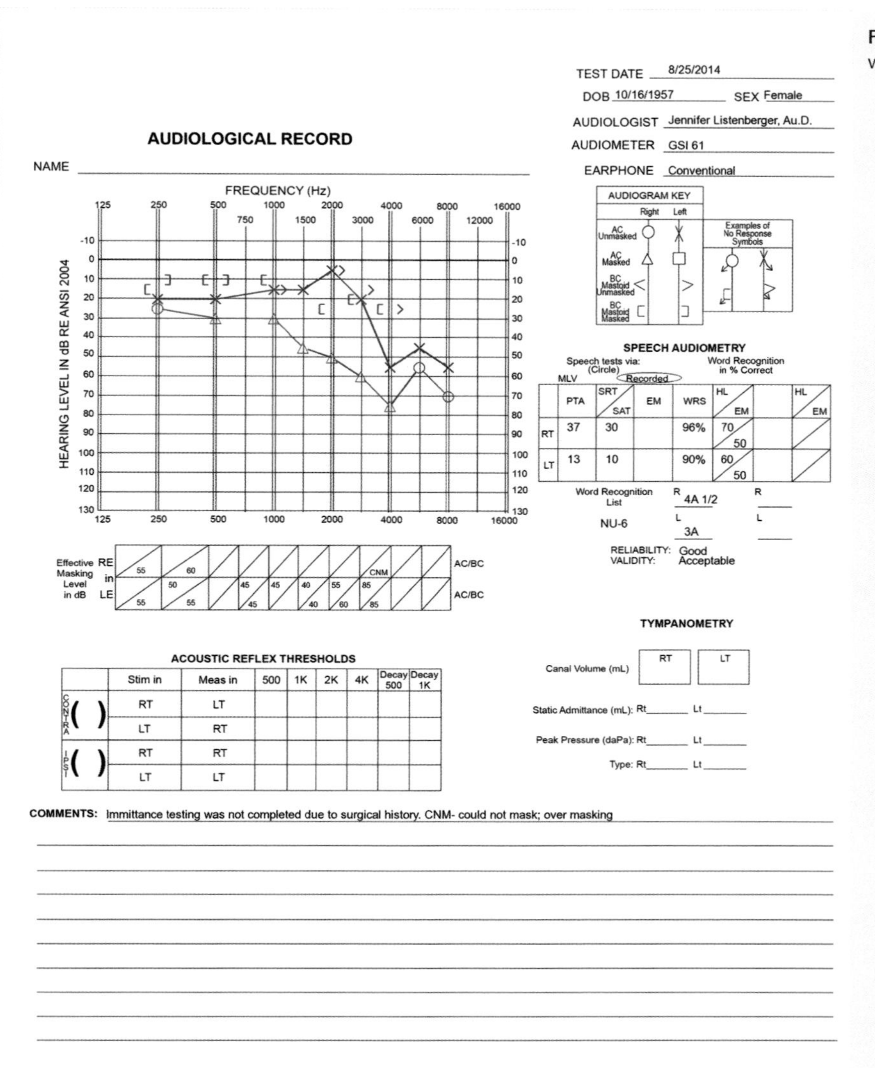

AUDIOLOGICAL RECORD

NAME

TEST DATE 8/25/2014

DOB 10/16/1957 SEX Female

AUDIOLOGIST Jennifer Listenberger, Au.D.

AUDIOMETER GSI 61

EARPHONE Conventional

SPEECH AUDIOMETRY

Speech tests via: (Circle) MLV Recorded

Word Recognition in % Correct

	PTA	SRT/SAT	EM	WRS	HL/EM		HL/EM
RT	37	30		96%	70/50		
LT	13	10		90%	60/50		

Word Recognition List NU-6: R 4A 1/2; L 3A

RELIABILITY: Good

VALIDITY: Acceptable

TYMPANOMETRY

Canal Volume (mL): RT LT

Static Admittance (mL): Rt____ Lt____

Peak Pressure (daPa): Rt____ Lt____

Type: Rt____ Lt____

ACOUSTIC REFLEX THRESHOLDS

	Stim in	Meas in	500	1K	2K	4K	Decay 500	Decay 1K
CONTRA ( )	RT	LT						
	LT	RT						
IPSI ( )	RT	RT						
	LT	LT						

COMMENTS: Immittance testing was not completed due to surgical history. CNM- could not mask; over masking

Fig. 7.9 Audiogram of a patient with otosclerosis who had a stapedectomy bilaterally.

7.9.2 Interpretation

Right ear—Pure-tone air and bone conduction thresholds revealed a slight sloping to mild mixed hearing loss at 250 to 1,000 Hz, sloping to moderate to severe at 2,000 to 4,000 Hz, and rising to moderate sloping to moderately severe at 6,000 and 8,000 Hz, respectively. The SRT revealed a mild loss in the ability to receive speech and was in agreement with the PTA. The WRS revealed a normal ability to recognize speech. Immittance testing was not measured due to a history of otosurgery.

Left ear—Pure-tone air and bone conduction thresholds revealed a slight sensorineural hearing loss at 250 to 500 Hz, rising to normal hearing sensitivity at 1,000 to 2,000 Hz, sloping to slight at 3,000 Hz, and steeply sloping to a moderate mixed hearing loss at 4,000 to 8,000 Hz. The SRT revealed a normal ability to receive speech and was in agreement with the PTA. The WRS revealed a normal ability to recognize speech. Immittance testing was not measured due to a history of otosurgery.

7.9.3 Intervention

The patient's primary reason for the visit was dizziness and not hearing loss. An ENT evaluation revealed symptoms that were consistent with left BPPV. The patient continued follow-up with an ENT specialist as recommended. Annual testing to monitor hearing stability was recommended, and to follow up with an audiologist when she became interested in amplification.

7.10 Case 10

7.10.1 Case History

A 61-year-old male entered the clinic for a hearing evaluation. He stated that he had a mass growing in his right ear canal. He reported intermittent bloody discharge from that ear. He stated that he had these symptoms for over a year and, due to a lack of insurance, could not seek help until now. He reported his hearing had decreased in the right ear over the last year. He reported extreme difficulty hearing and pain in the right ear. He noted that he heard well from the left ear.

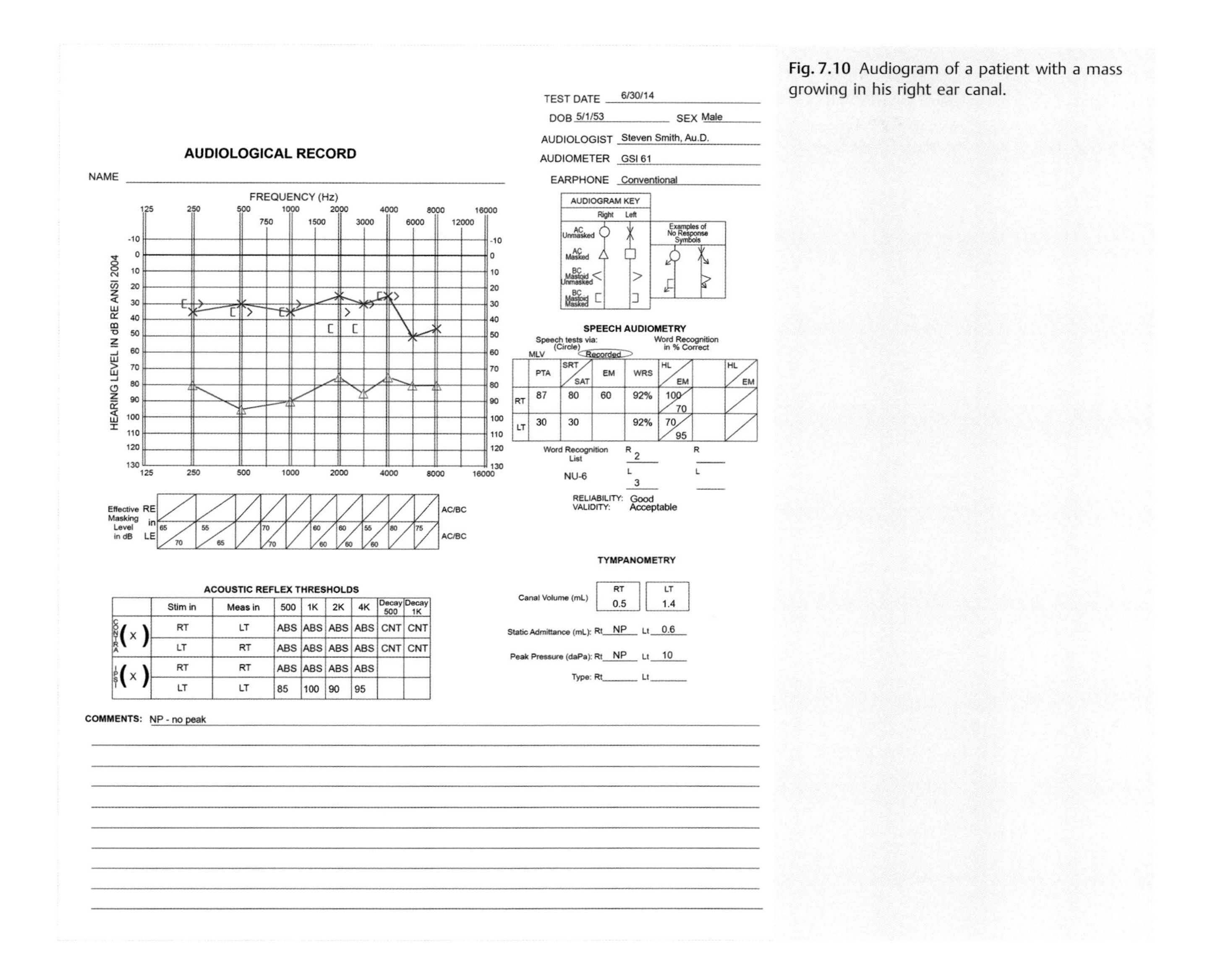

AUDIOLOGICAL RECORD

NAME

TEST DATE 6/30/14
DOB 5/1/53 SEX Male
AUDIOLOGIST Steven Smith, Au.D.
AUDIOMETER GSI 61
EARPHONE Conventional

Effective Masking Level in dB

	250	500	1000	2000	3000	4000	6000	8000	
RE in									AC/BC
LE	65 / 70	55 / 65	70 / 70	60 / 60	60 / 60	55 / 60	80	75	AC/BC

SPEECH AUDIOMETRY

Speech tests via: (Circle) MLV Recorded

Word Recognition in % Correct

	PTA	SRT/SAT	EM	WRS	HL/EM	HL/EM
RT	87	80	60	92%	100/70	
LT	30	30		92%	70/95	

Word Recognition List: NU-6 R 2 L 3 R ___ L ___

RELIABILITY: Good
VALIDITY: Acceptable

ACOUSTIC REFLEX THRESHOLDS

	Stim in	Meas in	500	1K	2K	4K	Decay 500	Decay 1K
CONTRA	RT	LT	ABS	ABS	ABS	ABS	CNT	CNT
	LT	RT	ABS	ABS	ABS	ABS	CNT	CNT
IPSI	RT	RT	ABS	ABS	ABS	ABS		
	LT	LT	85	100	90	95		

TYMPANOMETRY

	RT	LT
Canal Volume (mL)	0.5	1.4

Static Admittance (mL): Rt NP Lt 0.6
Peak Pressure (daPa): Rt NP Lt 10
Type: Rt ___ Lt ___

COMMENTS: NP - no peak

Fig. 7.10 Audiogram of a patient with a mass growing in his right ear canal.

7.10.2 Interpretation

Right ear—Severe mixed hearing loss at 250 through 8,000 Hz with a profound mixed hearing loss notch at 500 and 1,000 Hz. The SRT revealed a severe loss in the ability to receive speech and was in agreement with the PTA. The WRS was normal. Immittance testing revealed a flat tympanogram with a small ear canal volume. The acoustic reflex thresholds with ipsilateral and contralateral stimulation from 500 to 4,000 Hz were absent. Acoustic reflex decay could not be measured.

Left ear—Mild rising to slight sensorineural hearing loss from 250 to 4,000 Hz, sloping to a moderate sensorineural hearing loss from 6,000 to 8,000 Hz. The SRT revealed a mild loss in the ability to receive speech and was in agreement with the PTA. The WRS was normal. Immittance testing revealed a normal tympanogram. The acoustic reflex thresholds with ipsilateral stimulation from 500 to 4,000 Hz were within normal limits, and acoustic reflex thresholds were absent with contralateral stimulation from 500 to 4,000 Hz. Acoustic reflex decay could not be measured.

7.10.3 Intervention

The patient was referred to an ENT specialist for follow-up on the external ear mass. It was determined to be an external ear lesion and he was scheduled to have it surgically removed. The patient was recommended to follow up for a hearing evaluation to determine any improvement in hearing after surgery.

7.11 Case 11

7.11.1 Case History

The patient reported a sudden decrease of hearing in the left ear for the past several days. He was on a flight last week when he felt otalgia and a sensation of pressure in the left ear. At that time, he heard a loud pop in the left ear followed by decreased hearing and tinnitus. Prior to the airplane flight, he had an upper respiratory infection. His right ear had a pressure equalization tube for 1 to 2 months. He had intermittent ringing tinnitus in the right ear and constant ringing/roaring tinnitus in the left ear. He also occasionally had a sensation of feeling "whoozy." He did not report other otologic symptoms or history.

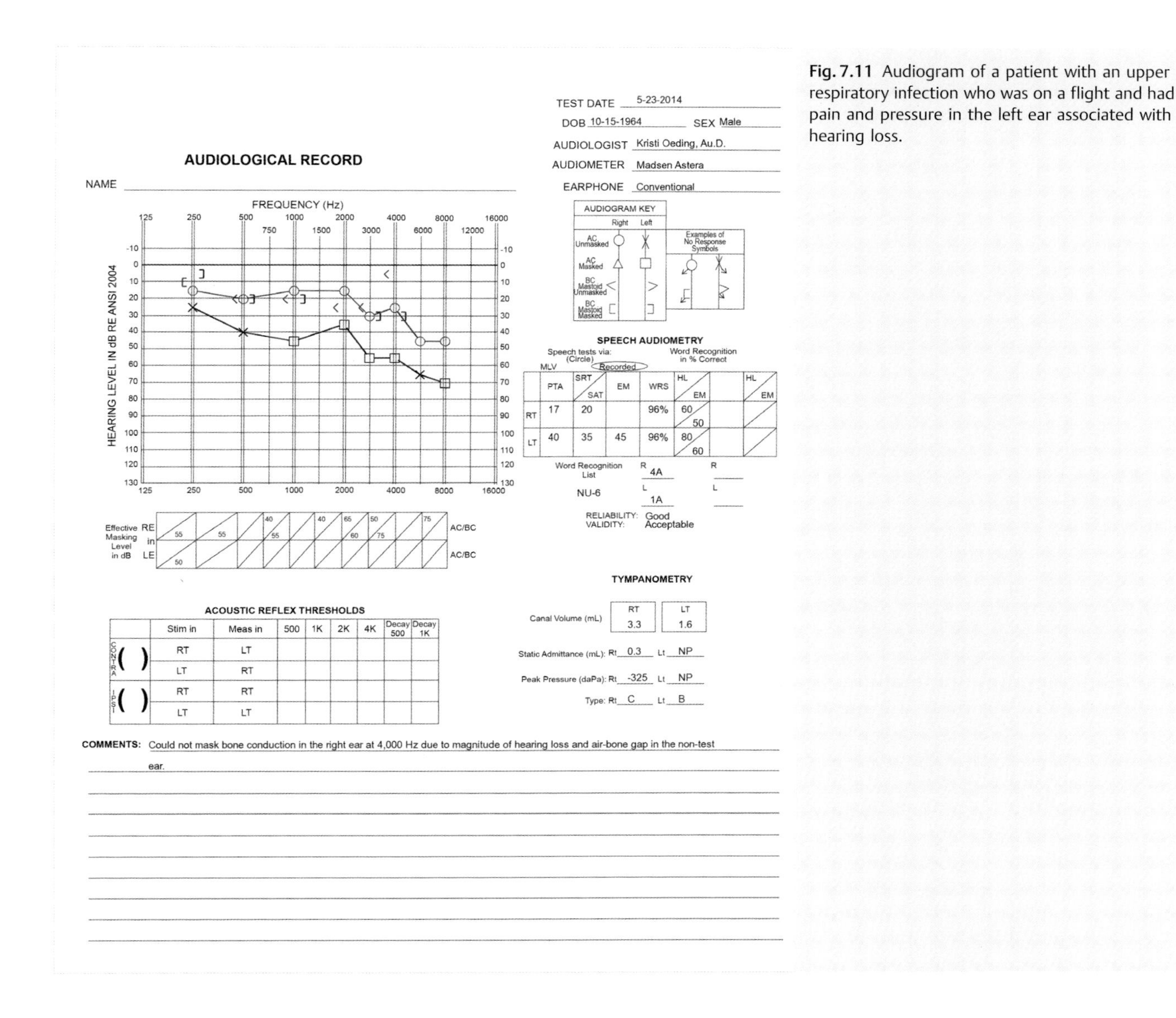

AUDIOLOGICAL RECORD

NAME

TEST DATE 5-23-2014

DOB 10-15-1964 SEX Male

AUDIOLOGIST Kristi Oeding, Au.D.

AUDIOMETER Madsen Astera

EARPHONE Conventional

SPEECH AUDIOMETRY

Speech tests via: (Circle) MLV Recorded (circled)

Word Recognition in % Correct

	PTA	SRT / SAT	EM	WRS	HL / EM		HL / EM
RT	17	20		96%	60 / 50		
LT	40	35	45	96%	80 / 60		

Word Recognition List NU-6: R 4A; L 1A

RELIABILITY: Good

VALIDITY: Acceptable

TYMPANOMETRY

	RT	LT
Canal Volume (mL)	3.3	1.6

Static Admittance (mL): Rt 0.3 Lt NP

Peak Pressure (daPa): Rt -325 Lt NP

Type: Rt C Lt B

ACOUSTIC REFLEX THRESHOLDS

		Stim in	Meas in	500	1K	2K	4K	Decay 500	Decay 1K
CONTRA	( )	RT	LT						
		LT	RT						
IPSI	( )	RT	RT						
		LT	LT						

COMMENTS: Could not mask bone conduction in the right ear at 4,000 Hz due to magnitude of hearing loss and air-bone gap in the non-test ear.

Fig. 7.11 Audiogram of a patient with an upper respiratory infection who was on a flight and had pain and pressure in the left ear associated with hearing loss.

7.11.2 Interpretation

Right ear—Pure-tone thresholds were within normal limits from 250 to 2,000 Hz, except for a slight sensorineural hearing loss at 500 Hz, sloping to a mild to slight possibly mixed hearing loss from 3,000 to 4,000 Hz, and sloping to a moderate hearing loss from 6,000 to 8,000 Hz. The SRT revealed a slight loss in the ability to receive speech and was in agreement with the PTA. The WRS revealed a normal ability to recognize speech. Immittance testing revealed excessive negative pressure and a large ear canal volume on the tympanogram. The ipsilateral and contralateral acoustic reflex thresholds and acoustic reflex decay were not measured at this appointment.

Left ear—Pure-tone thresholds were slight to moderate mixed hearing loss from 250 to 1,000 Hz, rising to a mild sensorineural hearing loss at 2,000 Hz, and sloping to a moderate to moderately severe mixed hearing loss from 3,000 to 8,000 Hz. The SRT revealed a mild loss in the ability to receive speech and was in agreement with the PTA. The WRS revealed a normal ability to recognize speech. Immittance testing revealed a flat tympanogram. The ipsilateral and contralateral acoustic reflex thresholds and acoustic reflex decay were not measured at this appointment.

7.11.3 Intervention

The otologist reported that the patient had serous otitis media in the left ear and eustachian tube dysfunction. He was prescribed Augmentin (GlaxoSmithKline) to help with his symptoms, and autoinsufflation was recommended to help resolve the effusion. If this did not help, a PE tube might be placed in the left ear.

7.12 Case 12

7.12.1 Case History

The patient had a history of bilateral otosclerosis. A left stapedectomy was completed over 10 years ago, and the patient reported difficulty with recovery, including dizziness for several days, a prolonged period of hyperacusis, and no significant improvement in hearing in the left ear. Per the ENT specialist's notes, the patient had a prolapsed left tympanic membrane, and it was touching the prosthesis. A right stapedectomy was completed approximately 5 years ago. The patient had used amplification in the right ear for many years, but perceived a significant improvement in hearing after surgery and now used amplification on the left side only. She no longer had hyperacusis. The last hearing test was completed approximately 3 years ago, and no significant changes had been reported. She denied tinnitus.

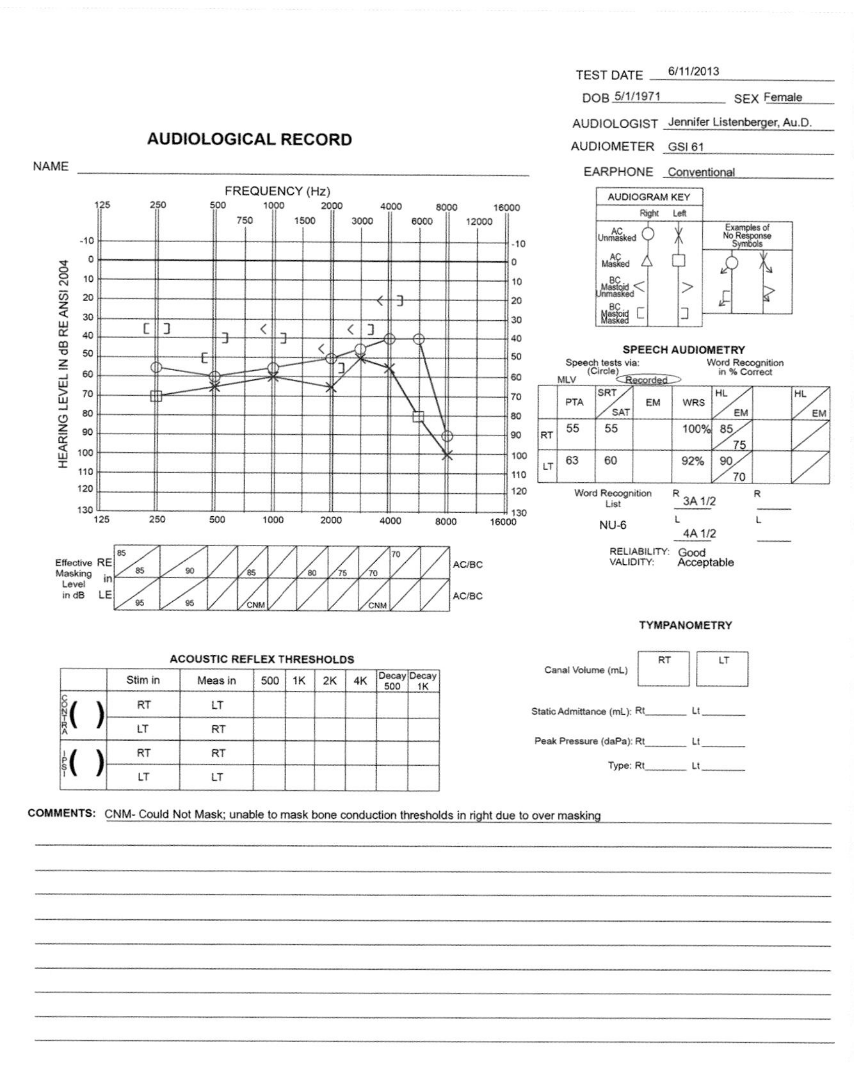

Fig. 7.12 Audiogram showing otosclerosis where stapedectomy surgery had been performed on each ear.

7.12.2 Interpretation

Right ear—Pure-tone air and bone conduction threshold testing revealed a moderate mixed hearing loss at 250 through 3,000 Hz, except for a moderately severe hearing loss at 500 Hz, rising to mild at 4,000 through 6,000 Hz, and steeply sloping to severe at 8,000 Hz. The SRT revealed a moderate loss in the ability to receive speech and was in agreement with the PTA. The WRS revealed a normal ability to recognize speech. Immittance testing was not measured due to a history of otosurgery.

Left ear—Pure-tone air and bone conduction threshold testing revealed a moderately severe mixed hearing loss at 250 through 2,000 Hz, rising to moderate at 3,000 and 4,000 Hz, and sloping to severe to profound at 6,000 and 8,000 Hz. The SRT revealed a moderately severe loss in the ability to receive speech and was in agreement with the PTA. The WRS revealed a normal ability to recognize speech. Immittance testing was not measured due to a history of otosurgery.

7.12.3 Intervention

It was recommended that the patient follow up with an otologist per the physician's recommendations. The audiological recommendations included follow-up with an audiologist for annual testing, a hearing aid evaluation for new technology and bilateral amplification, use of HAT, and hearing protection in noise.

7.13 Case 13

7.13.1 Case History

The patient was a 70-year-old female who stated that she had some hearing loss in the right ear that slowly progressed over years. She believed she heard well from the left ear. The patient reported tinnitus in the right ear. She denied aural pain, pressure, loud noise exposure, or a family history of hearing loss. She reported not being bothered by her hearing loss at this time.

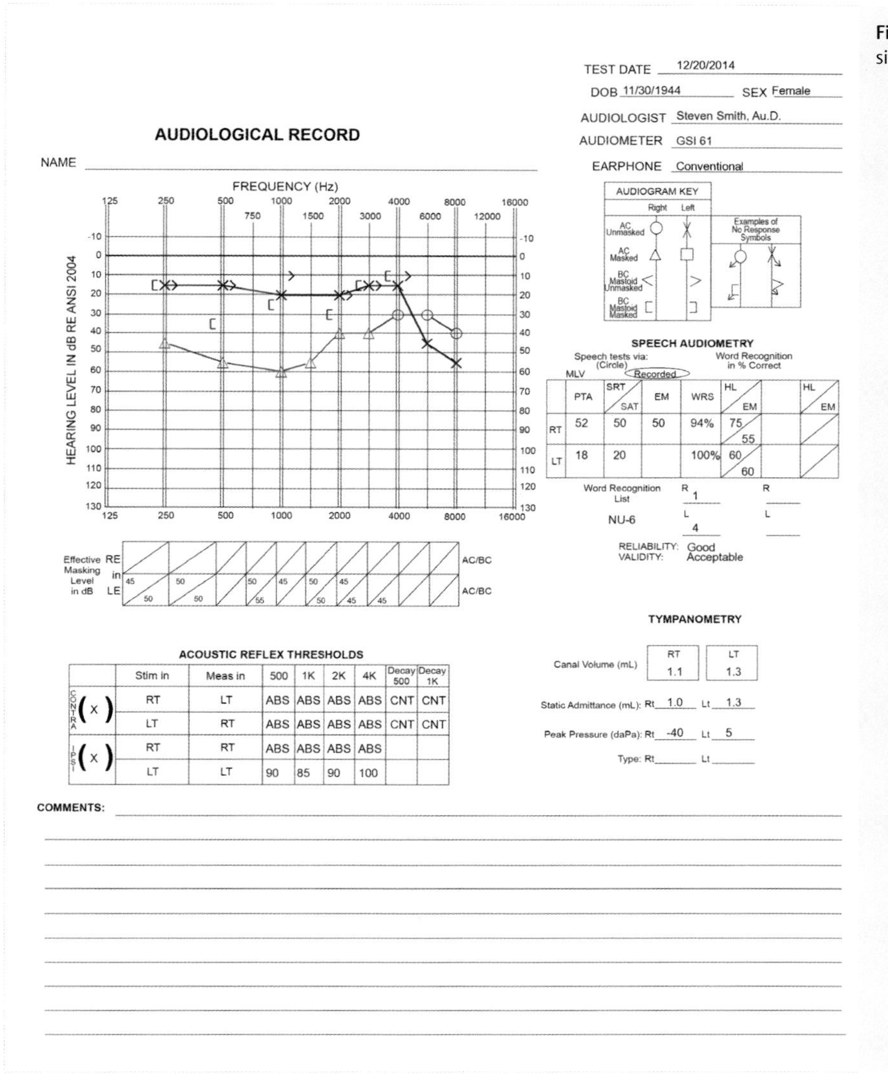

AUDIOLOGICAL RECORD

TEST DATE 12/20/2014
DOB 11/30/1944 SEX Female
AUDIOLOGIST Steven Smith, Au.D.
AUDIOMETER GSI 61
EARPHONE Conventional
NAME

Effective Masking Level in dB

	125	250	500	750	1000	1500	2000	3000	4000	6000	8000	
RE in												AC/BC
LE	45 / 50	50 / 50		50 / 55	45	50 / 50	45 / 45	45				AC/BC

SPEECH AUDIOMETRY

Speech tests via: (Circle) MLV Recorded (circled)

Word Recognition in % Correct

	PTA	SRT / SAT	EM	WRS	HL / EM		HL / EM
RT	52	50	50	94%	75 / 55		
LT	18	20		100%	60 / 60		

Word Recognition List NU-6 R 1 L 4 R ___ L ___

RELIABILITY: Good
VALIDITY: Acceptable

TYMPANOMETRY

	RT	LT
Canal Volume (mL)	1.1	1.3

Static Admittance (mL): Rt 1.0 Lt 1.3
Peak Pressure (daPa): Rt -40 Lt 5
Type: Rt ___ Lt ___

ACOUSTIC REFLEX THRESHOLDS

	Stim in	Meas in	500	1K	2K	4K	Decay 500	Decay 1K
CONTRA (X)	RT	LT	ABS	ABS	ABS	ABS	CNT	CNT
	LT	RT	ABS	ABS	ABS	ABS	CNT	CNT
IPSI (X)	RT	RT	ABS	ABS	ABS	ABS		
	LT	LT	90	85	90	100		

COMMENTS:

Fig. 7.13 Audiogram of a patient with progressive hearing loss in the right ear.

7.13.2 Interpretation

Right ear—Moderate to moderately severe mixed hearing loss from 250 to 1,500 Hz, rising to a mild hearing loss from 2,000 to 8,000 Hz. The SRT revealed a moderate loss in the ability to receive speech and was in agreement with the PTA. The WRS was normal. Immittance testing revealed a normal tympanogram. The acoustic reflex thresholds with ipsilateral and contralateral stimulation were absent from 500 to 4,000 Hz. Acoustic reflex decay could not be measured.

Left ear—Normal to slight sensorineural hearing loss from 250 to 4,000 Hz, sloping to a moderate hearing loss at 6,000 and 8,000 Hz. The SRT revealed a slight loss in the ability to receive speech and was in agreement with the PTA. The WRS was normal. Immittance testing revealed a normal tympanogram. The acoustic reflex thresholds with ipsilateral stimulation were normal at 500 to 4,000 Hz. The acoustic reflex thresholds with contralateral stimulation were absent at 500 to 4,000 Hz. Acoustic reflex decay could not be measured.

7.13.3 Intervention

The patient was referred to an ENT specialist due to the mixed hearing loss. It was determined that otosclerosis was causing the mixed hearing loss in the right ear. Surgery was recommended as well as amplification to help with her hearing loss. She declined both options because she feels, overall, she does well with her communication needs.

7.14 Case 14

7.14.1 Case History

The patient reported a long-standing history of a tympanic membrane perforation in the left ear. He reported that he had had chronic ear infections in the left ear since he was a child. He had occasional otalgia and a sensation of pressure in the left ear. He also reported hearing loss in the left ear. He had a tympanoplasty 3 years ago, but the procedure was not successful. He was here for a second opinion. He did not report other otologic symptoms or history.

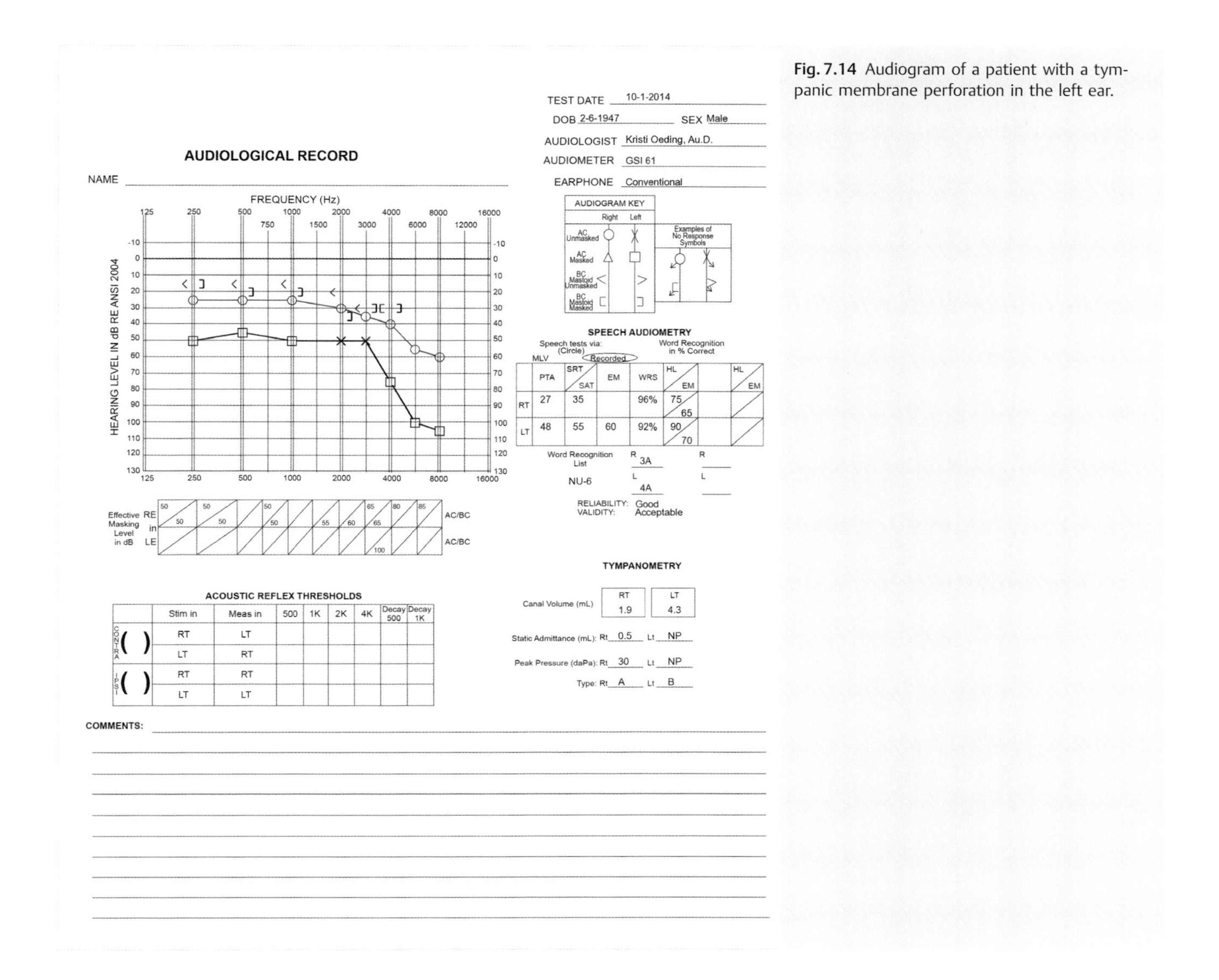

Fig. 7.14 Audiogram of a patient with a tympanic membrane perforation in the left ear.

7.14.2 Interpretation

Right ear—Pure-tone thresholds revealed a slight sensorineural hearing loss at 250 to 1,000 Hz, sloping to mild to moderately severe from 2,000 to 8,000 Hz. The SRT revealed a mild loss in the ability to receive speech and was in agreement with the PTA. The WRS revealed a normal ability to recognize speech. Immittance testing revealed a normal tympanogram. Acoustic reflex thresholds and decay were not measured at this appointment.

Left ear—Pure-tone thresholds revealed a moderate mixed hearing loss from 250 to 3,000 Hz and sloping to severe to profound from 4,000 to 8,000 Hz. The SRT revealed a moderate loss in the ability to receive speech and was in agreement with the PTA. The WRS revealed a normal ability to recognize speech. Immittance testing revealed a flat tympanogram with a large ear canal volume. Acoustic reflex thresholds and decay were not measured at this appointment.

7.14.3 Intervention

The otologist reported that he had otorrhea in the left ear, which was suctioned. The otologist prescribed antibiotic ear drops and said that if the left ear did not have another infection within 3 months a tympanoplasty could be tried again. The patient was told to keep water out of his left ear. The audiological recommendations included an annual hearing test and post medical management, a hearing aid evaluation pending medical clearance, HAT, and hearing protection in noise.

7.15 Case 15

7.15.1 Case History

The patient had a long-standing history of asymmetric hearing loss. The last hearing test was completed 2 years ago. She had Wegener's granulomatosis with cochlear and middle ear involvement with vasculitis and a tympanic membrane perforation in the right. She reported that all symptoms related to Wegener's granulomatosis had subsided over the past few years. She was not taking any medications at this time for the Wegener's granulomatosis.

She reported increased difficulty with hearing speech in noise and being fatigued due to the constant need to turn to the left. She denied any tinnitus or dizziness.

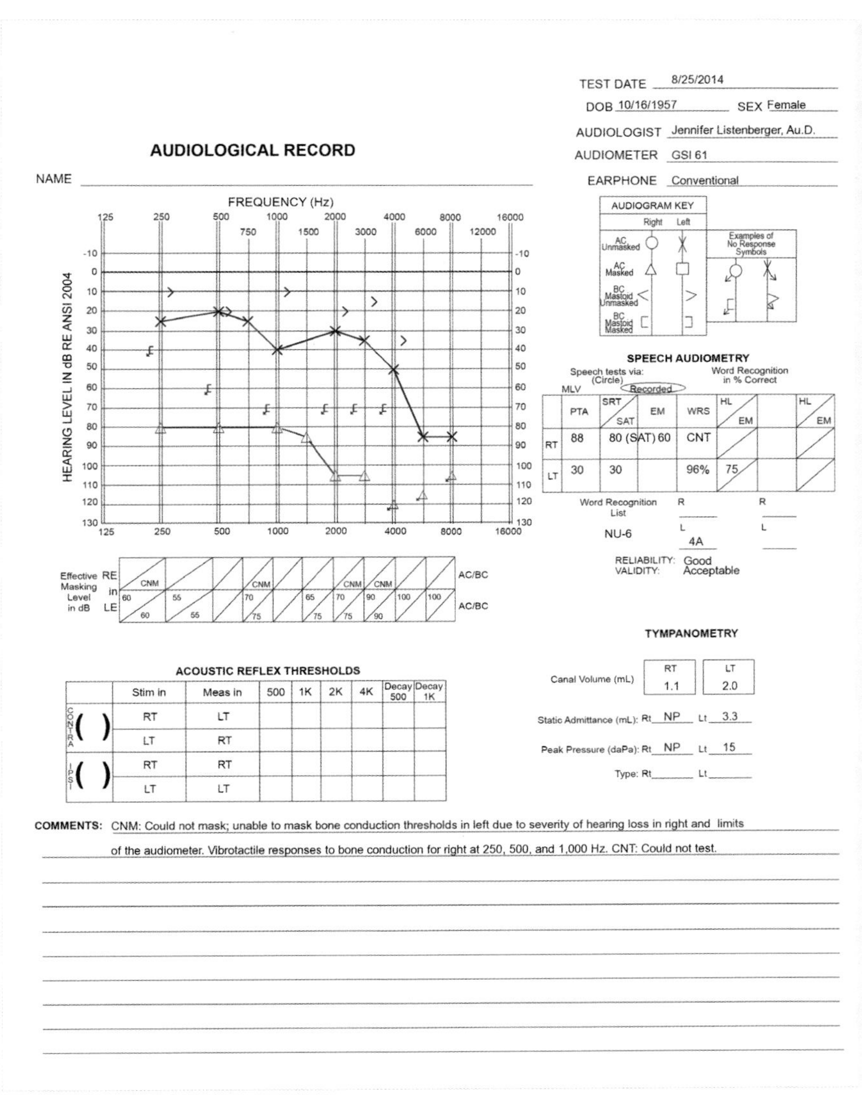

Fig. 7.15 Audiogram of a patient with Wegener's granulomatosis along with a perforation of the right tympanic membrane.

7.15.2 Interpretation

Right ear—Pure-tone air and bone conduction threshold testing revealed a severe sensorineural hearing loss at 250 through 1,500 Hz and sloping to profound at 2,000 through 8,000 Hz, with no measurable response within the limits of the audiometer at 4,000 through 8,000 Hz. No measurable response was obtained for the SRT, and the SAT revealed a severe loss in the ability to detect speech, which was in agreement with the PTA. WRS could not be completed due to a vibrotactile response with presentation levels over 100 dB HL and no measurable SRT. Immittance testing revealed a flat tympanogram with a normal ear canal volume. Acoustic reflex threshold and decay testing was not measured.

Left ear—Pure-tone air and bone conduction threshold testing revealed a slight sloping to mild mixed hearing loss at 250 through 3,000 Hz, sloping to moderate at 4,000 Hz, and steeply sloping to severe at 6,000 and 8,000 Hz. The SRT revealed a mild loss in the ability to receive speech and was in agreement with the PTA. The WRS revealed a normal ability to recognize speech. Immittance testing revealed a hypercompliant tympanogram. Acoustic reflex threshold and decay testing was not measured.

7.15.3 Intervention

The patient will follow up with an otologist as scheduled. Hearing test results were reviewed with the patient and the thresholds and WRS for the right ear had not changed since the previous test. Air conduction thresholds for the left ear had deteriorated slightly above 2,000 Hz. The audiological recommendations were to have the patient return annually for testing to monitor stability of hearing sensitivity, return for a hearing aid evaluation to discuss options for amplification and use of HAT, and use hearing protection in noise as needed.

7.16 Case 16

7.16.1 Case History

A 58-year-old female presented with a sudden decrease in hearing in the right ear. She stated that she had problems with her ears since childhood, with repeated infections and hearing loss in both ears. She reported using hearing aids bilaterally. She reported having a severe ear infection in her right ear last week, resulting in a spontaneous tympanic membrane rupture and decreased hearing. Hearing loss, aural pain, and aural pressure persist in the right ear.

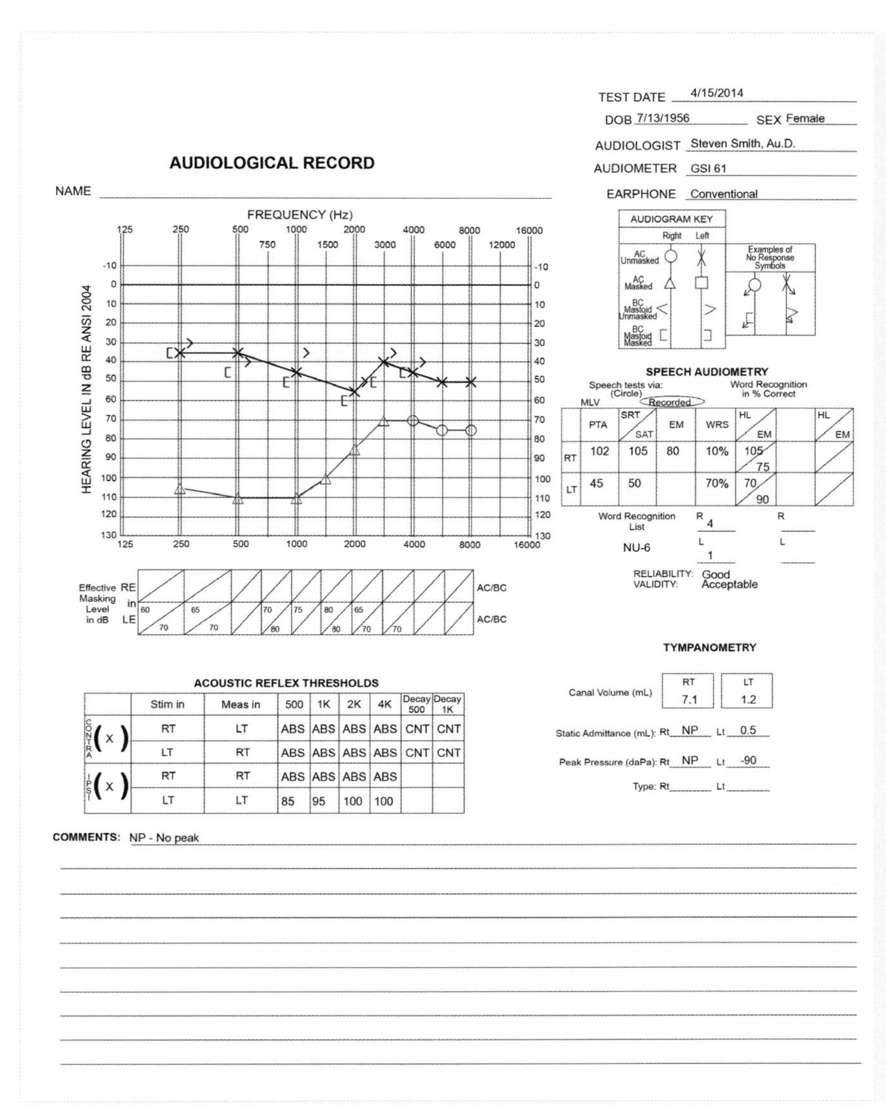

AUDIOLOGICAL RECORD

NAME

TEST DATE 4/15/2014
DOB 7/13/1956 SEX Female
AUDIOLOGIST Steven Smith, Au.D.
AUDIOMETER GSI 61
EARPHONE Conventional

SPEECH AUDIOMETRY

Speech tests via: (Circle) MLV Recorded
Word Recognition in % Correct

	PTA	SRT / SAT	EM	WRS	HL / EM		HL / EM
RT	102	105	80	10%	105 / 75		
LT	45	50		70%	70 / 90		

Word Recognition List NU-6: R 4, L 1

RELIABILITY: Good
VALIDITY: Acceptable

TYMPANOMETRY

Canal Volume (mL): RT 7.1, LT 1.2
Static Admittance (mL): Rt NP Lt 0.5
Peak Pressure (daPa): Rt NP Lt -90
Type: Rt____ Lt____

ACOUSTIC REFLEX THRESHOLDS

	Stim in	Meas in	500	1K	2K	4K	Decay 500	Decay 1K
CONTRA (x)	RT	LT	ABS	ABS	ABS	ABS	CNT	CNT
	LT	RT	ABS	ABS	ABS	ABS	CNT	CNT
IPSI (x)	RT	RT	ABS	ABS	ABS	ABS		
	LT	LT	85	95	100	100		

COMMENTS: NP - No peak

Fig. 7.16 Audiogram of a patient with long-standing hearing loss with an acute ear infection resulting in a perforated tympanic membrane in the right ear.

7.16.2 Interpretation

Right ear—Profound mixed hearing loss rising to moderately severe from 250 to 4,000 Hz, sloping to severe from 6,000 to 8,000 Hz. The SRT revealed a profound loss in the ability to receive speech and was in agreement with the PTA. The WRS was considered very poor ability to recognize speech. Immittance testing revealed a flat tympanogram with a large ear canal volume. Acoustic reflex thresholds with ipsilateral and contralateral stimulation from 500 to 4,000 Hz were absent. Acoustic reflex decay testing could not be measured due to absent reflexes.

Left ear—Flat mild sloping to moderate sensorineural hearing loss. The SRT revealed a moderate loss in the ability to receive speech and was in agreement with the PTA. The WRS revealed a moderate difficulty in the ability to recognize speech. Immittance testing revealed a normal tympanogram. Acoustic reflex thresholds with ipsilateral stimulation from 500 to 4,000 Hz were normal. Contralateral stimulation revealed absent acoustic reflex thresholds from 500 to 4,000 Hz. Acoustic reflex decay testing could not be measured due to absent reflexes.

7.16.3 Intervention

The patient was referred to an ENT specialist and prescribed antibiotic ear drops to clear the infection. She was instructed to return in 1 month to determine if the perforation was healing on its own or if surgical intervention was needed.

7.17 Case 17

7.17.1 Case History

The patient reported that 2 years ago he noted a static sound without hearing loss in the left ear. Six months later, he had decreased hearing in the left ear. If he yawned, his hearing seemed to improve for a few seconds. He had occasional twitching of the face, lip, nose, and eye on the left. He did notice hearing loss in the right ear. He did not report other otologic symptoms or history.

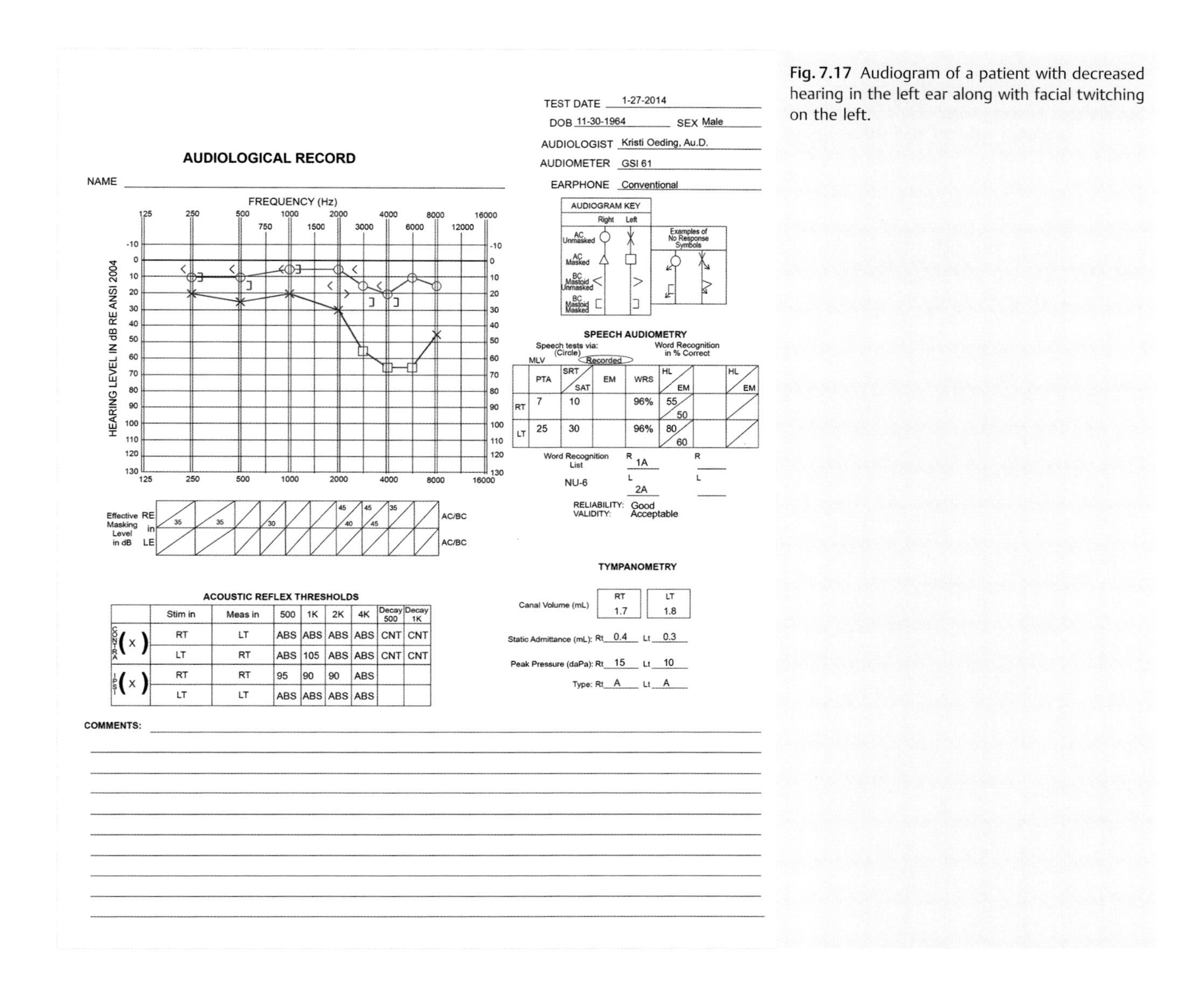

AUDIOLOGICAL RECORD

TEST DATE 1-27-2014
DOB 11-30-1964 SEX Male
AUDIOLOGIST Kristi Oeding, Au.D.
AUDIOMETER GSI 61
EARPHONE Conventional

NAME

SPEECH AUDIOMETRY

Speech tests via: (Circle) MLV Recorded

Word Recognition in % Correct

	PTA	SRT / SAT	EM	WRS	HL / EM		HL / EM
RT	7	10		96%	55 / 50		
LT	25	30		96%	80 / 60		

Word Recognition List: NU-6 — R 1A, L 2A

RELIABILITY: Good
VALIDITY: Acceptable

ACOUSTIC REFLEX THRESHOLDS

	Stim in	Meas in	500	1K	2K	4K	Decay 500	Decay 1K
CONTRA (X)	RT	LT	ABS	ABS	ABS	ABS	CNT	CNT
	LT	RT	ABS	105	ABS	ABS	CNT	CNT
IPSI (X)	RT	RT	95	90	90	ABS		
	LT	LT	ABS	ABS	ABS	ABS		

TYMPANOMETRY

	RT	LT
Canal Volume (mL)	1.7	1.8
Static Admittance (mL)	0.4	0.3
Peak Pressure (daPa)	15	10
Type	A	A

COMMENTS:

Fig. 7.17 Audiogram of a patient with decreased hearing in the left ear along with facial twitching on the left.

7.17.2 Interpretation

Right ear—Pure-tone thresholds were within normal limits from 250 to 3,000 Hz, sloping to a slight sensorineural hearing loss at 4,000 Hz, and rising to within normal limits from 6,000 to 8,000 Hz. The SRT revealed a normal ability to receive speech and was in agreement with the PTA. The WRS revealed a normal ability to recognize speech. Immittance testing revealed a normal tympanogram. The ipsilateral acoustic reflex thresholds were within normal limits from 500 to 2,000 Hz and absent at 4,000 Hz. Contralateral acoustic reflex thresholds were elevated at 1,000 Hz and absent at 500 and 2,000 to 4,000 Hz. Acoustic reflex decay could not be measured at 500 and 1,000 Hz due to elevated and absent contralateral acoustic reflex thresholds.

Left ear—Pure-tone thresholds revealed a slight to mild mixed hearing loss from 250 to 2,000 Hz, sloping to moderate to moderately severe from 3,000 to 6,000 Hz, and rising to moderate at 8,000 Hz. The SRT revealed a mild loss in the ability to receive speech and was in agreement with the PTA. The WRS revealed a normal ability to recognize speech. Immittance testing revealed a normal tympanogram. Ipsilateral and contralateral acoustic reflex thresholds were absent at 500 to 4,000 Hz. Acoustic reflex decay could not be measured at 500 and 1,000 Hz due to absent contralateral acoustic reflex thresholds.

7.17.3 Intervention

The otologist ordered MRI and CT scans, which revealed either a left facial nerve schwannoma or a hemangioma. Exploratory surgery revealed a left hemangioma, which was mostly removed, except for a part that was wrapped around the facial nerve. Decompression of the facial nerve was completed. His hearing decreased slightly after surgery, and the facial twitching slightly improved. The audiological recommendations included an annual hearing test, a hearing aid evaluation for the left ear pending medical clearance, use of HAT, and use of hearing protection in noise.

7.18 Case 18

7.18.1 Case History

The patient was a 76-year-old male with a long-standing history of mixed hearing loss in the left ear. He had a history of chronic otitis media and eustachian tube dysfunction in the left ear and four otosurgeries in that ear, including ossiculoplasty and PE tube replacement. He had not had a hearing test in 3 years. He reported a significant deterioration in his hearing in the left ear over the past few years as well as increased difficulty understanding speech in noise. The patient also reported an increased need for turning to the right and the need to place people on the right side to hear well, even in quiet. There was no report of tinnitus or dizziness. There was no reported history of familial hearing loss or noise exposure.

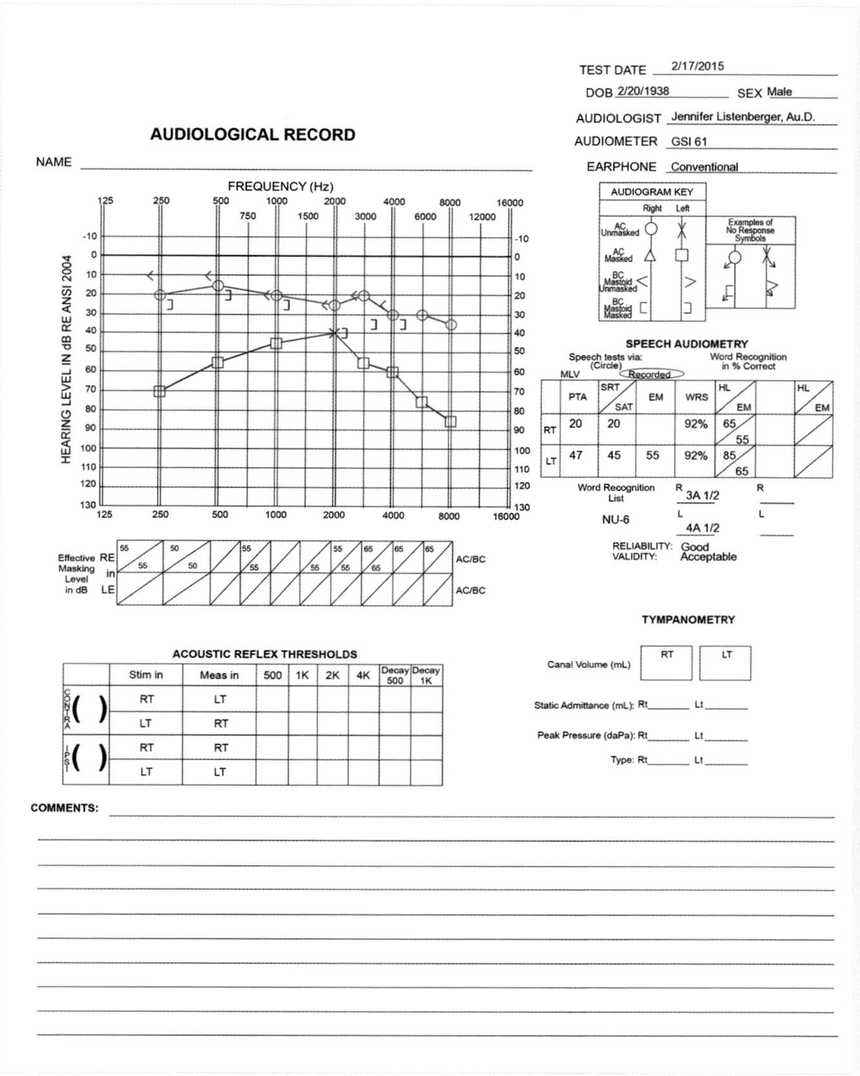

AUDIOLOGICAL RECORD

NAME

TEST DATE 2/17/2015
DOB 2/20/1938 SEX Male
AUDIOLOGIST Jennifer Listenberger, Au.D.
AUDIOMETER GSI 61
EARPHONE Conventional

SPEECH AUDIOMETRY

Speech tests via: (Circle) MLV Recorded — Word Recognition in % Correct

	PTA	SRT/SAT	EM	WRS	HL/EM		HL/EM
RT	20	20		92%	65/55		
LT	47	45	55	92%	85/65		

Word Recognition List NU-6: R 3A 1/2; L 4A 1/2

RELIABILITY: Good
VALIDITY: Acceptable

Fig. 7.18 Audiogram of a patient with a history of otitis media in the left that resulted in four otosurgeries, including ossiculoplasty.

7.18.2 Interpretation

Right ear—Pure-tone air and bone conduction threshold testing revealed a slight sensorineural hearing loss at 250 through 3,000 Hz, except for normal hearing at 500 Hz, sloping to mild at 4,000 through 8,000 Hz. The SRT revealed a slight loss in the ability to receive speech and was in agreement with the PTA. The WRS revealed a normal ability to recognize speech. Immittance testing was not measured.

Left ear—Pure-tone air and bone conduction threshold testing revealed a moderately severe gradually rising to mild mixed hearing loss at 250 through 2,000 Hz, then sloping to moderate to severe at 3,000 through 8,000 Hz. The SRT revealed a moderate loss in the ability to receive speech and was in agreement with the PTA. The WRS revealed a normal ability to recognize speech. Immittance testing was not measured.

7.18.3 Intervention

The patient will follow up with an otologist as scheduled. Hearing test results were reviewed with the patient and revealed minimal changes in thresholds in comparison to thresholds from the previous test. The audiological recommendations were to return for a hearing test annually to monitor stability of hearing sensitivity, to use hearing protection in noise as needed, and to schedule a hearing aid evaluation to discuss options for use of amplification and HAT.

7.19 Case 19

7.19.1 Case History

A 60-year-old male stated that he woke up one morning and his hearing had suddenly decreased bilaterally, and he was struggling to hear those around him. He reported the left ear as being poorer than the right ear. He had tinnitus prior to his decrease in hearing and the tinnitus had increased in intensity. He reported aural fullness bilaterally. He denied loud noise exposure or other ear problems prior to this. He stated that his allergies are very bad this year.

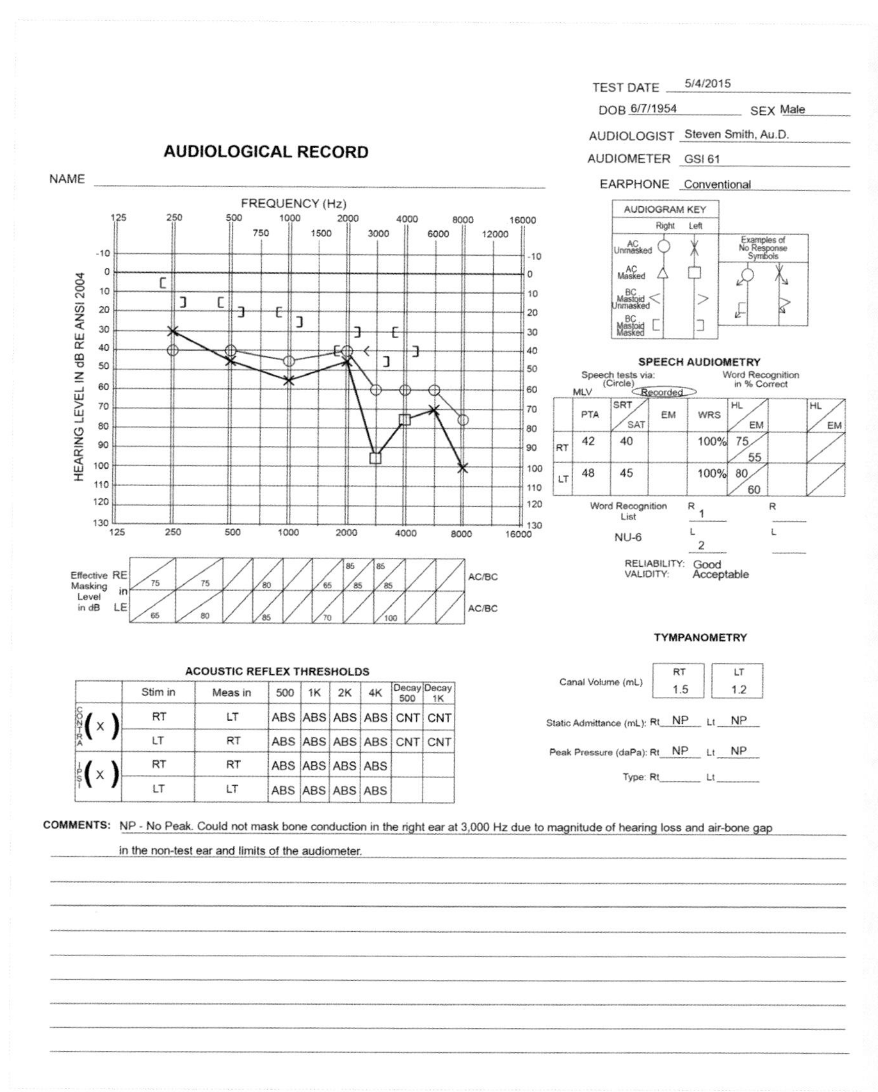

AUDIOLOGICAL RECORD

NAME

TEST DATE 5/4/2015
DOB 6/7/1954 SEX Male
AUDIOLOGIST Steven Smith, Au.D.
AUDIOMETER GSI 61
EARPHONE Conventional

Effective Masking Level in dB

RE	75	75	80	65	85/85	85/85				AC/BC
LE	65	80	85	70	100					AC/BC

SPEECH AUDIOMETRY

Speech tests via: (Circle) MLV Recorded

Word Recognition in % Correct

	PTA	SRT/SAT	EM	WRS	HL/EM	HL/EM
RT	42	40		100%	75/55	
LT	48	45		100%	80/60	

Word Recognition List: NU-6 — R 1, L 2

RELIABILITY: Good
VALIDITY: Acceptable

ACOUSTIC REFLEX THRESHOLDS

	Stim in	Meas in	500	1K	2K	4K	Decay 500	Decay 1K
CONTRA (X)	RT	LT	ABS	ABS	ABS	ABS	CNT	CNT
	LT	RT	ABS	ABS	ABS	ABS	CNT	CNT
IPSI (X)	RT	RT	ABS	ABS	ABS	ABS		
	LT	LT	ABS	ABS	ABS	ABS		

TYMPANOMETRY

	RT	LT
Canal Volume (mL)	1.5	1.2

Static Admittance (mL): Rt NP Lt NP
Peak Pressure (daPa): Rt NP Lt NP
Type: Rt Lt

COMMENTS: NP - No Peak. Could not mask bone conduction in the right ear at 3,000 Hz due to magnitude of hearing loss and air-bone gap in the non-test ear and limits of the audiometer.

Fig. 7.19 Audiogram showing the results for a patient with a sudden bilateral decrease in hearing with aural fullness.

7.19.2 Interpretation

Right ear—Mild sloping to moderate mixed hearing loss from 250 to 2,000 Hz, sloping to moderately severe to severe. The SRT revealed a mild loss in the ability to receive speech and was in agreement with the PTA. The WRS was normal. Immittance testing revealed a flat tympanogram with a normal ear canal volume. The acoustic reflexes with ipsilateral and contralateral stimulation from 500 to 4,000 Hz were absent. Acoustic reflex decay could not be measured.

Left ear—Mild sloping to moderate mixed hearing loss from 250 to 2,000 Hz, sloping to profound at 3,000 Hz, and rising to severe to moderately severe at 4,000 to 6,000 Hz, then sloping to profound. The SRT revealed a moderate loss in the ability to receive speech and was in agreement with the PTA. The WRS was normal. Immittance testing revealed a flat tympanogram with normal ear canal volume. The acoustic reflexes with ipsilateral and contralateral stimulation from 500 Hz to 4,000 Hz were absent. Acoustic reflex decay could not be measured.

7.19.3 Intervention

The patient was referred to an ENT specialist and was diagnosed with acute otitis media. He was prescribed a steroid nasal spray as well as allergy medication and was told to follow up in 1 month.

7.20 Case 20

7.20.1 Case History

The patient reported a long-standing history of bilateral hearing loss with the left ear being poorer than the right ear. He noticed increased difficulty hearing in background noise. He had a family history of hearing loss. He was interested in learning about his amplification options. He did not report other otologic symptoms or history.

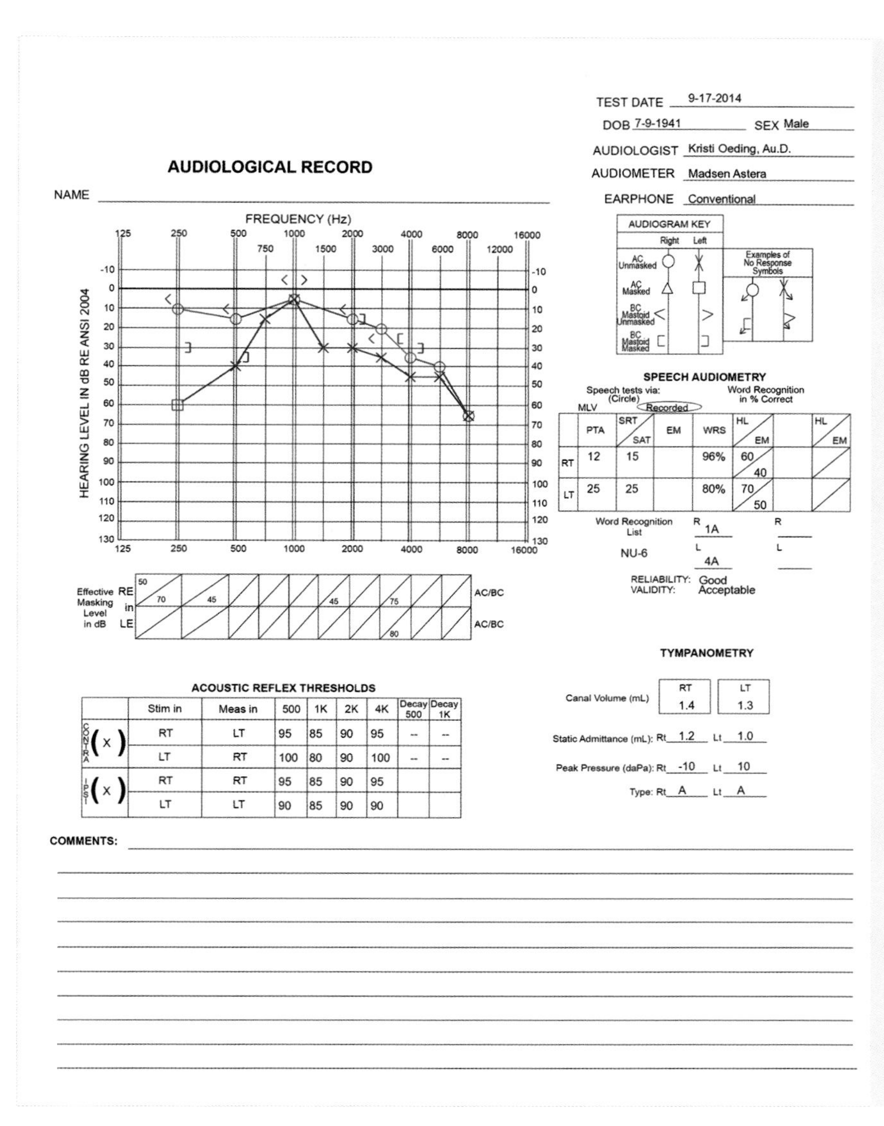

AUDIOLOGICAL RECORD

NAME

TEST DATE 9-17-2014

DOB 7-9-1941 SEX Male

AUDIOLOGIST Kristi Oeding, Au.D.

AUDIOMETER Madsen Astera

EARPHONE Conventional

Effective Masking Level in dB											
RE	50 / 70	45				45		75			AC/BC
LE								80			AC/BC

SPEECH AUDIOMETRY

Speech tests via: (Circle) MLV Recorded (circled)

Word Recognition in % Correct

	PTA	SRT / SAT	EM	WRS	HL / EM		HL / EM
RT	12	15		96%	60 / 40		
LT	25	25		80%	70 / 50		

Word Recognition List: NU-6 R 1A, L 4A; R ____, L ____

RELIABILITY: Good
VALIDITY: Acceptable

TYMPANOMETRY

	RT	LT
Canal Volume (mL)	1.4	1.3
Static Admittance (mL)	1.2	1.0
Peak Pressure (daPa)	-10	10
Type	A	A

ACOUSTIC REFLEX THRESHOLDS

	Stim in	Meas in	500	1K	2K	4K	Decay 500	Decay 1K
CONTRA (X)	RT	LT	95	85	90	95	--	--
	LT	RT	100	80	90	100	--	--
IPSI (X)	RT	RT	95	85	90	95		
	LT	LT	90	85	90	90		

COMMENTS:

Fig. 7.20 Audiogram of a patient with long-standing hearing loss, with the left ear being poorer than the right ear.

7.20.2 Interpretation

Right ear—Pure-tone thresholds were within normal limits from 250 to 2,000 Hz and sloping from a slight to moderately severe sensorineural hearing loss from 3,000 to 8,000 Hz. The SRT revealed a normal ability to receive speech and was in agreement with the PTA. The WRS revealed a normal ability to recognize speech. Immittance testing revealed a normal tympanogram and normal ipsilateral and contralateral acoustic reflex thresholds from 500 to 4,000 Hz. Acoustic reflex decay was negative at 500 and 1,000 Hz.

Left ear—Pure-tone thresholds revealed a moderately severe to mild mixed hearing loss from 250 to 500 Hz, rising to within normal limits from 750 to 1,000 Hz, and sloping to a mild to moderately severe mixed hearing loss from 1,500 to 8,000 Hz. The SRT revealed a slight loss in the ability to receive speech and was in agreement with the PTA. The WRS revealed slight difficulty in the ability to recognize speech. Immittance testing revealed a normal tympanogram and normal ipsilateral and contralateral acoustic reflex thresholds from 500 to 4,000 Hz. Acoustic reflex decay was negative at 500 and 1,000 Hz.

7.20.3 Intervention

The otologist ordered an ABR due to the asymmetric hearing loss. The results of the ABR were abnormal; therefore, an MRI was ordered. The MRI was normal. It was determined that the hearing loss was due to presbycusis and genetics. He was medically cleared for amplification and he obtained bilateral hearing aids.

7.21 Case 21

7.21.1 Case History

The patient was seen for follow-up testing to monitor a gradually progressive mixed hearing loss. The last test was completed 3 years ago. The hearing loss in the right ear had progressed and was poorer than the left ear and, even with the use of bilateral amplification, the patient was noticing increased difficulty understanding speech in most communication settings. There was no history of otosurgery or familial hearing.

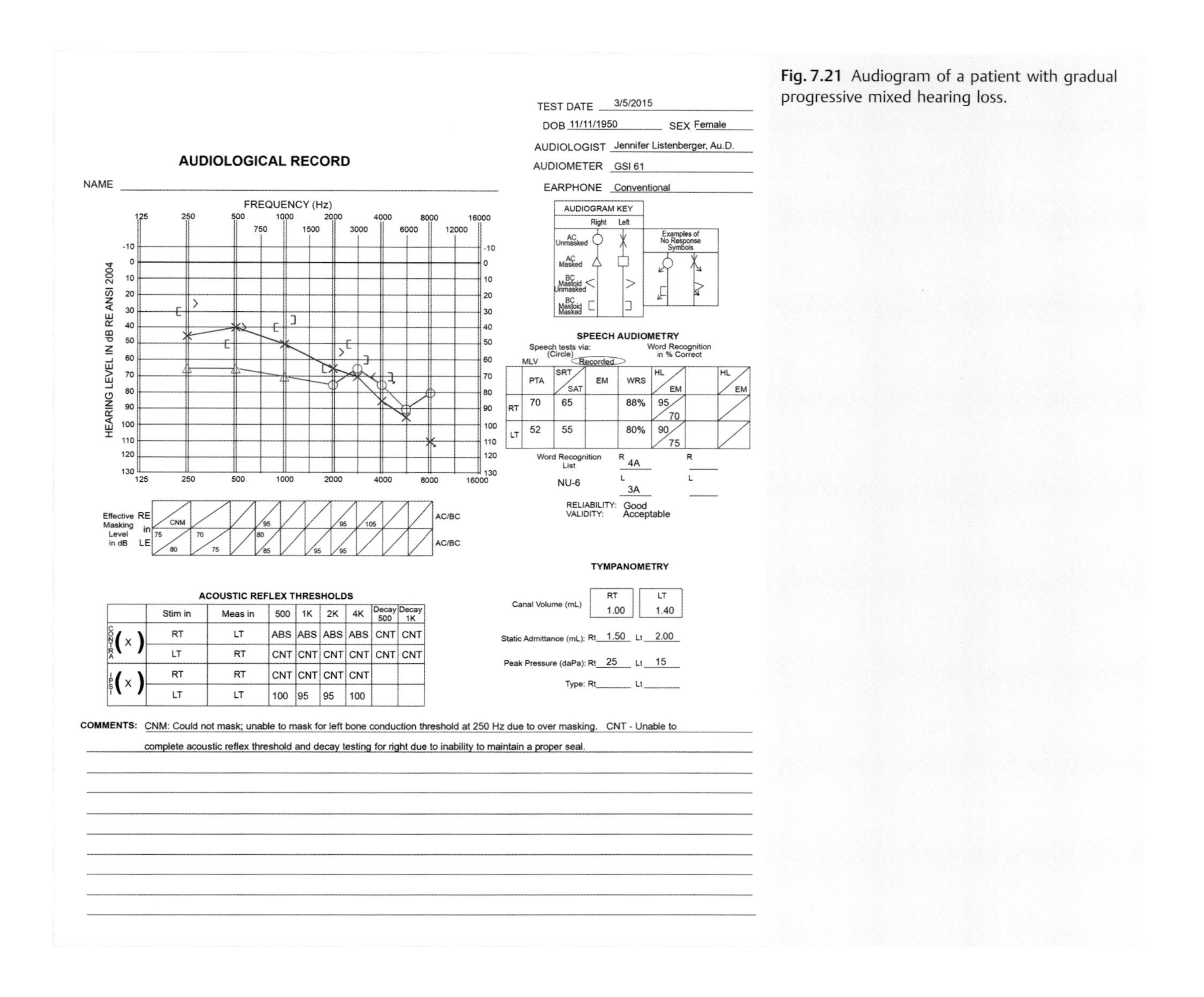
AUDIOLOGICAL RECORD

NAME

TEST DATE 3/5/2015
DOB 11/11/1950 SEX Female
AUDIOLOGIST Jennifer Listenberger, Au.D.
AUDIOMETER GSI 61
EARPHONE Conventional

Effective Masking Level in dB

RE in	CNM	75	70	95	80	95	105
LE in	80	75	85	95	95		

SPEECH AUDIOMETRY

Speech tests via: (Circle) MLV Recorded

	PTA	SRT / SAT	EM	WRS	HL / EM	HL / EM
RT	70	65		88%	95 / 70	
LT	52	55		80%	90 / 75	

Word Recognition List NU-6: R 4A, L 3A

RELIABILITY: Good
VALIDITY: Acceptable

TYMPANOMETRY

	RT	LT
Canal Volume (mL)	1.00	1.40

Static Admittance (mL): Rt 1.50 Lt 2.00

Peak Pressure (daPa): Rt 25 Lt 15

Type: Rt ___ Lt ___

ACOUSTIC REFLEX THRESHOLDS

	Stim in	Meas in	500	1K	2K	4K	Decay 500	Decay 1K
CONTRA (X)	RT	LT	ABS	ABS	ABS	ABS	CNT	CNT
	LT	RT	CNT	CNT	CNT	CNT	CNT	CNT
IPSI (X)	RT	RT	CNT	CNT	CNT	CNT		
	LT	LT	100	95	95	100		

COMMENTS: CNM: Could not mask; unable to mask for left bone conduction threshold at 250 Hz due to over masking. CNT - Unable to complete acoustic reflex threshold and decay testing for right due to inability to maintain a proper seal.

Fig. 7.21 Audiogram of a patient with gradual progressive mixed hearing loss.

7.21.2 Interpretation

Right ear—Pure-tone air and bone conduction threshold testing revealed an essentially flat moderately severe mixed hearing loss at 250 through 3,000 Hz, except for severe hearing loss at 2,000 Hz, and sloping to severe at 4,000 through 8,000 Hz. The SRT revealed a moderately severe loss in the ability to receive speech and was in agreement with the PTA. The WRS revealed a slight difficulty in the ability to recognize speech. Immittance testing revealed a normal tympanogram. Acoustic reflex threshold testing was not measured due to lack of ability to maintain a proper seal.

Left ear—Pure-tone air and bone conduction threshold testing revealed a mild, gradually sloping to moderately severe mixed hearing loss at 250 through 3,000 Hz, except for a moderate hearing loss at 250 Hz, and sloping to severe to profound at 4,000 through 8,000 Hz. No measurable response was obtained within the limits of the audiometer at 8,000 Hz. The SRT revealed a moderate loss in the ability to receive speech and was in agreement with the PTA. The WRS revealed a slight difficulty in the ability to recognize speech. Immittance testing revealed a hypercompliant tympanogram. The acoustic reflex thresholds were normal for ipsilateral stimulation at 500 to 4,000 Hz and absent for contralateral stimulation at 500 to 4,000 Hz. Acoustic reflex decay could not be measured due to absent contralateral acoustic reflex thresholds.

7.21.3 Intervention

Hearing test results were reviewed with the patient and it was noted that there was progression of hearing loss in the right ear and a larger air–bone gap. Otologic consultation was recommended regarding the increased mixed hearing loss. The audiological recommendations included continued use of amplification, use of HAT, and annual testing to monitor stability of hearing sensitivity.

7.22 Case 22

7.22.1 Case History

A 64-year-old male reported that his hearing had decreased bilaterally, with the right being poorer than the left. He reported that this decline had started soon after his having received radiation and chemotherapy. He stated that his chemotherapy included three doses of cisplatin, and he received radiation to his nasal passageways due to cancer. He denied tinnitus as well as pain or pressure in his ears. He reported that his hearing was good prior to treatment.

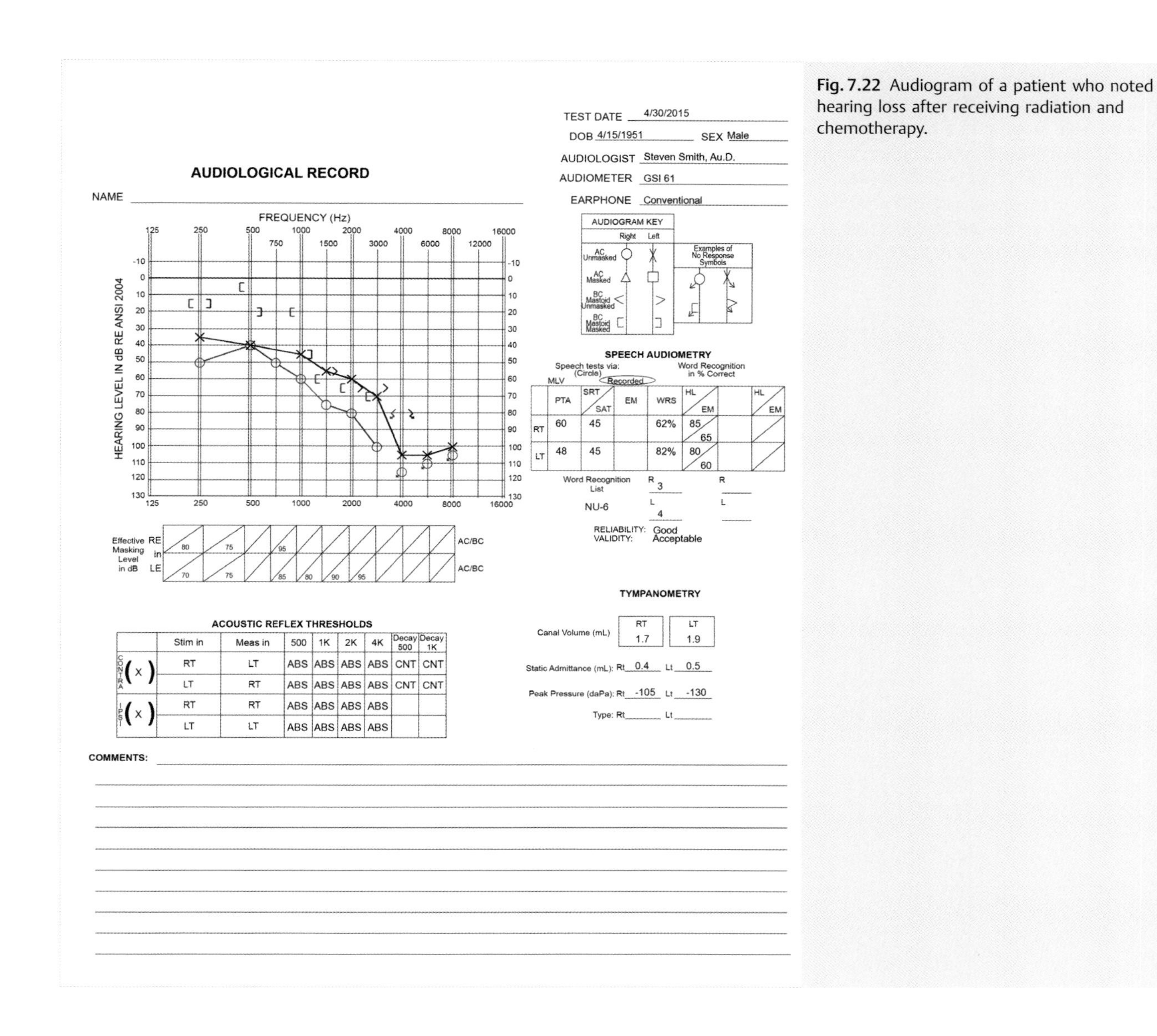

AUDIOLOGICAL RECORD

TEST DATE 4/30/2015

DOB 4/15/1951 SEX Male

AUDIOLOGIST Steven Smith, Au.D.

AUDIOMETER GSI 61

EARPHONE Conventional

NAME

Effective Masking Level in dB

RE	80	75		95							AC/BC
LE	70	75		85	80	90	95				AC/BC

SPEECH AUDIOMETRY

Speech tests via: (Circle) MLV Recorded

Word Recognition in % Correct

	PTA	SRT / SAT	EM	WRS	HL / EM		HL / EM
RT	60	45		62%	85 / 65		
LT	48	45		82%	80 / 60		

Word Recognition List NU-6: R 3, L 4; R ___, L ___

RELIABILITY: Good

VALIDITY: Acceptable

TYMPANOMETRY

	RT	LT
Canal Volume (mL)	1.7	1.9

Static Admittance (mL): Rt 0.4 Lt 0.5

Peak Pressure (daPa): Rt -105 Lt -130

Type: Rt ___ Lt ___

ACOUSTIC REFLEX THRESHOLDS

	Stim in	Meas in	500	1K	2K	4K	Decay 500	Decay 1K
CONTRA (x)	RT	LT	ABS	ABS	ABS	ABS	CNT	CNT
	LT	RT	ABS	ABS	ABS	ABS	CNT	CNT
IPSI (x)	RT	RT	ABS	ABS	ABS	ABS		
	LT	LT	ABS	ABS	ABS	ABS		

COMMENTS:

Fig. 7.22 Audiogram of a patient who noted hearing loss after receiving radiation and chemotherapy.

7.22.2 Interpretation

Right ear—Moderate rising to mild mixed hearing loss at 250 to 500 Hz, and sloping to moderately severe to profound at 1,000 to 8,000 Hz, with no measurable response within audiometer limits at 4,000 to 8,000 Hz. The SRT revealed a moderate loss in the ability to receive speech and was not in agreement with the PTA, which may be due to the sloping hearing loss. The WRS revealed moderate difficulty in the ability to recognize speech. Immittance testing revealed excessive negative pressure for tympanometry. The acoustic reflex thresholds with ipsilateral and contralateral stimulation from 500 to 4,000 Hz were absent. Acoustic reflex decay could not be measured.

Left ear—Mild sloping to a moderately severe mixed hearing loss at 250 to 3,000 Hz, and sloping to profound at 4,000 to 8,000 Hz. The hearing loss is predominantly sensorineural with air–bone gaps present only at 250 to 500 Hz. The SRT revealed a moderate loss in the ability to receive speech and was in agreement with the PTA. The WRS revealed slight difficulty in the ability to recognize speech. Immittance testing revealed excessive negative pressure for tympanometry. Acoustic reflex thresholds with ipsilateral and contralateral stimulation from 500 to 4,000 Hz were absent. Acoustic reflex decay could not be measured.

7.22.3 Intervention

The patient was referred to an ENT specialist due to the mixed hearing loss. He was counseled that he may receive benefit from hearing aids after receiving medical treatment. The ENT specialist determined that the sensorineural portion of his hearing loss was due to the administration of cisplatin, and the conductive portion of his hearing loss was due to eustachian tube dysfunction secondary to radiation. He was referred for a hearing aid evaluation.

7.23 Case 23

7.23.1 Case History

The patient reported a right sudden hearing loss about 2 weeks ago. A popping sound occurred in the right ear followed by decreased hearing, static, and distortion in that ear. She had had this happen in the past, but typically her hearing had returned. Her hearing still seemed decreased in the right ear. She had a long-standing history of mixed hearing loss in the left ear from chronic ear infections and a mastoidectomy. She also noted that both ears itch due to eczema. She did not report other otologic symptoms or history.

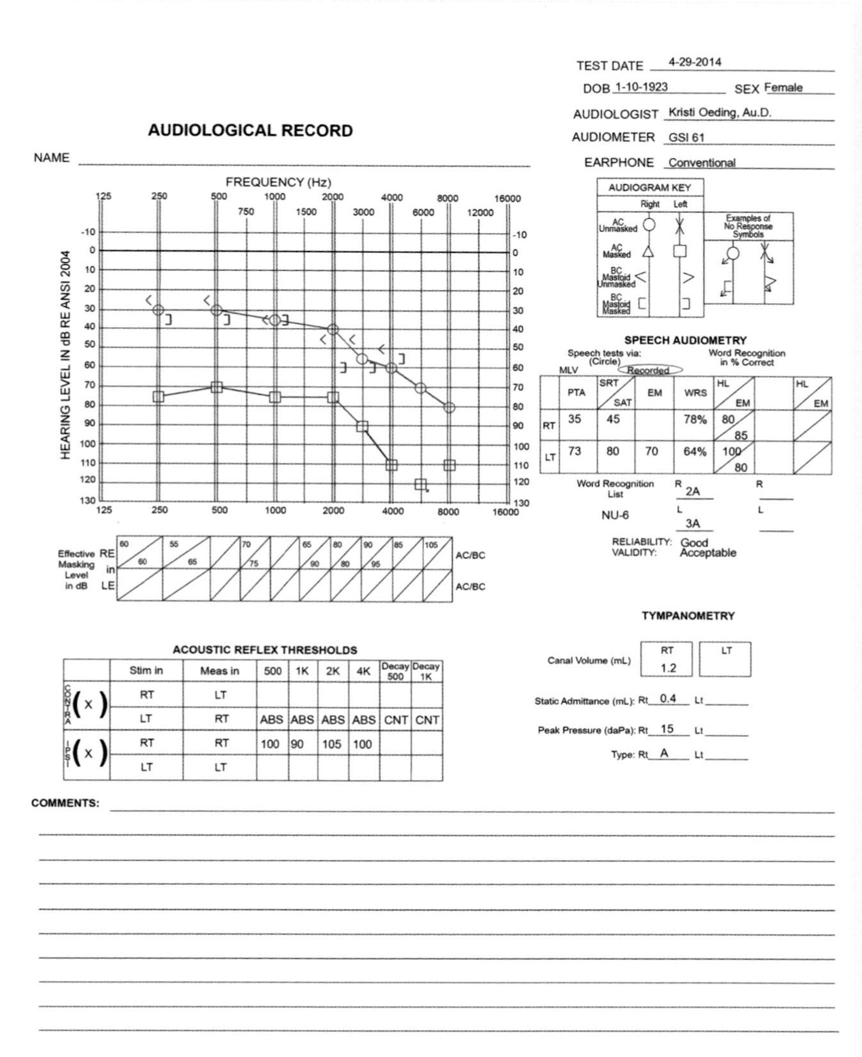

AUDIOLOGICAL RECORD

NAME

TEST DATE 4-29-2014
DOB 1-10-1923 SEX Female
AUDIOLOGIST Kristi Oeding, Au.D.
AUDIOMETER GSI 61
EARPHONE Conventional

SPEECH AUDIOMETRY

Speech tests via: (Circle) MLV Recorded

Word Recognition in % Correct

	PTA	SRT / SAT	EM	WRS	HL / EM		HL / EM
RT	35	45		78%	80 / 85		
LT	73	80	70	64%	100 / 80		

Word Recognition List NU-6: R 2A, L 3A; R ___, L ___

RELIABILITY: Good
VALIDITY: Acceptable

Effective Masking Level in dB

RE	60 / 60	55 / 65		70 / 75		65 / 90	80 / 80	90 / 95	85	105	AC/BC
LE											AC/BC

ACOUSTIC REFLEX THRESHOLDS

	Stim in	Meas in	500	1K	2K	4K	Decay 500	Decay 1K
CONTRA (X)	RT	LT						
	LT	RT	ABS	ABS	ABS	ABS	CNT	CNT
IPSI (X)	RT	RT	100	90	105	100		
	LT	LT						

TYMPANOMETRY

Canal Volume (mL): RT 1.2, LT
Static Admittance (mL): Rt 0.4 Lt ___
Peak Pressure (daPa): Rt 15 Lt ___
Type: Rt A Lt ___

COMMENTS:

Fig. 7.23 Audiogram of a patient with a chronic ear infection and a mastoidectomy who had a sudden decrease in hearing in the right ear.

7.23.2 Interpretation

Right ear—Pure-tone thresholds revealed a mild sensorineural hearing loss from 250 to 2,000 Hz then sloping to moderate to severe from 3,000 to 8,000 Hz. The SRT revealed a moderate loss in the ability to receive speech and was in agreement with the PTA. The WRS revealed a slight difficulty in the ability to recognize speech. Immittance testing revealed a normal tympanogram. The ipsilateral acoustic reflex thresholds were normal at 500, 1,000, and 4,000 Hz and elevated at 2,000 Hz. The contralateral acoustic reflex thresholds were absent from 500 to 4,000 Hz. Acoustic reflex decay could not be measured due to absent contralateral acoustic reflex thresholds.

Left ear—Pure-tone thresholds revealed a severe mixed hearing loss from 250 to 3,000 Hz, except for a moderately severe hearing loss at 500 Hz, and sloping to profound from 4,000 to 8,000 Hz. The SRT revealed a severe loss in the ability to receive speech and was in agreement with the PTA. The WRS revealed moderate difficulty in the ability to recognize speech. Immittance testing could not be measured due to previous otosurgery.

7.23.3 Intervention

The otologist prescribed a short course of oral steroids for 12 days. When she returned for follow-up, the pure-tone thresholds did not improve; however, the WRS had increased to 96%. Further medical management was not recommended. The audiological recommendations included an annual hearing test, an evaluation for hearing aids, use of HAT, and use of hearing protection in noise.

7.24 Case 24

7.24.1 Case History

Patient was a 76-year-old male with a long-standing history of asymmetric hearing loss and multiple otosurgeries on the left. First surgery was completed approximately 50 years ago and then a modified radical mastoidectomy was performed approximately 30 years ago. The patient was followed every six months by otology for cleaning of the mastoid cavity bowl. Hearing testing was completed regularly to monitor hearing sensitivity with the last hearing test being completed two years ago. Patient used amplification in the better hearing right ear and tried amplification in the left ear approximately ten years ago, but the trial was unsuccessful due to physical and auditory discomfort.

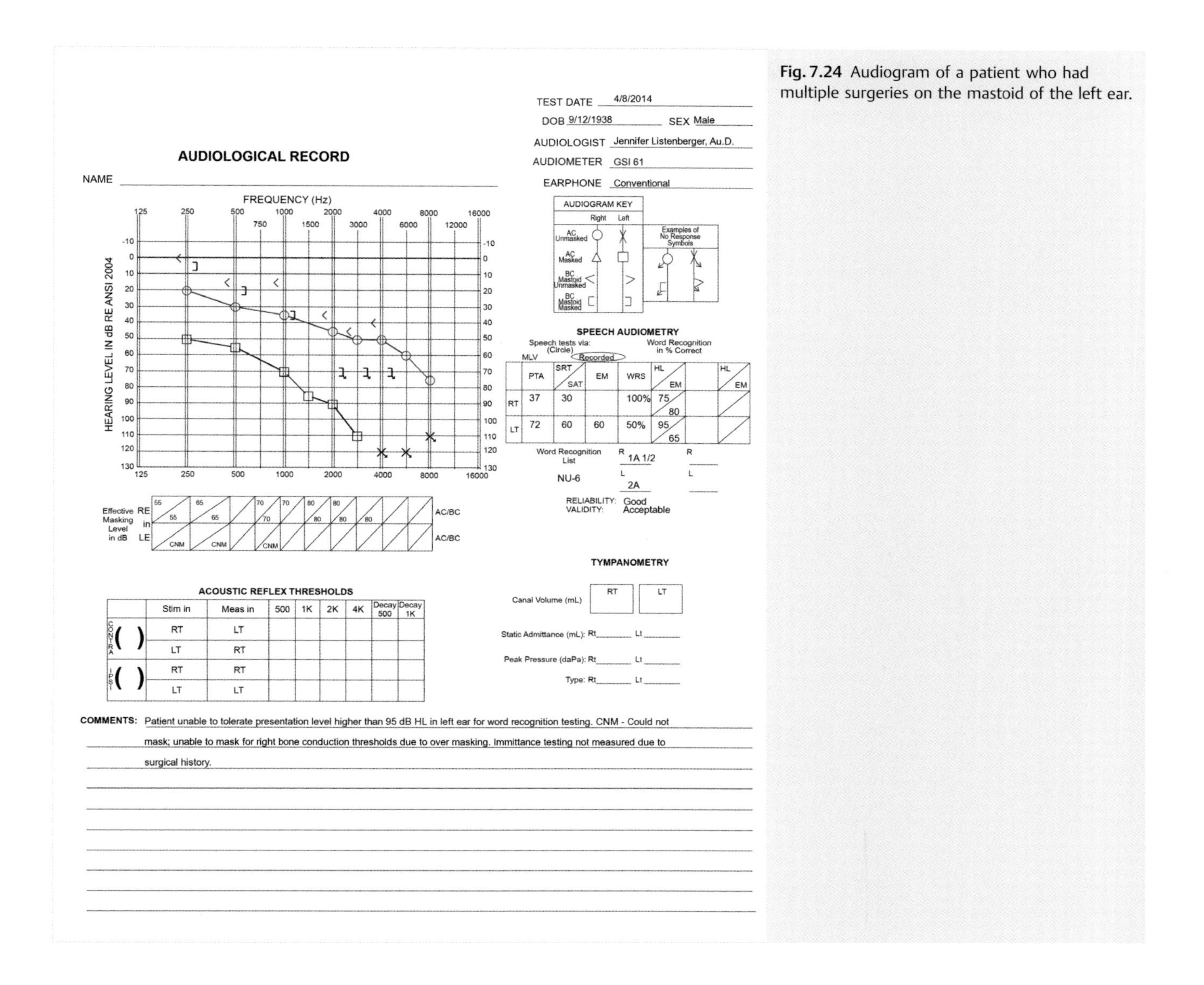

AUDIOLOGICAL RECORD

NAME

TEST DATE 4/8/2014

DOB 9/12/1938 SEX Male

AUDIOLOGIST Jennifer Listenberger, Au.D.

AUDIOMETER GSI 61

EARPHONE Conventional

Effective Masking Level in dB

	250	500	750	1000	1500	2000	3000	4000	6000	8000	
RE in	55 / 55	65 / 65		70 / 70	70	80 / 80	80 / 80	80			AC/BC
LE in	CNM	CNM		CNM							AC/BC

SPEECH AUDIOMETRY

Speech tests via: (Circle) MLV Recorded

Word Recognition in % Correct

	PTA	SRT/SAT	EM	WRS	HL/EM		HL/EM
RT	37	30		100%	75/80		
LT	72	60	60	50%	95/65		

Word Recognition List NU-6: R 1A 1/2; L 2A; R ___; L ___

RELIABILITY: Good
VALIDITY: Acceptable

ACOUSTIC REFLEX THRESHOLDS

	Stim in	Meas in	500	1K	2K	4K	Decay 500	Decay 1K
CONTRA ( )	RT	LT						
	LT	RT						
IPSI ( )	RT	RT						
	LT	LT						

TYMPANOMETRY

Canal Volume (mL): RT ___ LT ___

Static Admittance (mL): Rt___ Lt___

Peak Pressure (daPa): Rt___ Lt___

Type: Rt___ Lt___

COMMENTS: Patient unable to tolerate presentation level higher than 95 dB HL in left ear for word recognition testing. CNM - Could not mask; unable to mask for right bone conduction thresholds due to over masking. Immittance testing not measured due to surgical history.

Fig. 7.24 Audiogram of a patient who had multiple surgeries on the mastoid of the left ear.

7.24.2 Interpretation

Right ear—Pure-tone air and bone conduction threshold testing revealed a slight sloping to mild mixed hearing loss at 250 through 1,000 Hz, then sloping to a moderate to severe sensorineural hearing loss at 2,000 through 8,000 Hz. The SRT revealed a mild loss in the ability to receive speech and was in agreement with the PTA. The WRS revealed a normal ability to recognize speech. Immittance testing was not measured. The thresholds and WRS remained unchanged in comparison to previous hearing tests.

Left ear—Pure-tone air and bone conduction threshold testing revealed a moderate sloping to severe mixed hearing loss at 250 through 2,000 Hz, and sloping to profound at 3,000 through 8,000 Hz, with no measurable response within the limits of the audiometer at 4,000 through 8,000 Hz. The SRT revealed a moderately severe loss in the ability to receive speech and was in agreement with the PTA. The WRS revealed a poor ability to recognize speech. Immittance testing was not measured.

7.24.3 Intervention

The hearing test results were reviewed. The hearing loss had progressed gradually bilaterally. The patient will follow up with the otologist as scheduled. The audiological recommendations were to return for hearing testing annually to monitor the stability of hearing sensitivity, to continue use of amplification in the right ear and reconsider a trial of amplification in the left ear, and to use HAT.

7.25 Case 25

7.25.1 Case History

A 78-year-old female stated that she had noticed hearing loss for the last 10 years. More recently she stated that the hearing in the right ear started to decline more than the left ear. She reported tinnitus bilaterally with equal loudness. She did not report any symptoms of pain or pressure in her ears. She stated she may be considering hearing aids because she is having difficulty following conversations.

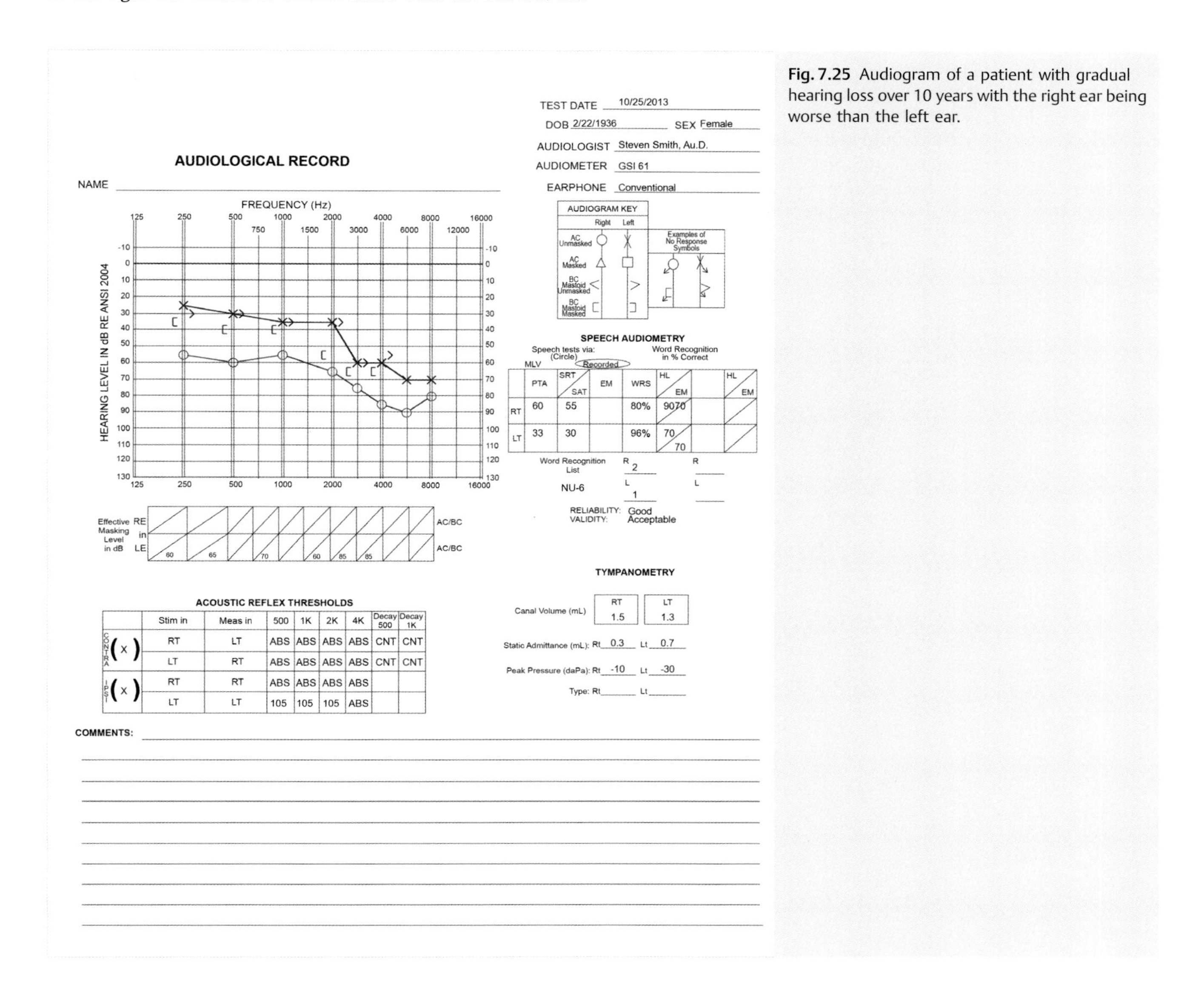

AUDIOLOGICAL RECORD

NAME

TEST DATE 10/25/2013

DOB 2/22/1936 SEX Female

AUDIOLOGIST Steven Smith, Au.D.

AUDIOMETER GSI 61

EARPHONE Conventional

SPEECH AUDIOMETRY

Speech tests via: (Circle) MLV Recorded

Word Recognition in % Correct

	PTA	SRT / SAT	EM	WRS	HL / EM		HL / EM
RT	60	55		80%	90 70		
LT	33	30		96%	70 / 70		

Word Recognition List NU-6: R 2, L 1

RELIABILITY: Good

VALIDITY: Acceptable

ACOUSTIC REFLEX THRESHOLDS

	Stim in	Meas in	500	1K	2K	4K	Decay 500	Decay 1K
CONTRA (x)	RT	LT	ABS	ABS	ABS	ABS	CNT	CNT
	LT	RT	ABS	ABS	ABS	ABS	CNT	CNT
IPSI (x)	RT	RT	ABS	ABS	ABS	ABS		
	LT	LT	105	105	105	ABS		

TYMPANOMETRY

	RT	LT
Canal Volume (mL)	1.5	1.3

Static Admittance (mL): Rt 0.3 Lt 0.7

Peak Pressure (daPa): Rt -10 Lt -30

Type: Rt____ Lt____

COMMENTS:

Fig. 7.25 Audiogram of a patient with gradual hearing loss over 10 years with the right ear being worse than the left ear.

7.25.2 Interpretation

Right ear—Moderate sloping to a severe mixed hearing loss from 250 to 8,000 Hz. The SRT revealed a moderate loss in the ability to receive speech and was in agreement with the PTA. The WRS revealed a slight difficulty in speech recognition. Immittance testing revealed a normal tympanogram. The acoustic reflex thresholds with ipsilateral and contralateral stimulation were absent from 500 to 4,000 Hz. Acoustic reflex decay could not be measured.

Left ear—Slight sloping to a mild sensorineural hearing loss at 250 to 2,000 Hz, sloping to moderately severe at 3,000 to 8,000 Hz. The SRT revealed a mild loss in the ability to receive speech and was in agreement with the PTA. The WRS was normal. Immittance testing revealed a normal tympanogram. The acoustic reflex thresholds with ipsilateral stimulation were elevated from 500 to 2,000 Hz and absent at 4,000 Hz. The acoustic reflex thresholds with contralateral stimulation from 500 to 4,000 Hz were absent. Acoustic reflex decay could not be measured.

7.25.3 Intervention

Due to the mixed hearing loss and the asymmetry, the patient was referred to an ENT specialist for evaluation. Tympanosclerosis was determined to be the cause of the conductive component of her hearing loss in the right ear. No medical or surgical intervention was recommended. She was referred to audiology for a hearing aid evaluation, where she purchased and was fit with bilateral amplification.

7.26 Case 26

7.26.1 Case History

The patient reported that his hearing had recently decreased bilaterally. The ears seemed to be equal in hearing. He had to increase the volume of his hearing aids to hear well. Sound was also distorted bilaterally. He had some dizziness, but this was mainly when he stood up. He also had dizziness when he laid in bed at night and quickly turned his head. He had otosurgery for otosclerosis bilaterally. He was concerned about being able to drive a car. He had bilateral, constant tinnitus that was bothersome only when he removed his hearing aids at night. He had an intermittent sensation of pressure and fluid bilaterally. He did not report other otologic symptoms or history.

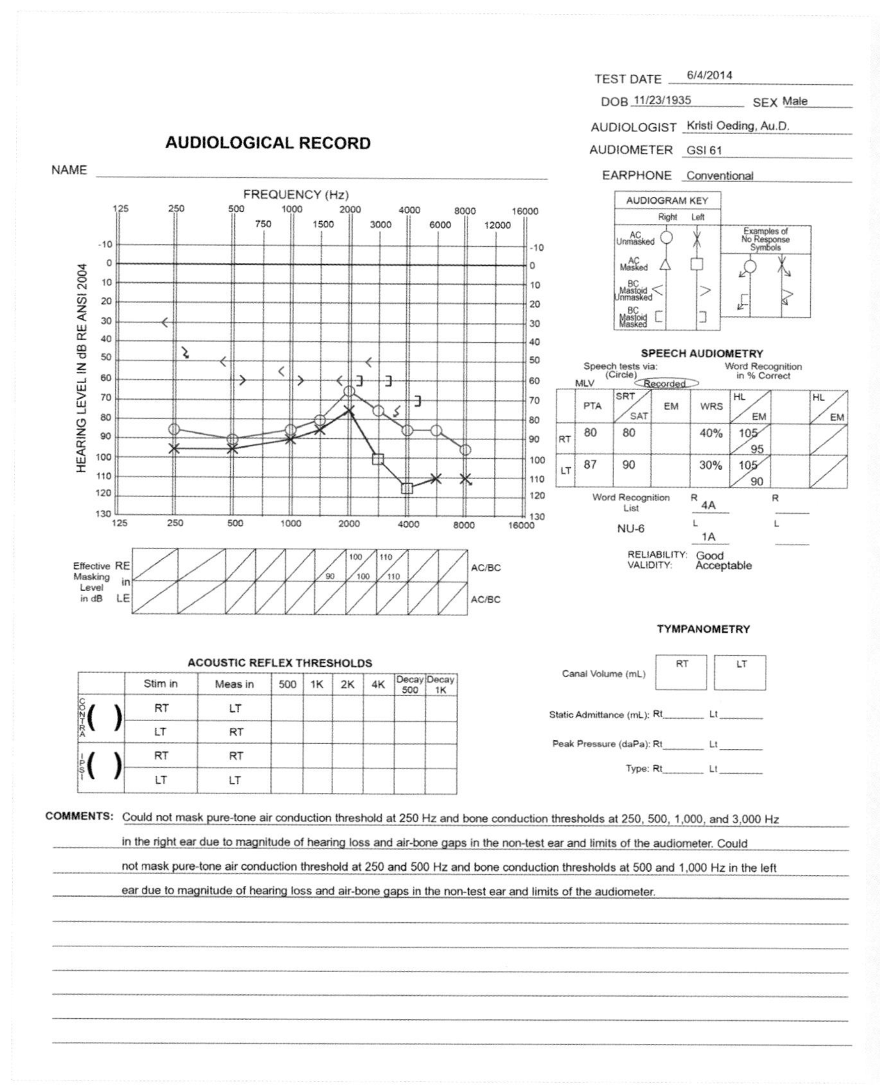

AUDIOLOGICAL RECORD

NAME

TEST DATE 6/4/2014
DOB 11/23/1935 SEX Male
AUDIOLOGIST Kristi Oeding, Au.D.
AUDIOMETER GSI 61
EARPHONE Conventional

SPEECH AUDIOMETRY

Speech tests via: (Circle) MLV Recorded

Word Recognition in % Correct

	PTA	SRT / SAT	EM	WRS	HL / EM	HL / EM
RT	80	80		40%	105 / 95	
LT	87	90		30%	105 / 90	

Word Recognition List: NU-6 R 4A L 1A; R ___ L ___

RELIABILITY: Good
VALIDITY: Acceptable

TYMPANOMETRY

	RT	LT
Canal Volume (mL)		

Static Admittance (mL): Rt____ Lt____
Peak Pressure (daPa): Rt____ Lt____
Type: Rt____ Lt____

ACOUSTIC REFLEX THRESHOLDS

	Stim in	Meas in	500	1K	2K	4K	Decay 500	Decay 1K
CONTRA ( )	RT	LT						
	LT	RT						
IPSI ( )	RT	RT						
	LT	LT						

COMMENTS: Could not mask pure-tone air conduction threshold at 250 Hz and bone conduction thresholds at 250, 500, 1,000, and 3,000 Hz in the right ear due to magnitude of hearing loss and air-bone gaps in the non-test ear and limits of the audiometer. Could not mask pure-tone air conduction threshold at 250 and 500 Hz and bone conduction thresholds at 500 and 1,000 Hz in the left ear due to magnitude of hearing loss and air-bone gaps in the non-test ear and limits of the audiometer.

Fig. 7.26 Audiogram of a patient who has had otosurgery for otosclerosis bilaterally and is now starting to have dizziness.

7.26.2 Interpretation

Right ear—Pure-tone thresholds revealed a severe mixed hearing loss from 250 to 1,500 Hz, rising to a moderately severe sensorineural hearing loss at 2,000 Hz, and sloping to a severe to profound mixed hearing loss from 3,000 to 8,000 Hz. The SRT revealed a severe loss in the ability to receive speech and was in agreement with the PTA. The WRS revealed a very poor ability to recognize speech. Immittance testing was not measured due to previous otosurgery.

Left ear—Pure-tone thresholds revealed a profound mixed hearing loss from 250 to 500 Hz, rising to severe from 1,000 to 2,000 Hz, and sloping to profound from 3,000 to 8,000 Hz. The SRT revealed a severe loss in the ability to receive speech and was in agreement with the PTA. The WRS revealed a very poor ability to recognize speech. Immittance testing was not measured due to previous otosurgery.

7.26.3 Intervention

The patient was diagnosed with BPPV and was counseled on performing the Epley maneuver. The otologist reported that the otosclerosis had progressed. The patient was counseled on considering a cochlear implant given that his hearing had steadily decreased. Other audiological recommendations included an annual hearing test, HAT, and hearing protection in noise.

7.27 Case 27

7.27.1 Case History

The patient was a 92-year-old female with a 60-year history of hearing loss. The patient's daughter attended the appointment and acted as her historian. The patient had used amplification in the right ear for approximately 20 years. She perceived balanced hearing loss, but reported that amplification was never recommended for the left ear. There was a report of only one other family member, the patient's maternal aunt, having had significant hearing loss early in life. The patient denied any tinnitus or dizziness. There was no reported history of known ear pathology, otosurgery, or noise exposure.

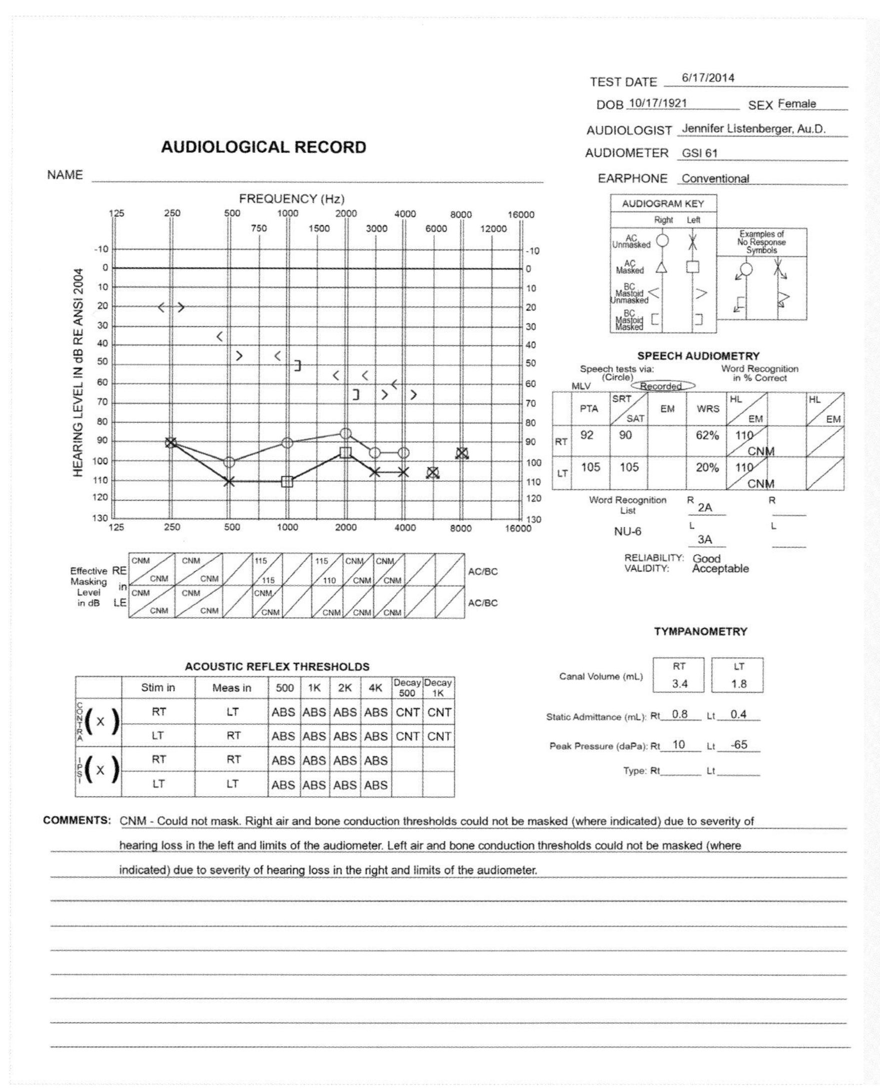

AUDIOLOGICAL RECORD

NAME

TEST DATE 6/17/2014
DOB 10/17/1921 SEX Female
AUDIOLOGIST Jennifer Listenberger, Au.D.
AUDIOMETER GSI 61
EARPHONE Conventional

Effective Masking Level in dB

RE	AC/BC	CNM / CNM	CNM / CNM		115 / 115		115 / 110	CNM / CNM	CNM / CNM		
LE	AC/BC	CNM / CNM	CNM / CNM		CNM / CNM		/ CNM	/ CNM	/ CNM		

SPEECH AUDIOMETRY

Speech tests via: (Circle) MLV Recorded

Word Recognition in % Correct

	PTA	SRT / SAT	EM	WRS	HL / EM	HL / EM
RT	92	90		62%	110 / CNM	
LT	105	105		20%	110 / CNM	

Word Recognition List: NU-6 R 2A L 3A; R L

RELIABILITY: Good
VALIDITY: Acceptable

ACOUSTIC REFLEX THRESHOLDS

	Stim in	Meas in	500	1K	2K	4K	Decay 500	Decay 1K
CONTRA (X)	RT	LT	ABS	ABS	ABS	ABS	CNT	CNT
	LT	RT	ABS	ABS	ABS	ABS	CNT	CNT
IPSI (X)	RT	RT	ABS	ABS	ABS	ABS		
	LT	LT	ABS	ABS	ABS	ABS		

TYMPANOMETRY

	RT	LT
Canal Volume (mL)	3.4	1.8

Static Admittance (mL): Rt 0.8 Lt 0.4
Peak Pressure (daPa): Rt 10 Lt -65
Type: Rt ____ Lt ____

COMMENTS: CNM - Could not mask. Right air and bone conduction thresholds could not be masked (where indicated) due to severity of hearing loss in the left and limits of the audiometer. Left air and bone conduction thresholds could not be masked (where indicated) due to severity of hearing loss in the right and limits of the audiometer.

Fig. 7.27 Audiogram of a patient with a 60-year history of hearing loss with the use of amplification in the right ear for the last 20 years.

7.27.2 Interpretation

Right ear—Pure-tone air and bone conduction threshold testing revealed a flat severe and profound mixed hearing loss at 250 to 8,000 Hz, with no measurable response within the limits of the audiometer at 6,000 and 8,000 Hz. The SRT revealed a severe loss in the ability to receive speech and was in agreement with the PTA. The WRS revealed a moderate difficulty in the ability to recognize speech. Immittance testing revealed a normal tympanogram with a large ear canal volume. The acoustic reflex thresholds were absent for ipsilateral and contralateral stimulation at all frequencies. Acoustic reflex decay could not be measured due to absent reflex thresholds.

Left ear—Pure-tone air and bone conduction threshold testing revealed a severe mixed hearing loss at 250 Hz sloping to profound at 500 to 8,000 Hz, with no measurable response within the limits of the audiometer at 6,000 and 8,000 Hz. The SRT revealed a profound loss in the ability to receive speech and was in agreement with the PTA. The WRS revealed a very poor ability to recognize speech. Immittance testing revealed a normal tympanogram. The acoustic reflex thresholds were absent for ipsilateral and contralateral stimulation at all frequencies. Acoustic reflex decay could not be measured due to absent reflex thresholds.

7.27.3 Intervention

The patient will follow up with the otologist as scheduled. The audiological recommendations were to continue use of amplification for the right ear and consider options for alternative amplification, such as a BAHA, as well as amplification for the left ear, evaluation for HAT, and return for hearing testing as needed.

7.28 Case 28

7.28.1 Case History

The patient was a 68-year-old male stating that his hearing had recently decreased in the right ear. He reported that he felt congested, with fullness in his right ear. He stated that for years he had always felt the hearing in the right ear was poorer than in the left ear. He had tinnitus bilaterally. He had been around noise throughout his life when he was racing cars. He reported this hearing decrease happened in the past few weeks as his seasonal allergies worsened.

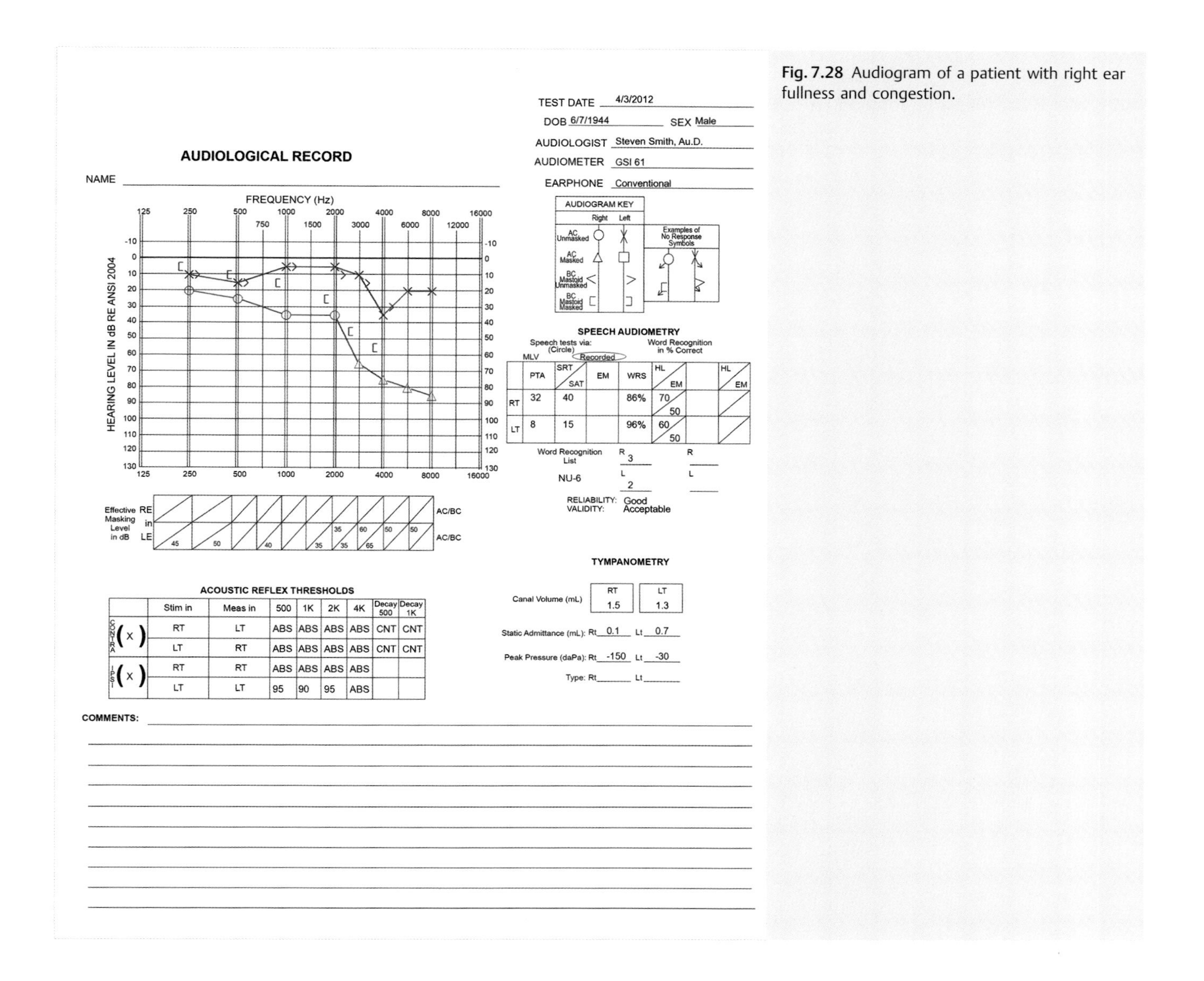

AUDIOLOGICAL RECORD

NAME

TEST DATE 4/3/2012

DOB 6/7/1944 SEX Male

AUDIOLOGIST Steven Smith, Au.D.

AUDIOMETER GSI 61

EARPHONE Conventional

SPEECH AUDIOMETRY

Speech tests via: (Circle) MLV Recorded

Word Recognition in % Correct

	PTA	SRT / SAT	EM	WRS	HL / EM		HL / EM
RT	32	40		86%	70 / 50		
LT	8	15		96%	60 / 50		

Word Recognition List NU-6: R 3, L 2

RELIABILITY: Good

VALIDITY: Acceptable

TYMPANOMETRY

	RT	LT
Canal Volume (mL)	1.5	1.3

Static Admittance (mL): Rt 0.1 Lt 0.7

Peak Pressure (daPa): Rt -150 Lt -30

Type: Rt ____ Lt ____

ACOUSTIC REFLEX THRESHOLDS

	Stim in	Meas in	500	1K	2K	4K	Decay 500	Decay 1K
CONTRA (x)	RT	LT	ABS	ABS	ABS	ABS	CNT	CNT
	LT	RT	ABS	ABS	ABS	ABS	CNT	CNT
IPSI (x)	RT	RT	ABS	ABS	ABS	ABS		
	LT	LT	95	90	95	ABS		

COMMENTS:

Fig. 7.28 Audiogram of a patient with right ear fullness and congestion.

7.28.2 Interpretation

Right ear—Slight to mild mixed hearing loss from 250 to 2,000 Hz, sloping to moderately severe to severe at 3,000 to 8,000 Hz. The SRT revealed a mild loss in the ability to receive speech and was in agreement with the PTA. The WRS revealed a slight difficulty in the ability to recognize speech. Immittance testing revealed excessive negative pressure and a hypocompliant tympanogram. The acoustic reflex thresholds with ipsilateral and contralateral stimulation were absent from 500 to 4,000 Hz. Acoustic reflex decay could not be measured.

Left ear—Normal hearing from 250 to 3,000 Hz, sloping to a mild sensorineural hearing loss at 4,000 Hz, and rising to slight at 6,000 to 8,000 Hz. The SRT was normal and was in agreement with the PTA. The WRS was normal. Immittance testing revealed a normal tympanogram. The acoustic reflex thresholds with ipsilateral stimulation were normal from 500 to 2,000 Hz and absent at 4,000 Hz. The acoustic reflex thresholds with contralateral stimulation from 500 to 4,000 Hz were absent. Acoustic reflex decay could not be measured.

7.28.3 Intervention

The patient was referred to an ENT specialist regarding his mixed and asymmetric hearing loss. He was prescribed allergy medication to help with his eustachian tube dysfunction. After this was cleared he was referred for an ABR to rule out retrocochlear pathology.

7.29 Case 29

7.29.1 Case History

The patient reported progression of hearing loss and increased tinnitus, particularly in the right ear, over the past 4 months. The tinnitus was described as insect sounds and was affecting her ability to sleep. She had bilateral intermittent otalgia. She had dizziness every day, with and without head movement, that lasted for a few seconds. She had a history of chronic ear disease. She had white otorrhea from the right ear over the last few months. She had had a tympanomastoidectomy and ossicular chain reconstruction in the right ear and a tympanoplasty in the left ear. She did not report other otologic symptoms or history.

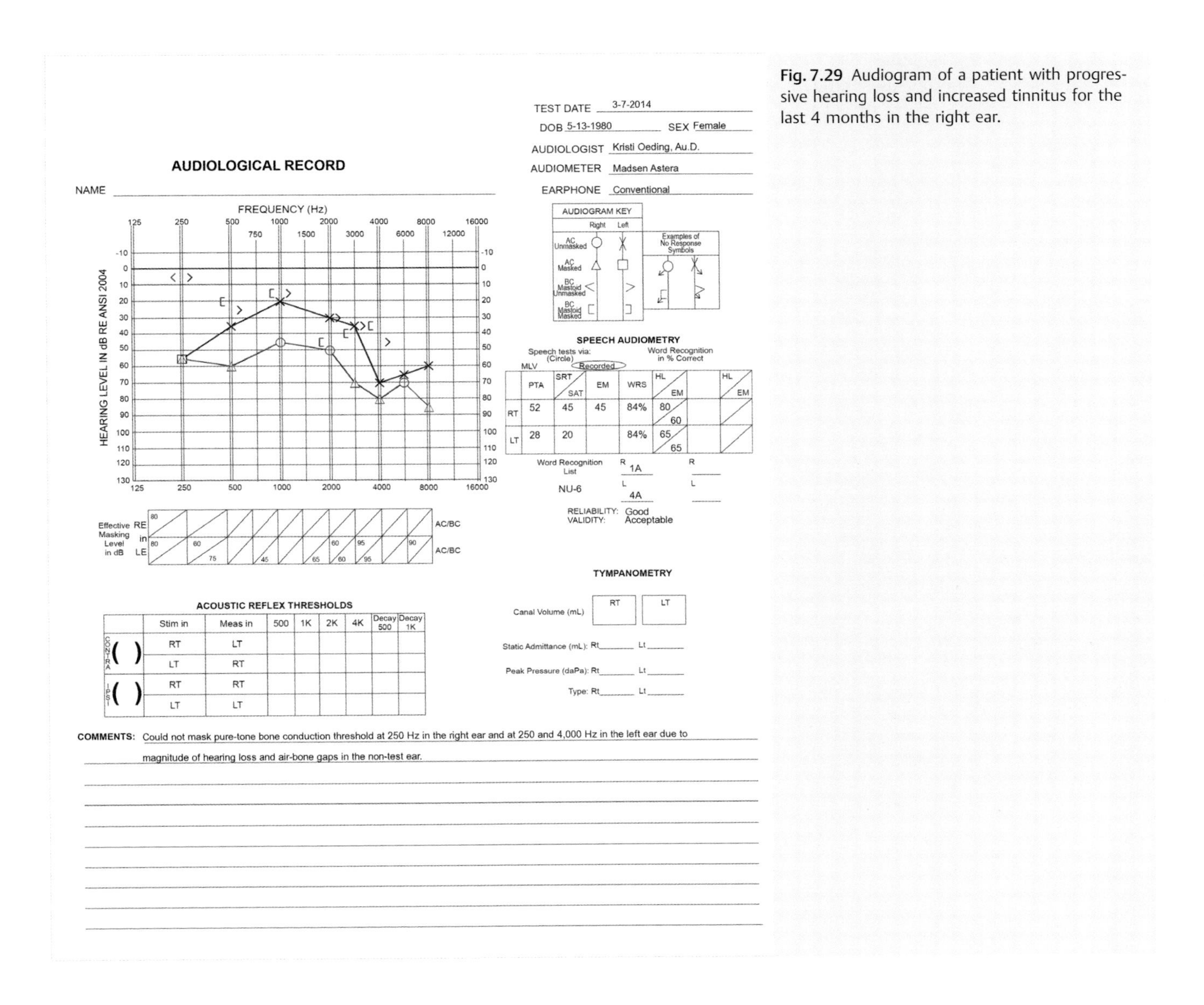

Fig. 7.29 Audiogram of a patient with progressive hearing loss and increased tinnitus for the last 4 months in the right ear.

7.29.2 Interpretation

Right ear—Pure-tone thresholds revealed a moderate to moderately severe mixed hearing loss from 250 to 500 Hz, rising to moderate from 1,000 to 2,000 Hz, and sloping to moderately severe to severe from 3,000 to 8,000 Hz. The SRT revealed a moderate loss in the ability to receive speech and was in agreement with the PTA. The WRS revealed a slight difficulty in the ability to recognize speech. Immittance testing could not be measured due to previous otosurgery.

Left ear—Pure-tone thresholds revealed a moderate rising to a slight mixed hearing loss from 250 to 1,000 Hz, sloping to a mild sensorineural hearing loss from 2,000 to 3,000 Hz, and sloping to a moderately severe mixed hearing loss from 4,000 to 8,000 Hz. The SRT revealed a slight loss in the ability to receive speech and was in agreement with the PTA. The WRS revealed a slight difficulty in the ability to recognize speech. Immittance testing could not be measured due to previous otosurgery.

7.29.3 Intervention

The otologist reported an ear infection in the right ear. The patient was provided with medication and told to follow up in 1 month. At that time, further surgery will be considered. The audiological recommendations included an annual hearing test, a hearing aid evaluation pending medical clearance, HAT, and hearing protection in noise.

7.30 Case 30

7.30.1 Case History

The patient had returned for testing to monitor hearing sensitivity. There was a long-standing history of mixed hearing loss in the left ear. The patient had a history of chronic otitis media, cholesteatoma, and multiple surgeries, including mastoidectomy and ossiculoplasty. There was a history of constant bilateral tinnitus. The patient reported no significant changes in hearing over the past few years. The last hearing test was completed 1 year ago.

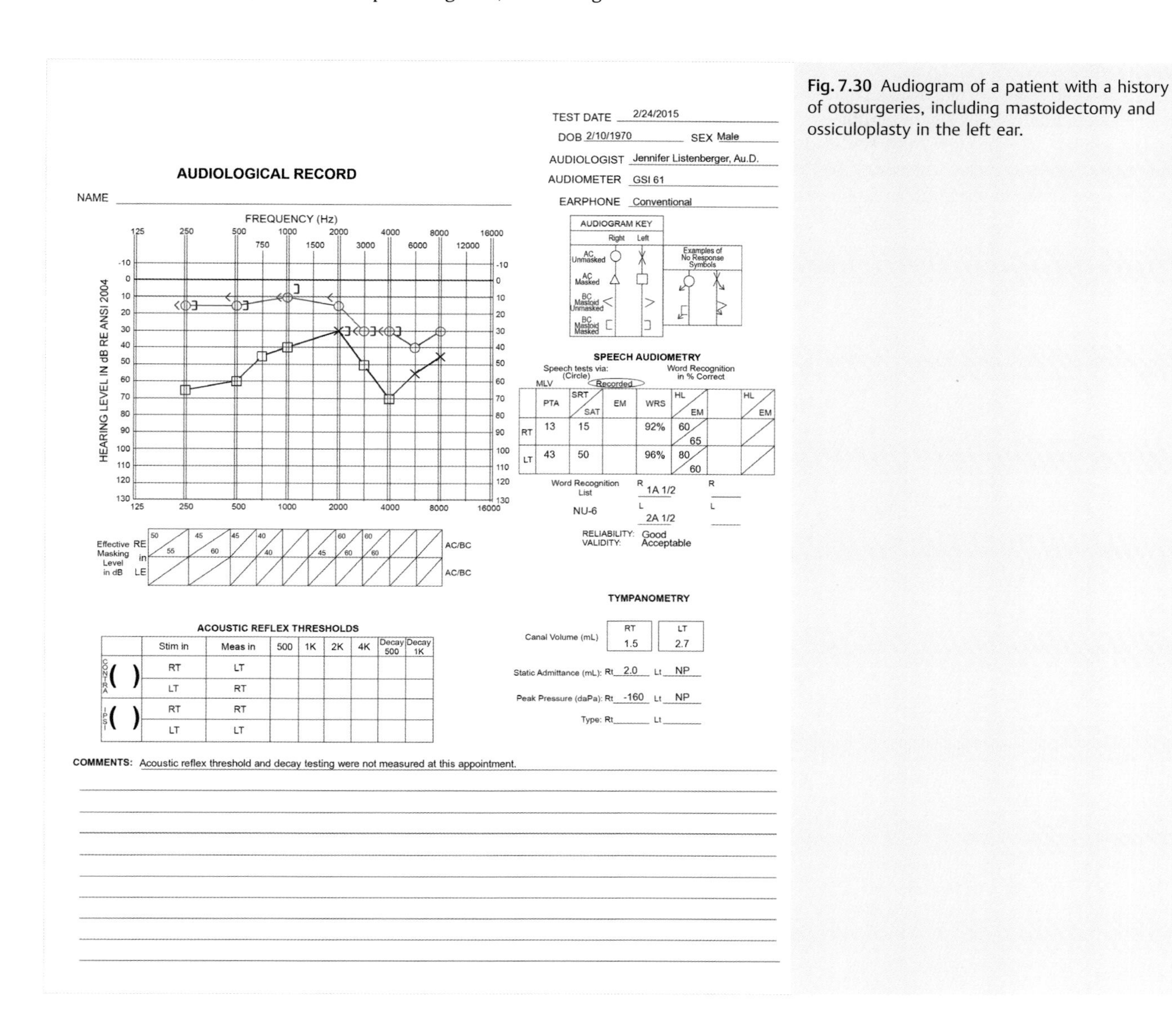

AUDIOLOGICAL RECORD

NAME

TEST DATE 2/24/2015
DOB 2/10/1970 SEX Male
AUDIOLOGIST Jennifer Listenberger, Au.D.
AUDIOMETER GSI 61
EARPHONE Conventional

Effective Masking Level in dB: RE in AC/BC: 50, 55, 45, 60, 45, 40, 40, 45, 60, 60, 60, 60; LE in AC/BC

SPEECH AUDIOMETRY

Speech tests via: (Circle) MLV Recorded — Word Recognition in % Correct

	PTA	SRT/SAT	EM	WRS	HL/EM		HL/EM
RT	13	15		92%	60/65		
LT	43	50		96%	80/60		

Word Recognition List NU-6: R 1A 1/2; L 2A 1/2

RELIABILITY: Good
VALIDITY: Acceptable

TYMPANOMETRY

Canal Volume (mL): RT 1.5; LT 2.7
Static Admittance (mL): Rt 2.0 Lt NP
Peak Pressure (daPa): Rt -160 Lt NP
Type: Rt ___ Lt ___

ACOUSTIC REFLEX THRESHOLDS

	Stim in	Meas in	500	1K	2K	4K	Decay 500	Decay 1K
CONTRA ( )	RT	LT						
	LT	RT						
IPSI ( )	RT	RT						
	LT	LT						

COMMENTS: Acoustic reflex threshold and decay testing were not measured at this appointment.

Fig. 7.30 Audiogram of a patient with a history of otosurgeries, including mastoidectomy and ossiculoplasty in the left ear.

7.30.2 Interpretation

Right ear—Pure-tone air and bone conduction threshold testing revealed normal hearing sensitivity at 250 through 2,000 Hz, then sloping to mild sensorineural hearing loss at 3,000 through 8,000 Hz. The SRT revealed a normal ability to receive speech and was in agreement with the PTA. The WRS revealed a normal ability to recognize speech. Immittance testing revealed a hypercompliant tympanic membrane with excessive negative pressure. Acoustic reflex threshold and decay testing were not measured.

Left ear—Pure-tone air and bone conduction threshold testing revealed a moderately severe gradually rising to mild mixed hearing loss at 250 through 2,000 Hz, sloping to moderate to moderately severe mixed hearing loss at 3,000 through 4,000 Hz, and rising to moderate at 6,000 and 8,000 Hz. The SRT revealed a moderate loss in the ability to receive speech and was in agreement with the PTA. The WRS revealed a normal ability to recognize speech. Immittance testing revealed a flat tympanogram with a large ear canal volume. Acoustic reflex threshold and decay testing were not measured.

7.30.3 Intervention

Test results were reviewed with the patient, and it was explained that his hearing had remained stable with no significant changes in the measured thresholds or WRS. The patient will follow up with an otologist as scheduled. The audiological recommendations were to return for a hearing test after medical management and as needed and to discuss amplification for the left ear as well as the use of HAT technology.

8 Nonorganic Hearing Loss Cases

8.1 Case 1

8.1.1 Case History

A 53-year-old female entered the clinic for a hearing evaluation. She stated that a few months ago she had had pain in her left ear that was caused by an ear infection. She went to the emergency department and reported that her ear was drained several times. Since that time, she continued to have pain in that ear and reported some drainage from that ear. She reported that she cannot hear anything from the left ear.

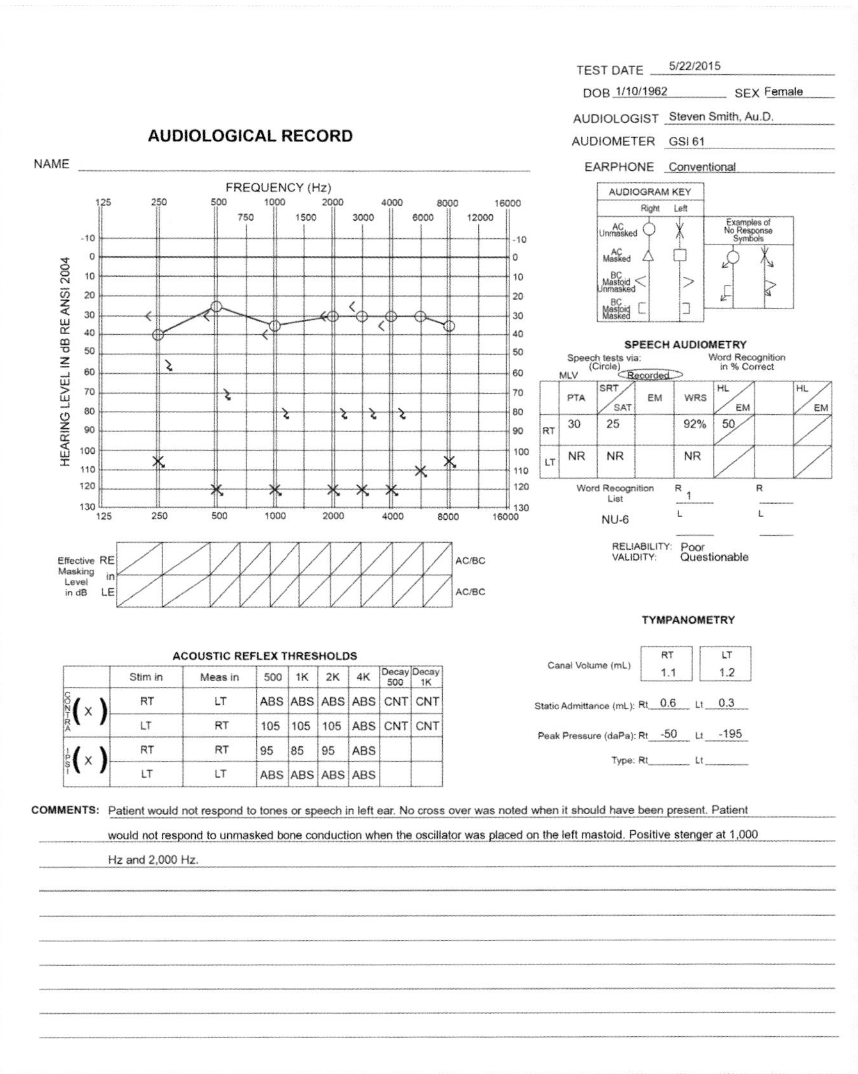

AUDIOLOGICAL RECORD

TEST DATE 5/22/2015
DOB 1/10/1962 SEX Female
AUDIOLOGIST Steven Smith, Au.D.
AUDIOMETER GSI 61
EARPHONE Conventional
NAME

SPEECH AUDIOMETRY

	PTA	SRT/SAT	EM	WRS	HL/EM		HL/EM
RT	30	25		92%	50		
LT	NR	NR		NR			

Speech tests via: (Circle) MLV Recorded
Word Recognition List: NU-6, R 1

RELIABILITY: Poor
VALIDITY: Questionable

ACOUSTIC REFLEX THRESHOLDS

	Stim in	Meas in	500	1K	2K	4K	Decay 500	Decay 1K
CONTRA	RT	LT	ABS	ABS	ABS	ABS	CNT	CNT
CONTRA	LT	RT	105	105	105	ABS	CNT	CNT
IPSI	RT	RT	95	85	95	ABS		
IPSI	LT	LT	ABS	ABS	ABS	ABS		

TYMPANOMETRY

	RT	LT
Canal Volume (mL)	1.1	1.2
Static Admittance (mL)	0.6	0.3
Peak Pressure (daPa)	-50	-195
Type		

COMMENTS: Patient would not respond to tones or speech in left ear. No cross over was noted when it should have been present. Patient would not respond to unmasked bone conduction when the oscillator was placed on the left mastoid. Positive stenger at 1,000 Hz and 2,000 Hz.

Fig. 8.1 Audiogram of a patient with left otalgia and otorrhea caused by an ear infection and no hearing in the left ear.

8.1.2 Interpretation

Right ear—Flat mild sensorineural hearing loss from 250 to 8,000 Hz, with slight hearing loss at 2,000 Hz. The SRT revealed a slight loss in the ability to receive speech and was in agreement with the PTA. The WRS was normal. Immittance testing revealed a normal tympanogram. The acoustic reflex thresholds with ipsilateral stimulation were normal from 500 to 2,000 Hz and absent at 4,000 Hz. The acoustic reflex thresholds with contralateral stimulation were elevated from 500 to 2,000 Hz and absent at 4,000 Hz. Acoustic reflex decay could not be measured.

Left ear—No response was obtained for unmasked pure-tone air conduction or bone conduction testing. No crossover was noted when this should have been present without masking. The patient did not respond to unmasked speech testing. A Stenger test was positive at 1,000 and 2,000 Hz. Immittance testing revealed a tympanogram with excessive negative pressure. The acoustic reflexes with ipsilateral and contralateral stimulation were absent at all frequencies. Acoustic reflex decay could not be measured.

8.1.3 Intervention

The patient was counseled regarding the lack of consistent results. She was referred to an ENT specialist regarding the possible ear infection. It was also recommended that she receive a latency intensity function ABR to obtain further information on possible hearing thresholds.

8.2 Case 2

8.2.1 Case History

A 57-year-old female reported an 11-year history of chronic left ear infections that started while she was in Iraq for 14 months in 2003 and 2004. She also reported excessive noise exposure during that time due to frequent cannon fire outside the medical tent where she worked. She reported continued pain and fullness in the left ear. There was a report of constant bilateral tinnitus that started after one explosion. The tinnitus was reported to be worse and louder in the left ear. She described the tinnitus to be a loud, steady ringing sound that caused great stress and caused her not to hear well. She reported no otosurgery or familial hearing loss and denied any dizziness.

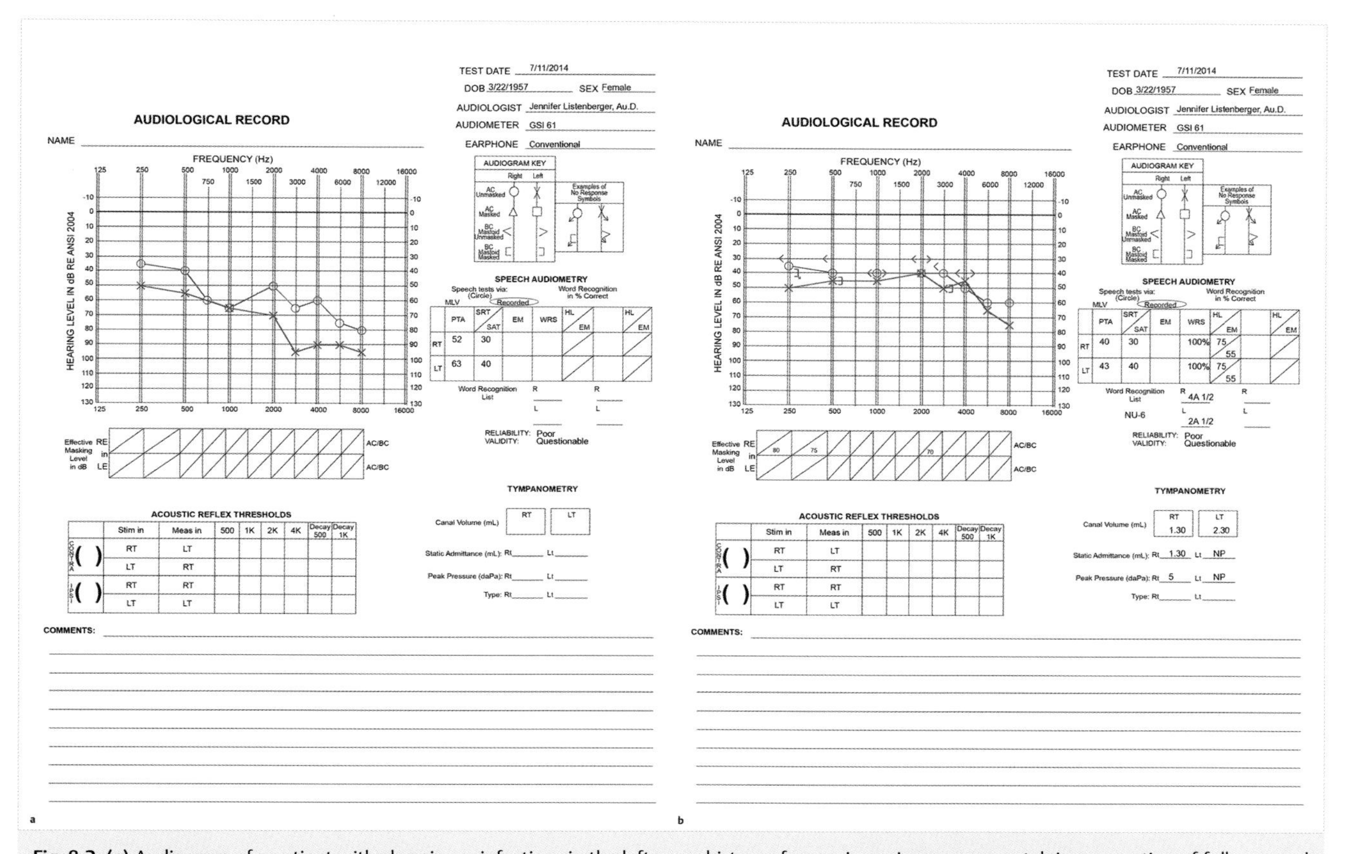

Fig. 8.2 **(a)** Audiogram of a patient with chronic ear infections in the left ear, a history of excessive noise exposure, otalgia, a sensation of fullness, and tinnitus in the left ear. **(b)** Audiogram of the same patient after significant reinstruction.

8.2.2 Interpretation 1

Right ear—Pure-tone air conduction testing originally revealed a mild hearing loss at 250 to 500 Hz, sloping to moderately severe at 750 to 4,000 Hz, with a rise to moderate at 2,000 Hz, and sloping to severe at 6,000 to 8,000 Hz. The SRT revealed a mild loss in the ability to receive speech and was not in agreement with the PTA; there was a 22 dB HL difference between the PTA and the SRT.

Left ear—Pure-tone air conduction testing originally revealed a moderate sloping to moderately severe hearing loss at 250 to 2,000 Hz, sloping to profound at 3,000 Hz, rising to severe at 4,000 to 6,000 Hz, and sloping to profound at 8,000 Hz. The SRT revealed a mild loss in the ability to receive speech and was not in agreement with the PTA; there was a 23 dB HL difference between the PTA and the SRT.

Due to a significant difference between the SRT and PTA bilaterally and due to inconsistencies in responses and behaviors during testing, the pure-tone audiogram was repeated during the same visit. A significant amount of repeated reinstruction was given during testing.

8.2.3 Interpretation 2

Right ear—Pure-tone air and bone conduction testing revealed a mild sensorineural hearing loss at 250 to 3,000 Hz, sloping to moderate to moderately severe at 4,000 to 8,000 Hz. A significant improvement in air conduction thresholds was noted. The SRT revealed a mild loss in the ability to receive speech and was now in agreement with the PTA. The WRS revealed a normal ability to recognize speech. Immittance testing revealed a normal tympanogram. Acoustic reflex threshold and decay testing were not measured.

Left ear—Pure-tone air and bone conduction testing revealed a moderate sensorineural hearing loss at 250 to 4,000 Hz, except for mild hearing loss at 2,000 Hz, sloping to moderately severe to severe at 6,000 and 8,000 Hz. A significant improvement in air conduction thresholds was noted. The SRT revealed a mild loss in the ability to receive speech and was now in agreement with the PTA. Immittance testing revealed a flat tympanogram with a large ear canal volume. Acoustic reflex threshold and decay testing were not measured.

8.2.4 Intervention

The patient was encouraged to follow up with an otologist as scheduled. The audiological recommendations were to return for a hearing test after medical management and annually to monitor the stability of her hearing.

8.3 Case 3

8.3.1 Case History

The patient reported hearing loss and tinnitus in the right ear since radiation to the neck in 2009 for carcinoma of the right tonsil. She also reported sensitivity to loud, high-pitched sounds in the right that started after radiation therapy. Tinnitus and hearing loss were reported to be greater. There was no reported noise exposure. A family history of hearing loss was unknown.

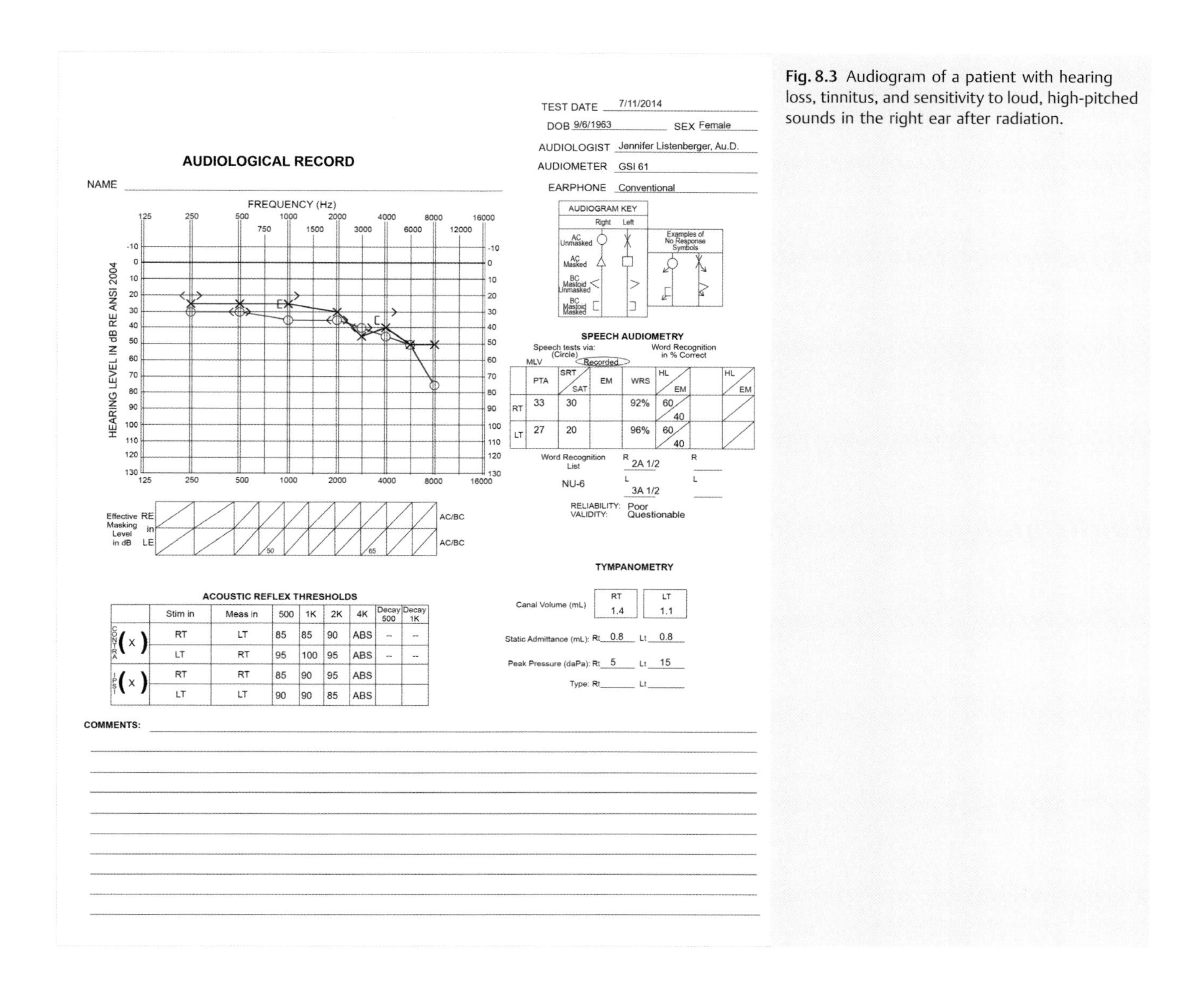

AUDIOLOGICAL RECORD

NAME

TEST DATE 7/11/2014
DOB 9/6/1963 SEX Female
AUDIOLOGIST Jennifer Listenberger, Au.D.
AUDIOMETER GSI 61
EARPHONE Conventional

SPEECH AUDIOMETRY

Speech tests via: (Circle) MLV Recorded

Word Recognition in % Correct

	PTA	SRT/SAT	EM	WRS	HL/EM
RT	33	30		92%	60/40
LT	27	20		96%	60/40

Word Recognition List: NU-6; R 2A 1/2; L 3A 1/2

RELIABILITY: Poor
VALIDITY: Questionable

ACOUSTIC REFLEX THRESHOLDS

	Stim in	Meas in	500	1K	2K	4K	Decay 500	Decay 1K
CONTRA (x)	RT	LT	85	85	90	ABS	--	--
	LT	RT	95	100	95	ABS	--	--
IPSI (x)	RT	RT	85	90	95	ABS		
	LT	LT	90	90	85	ABS		

TYMPANOMETRY

	RT	LT
Canal Volume (mL)	1.4	1.1

Static Admittance (mL): Rt 0.8 Lt 0.8
Peak Pressure (daPa): Rt 5 Lt 15
Type: Rt Lt

COMMENTS:

Fig. 8.3 Audiogram of a patient with hearing loss, tinnitus, and sensitivity to loud, high-pitched sounds in the right ear after radiation.

8.3.2 Interpretation

Right ear—Pure-tone air and bone conduction threshold testing revealed a mild sensorineural hearing loss at 250 through 3,000 Hz, sloping to moderate at 4,000 through 6,000 Hz, then sloping to severe at 8,000 Hz. The SRT revealed a mild loss in the ability to receive speech and was in agreement with the PTA. The WRS revealed a normal ability to recognize speech. Immittance testing revealed a normal tympanogram. The acoustic reflex thresholds were present and normal for ipsilateral and contralateral stimulation at 500, 1,000, and 2,000 Hz and absent at 4,000 Hz. Acoustic reflex decay was negative for contralateral stimulation at 500 and 1,000 Hz. Initially, the SRT and PTA were not in agreement, with the PTA being 20 dB HL poorer than the SRT. Repeated reinstruction was needed for pure-tone air conduction threshold testing for the right ear.

Left ear—Pure-tone air and bone conduction threshold testing revealed a slight sloping to mild sensorineural hearing loss at 250 through 4,000 Hz with a moderate notch at 3,000 Hz, then sloping to moderate at 6,000 through 8,000 Hz. The SRT revealed a slight loss in the ability to receive speech and was in agreement with the PTA. The WRS revealed a normal ability to recognize speech. Immittance testing revealed a normal tympanogram. The acoustic reflex thresholds were present and normal for ipsilateral and contralateral stimulation at 500, 1,000, and 2,000 Hz and absent at 4,000 Hz. Acoustic reflex decay was negative for contralateral stimulation at 500 and 1,000 Hz. Initially, the SRT and PTA were not in agreement, with the PTA being 20 dB HL worse than the SRT. Repeated reinstruction was needed for pure-tone air conduction threshold testing for the left ear.

8.3.3 Intervention

The patient was referred to the otologist. The audiological recommendations were to return annually for hearing testing to monitor hearing sensitivity, use hearing protection when exposed to noise, return for an evaluation for management options for tinnitus and hyperacusis, and return for an evaluation for use of amplification and HAT.

8.4 Case 4

8.4.1 Case History

The patient arrived reporting hearing loss in the left ear since 2004 when a tumor was removed; although, the ENT physician's note stated that it was likely a mastoidectomy that had been completed. She reported that she could not hear from her left ear. She did not report hearing loss in the right ear. She reported a perforation in the left tympanic membrane. Initially, she did not report otalgia, but later reported otalgia that was greater in intensity in the left ear than in the right ear. She had a history of ear infections in childhood. She did not report other otologic symptoms or history.

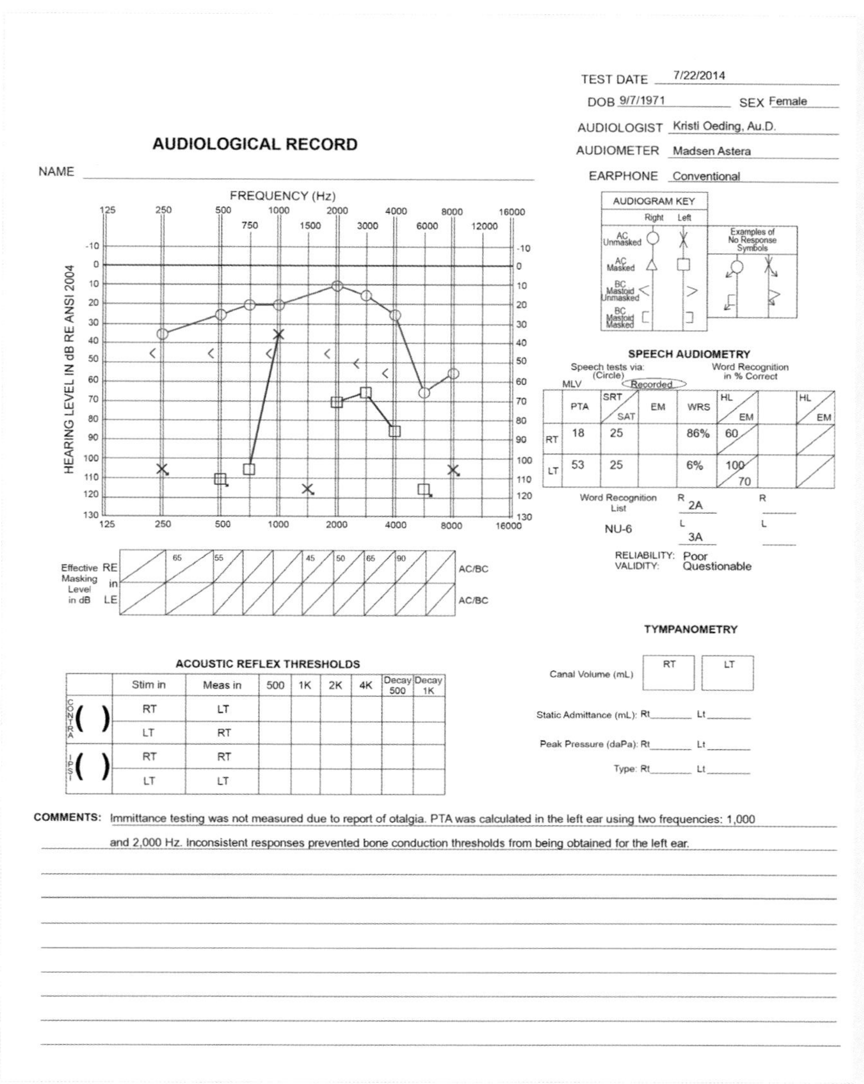

AUDIOLOGICAL RECORD

NAME

TEST DATE 7/22/2014
DOB 9/7/1971 SEX Female
AUDIOLOGIST Kristi Oeding, Au.D.
AUDIOMETER Madsen Astera
EARPHONE Conventional

SPEECH AUDIOMETRY

Speech tests via: (Circle) MLV Recorded

	PTA	SRT/SAT	EM	WRS	HL/EM	HL/EM
RT	18	25		86%	60	
LT	53	25		6%	100 / 70	

Word Recognition List: NU-6 — R 2A; L 3A

RELIABILITY: Poor
VALIDITY: Questionable

ACOUSTIC REFLEX THRESHOLDS

	Stim in	Meas in	500	1K	2K	4K	Decay 500	Decay 1K
CONTRA	RT	LT						
	LT	RT						
IPSI	RT	RT						
	LT	LT						

TYMPANOMETRY

Canal Volume (mL): RT ___ LT ___
Static Admittance (mL): Rt ___ Lt ___
Peak Pressure (daPa): Rt ___ Lt ___
Type: Rt ___ Lt ___

COMMENTS: Immittance testing was not measured due to report of otalgia. PTA was calculated in the left ear using two frequencies: 1,000 and 2,000 Hz. Inconsistent responses prevented bone conduction thresholds from being obtained for the left ear.

Fig. 8.4 Audiogram of a patient with hearing loss in the left ear likely due to a mastoidectomy. She reported a perforation in the left tympanic membrane and otalgia in the left ear.

8.4.2 Interpretation

Right ear—Pure-tone thresholds revealed a mild sensorineural hearing loss at 250 Hz gradually rising to within normal limits at 2,000 to 3000 Hz, sloping from a slight to moderately severe sensorineural hearing loss from 4,000 to 6,000 Hz, and rising to moderate at 8,000 Hz. The SRT revealed a slight loss in the ability to receive speech and was in agreement with the PTA. The WRS revealed a slight difficulty in the ability to recognize speech. Immittance testing was not measured due to the patient's report of otalgia.

Left ear—Pure-tone thresholds were profound from 250 to 750 Hz, steeply rising to mild at 1,000 Hz, steeply sloping to profound at 1,500 Hz, rising to moderately severe at 2,000 to 3,000 Hz, and sloping from severe to profound at 4,000 to 8,000 Hz. No measurable response was obtained within the limits of the audiometer at 250, 500, 1,500, 6,000, and 8,000 Hz.

Patient responses were very inconsistent after 4,000 Hz. After reinstruction and rechecking these thresholds, she was inconsistent at all frequencies bilaterally (thresholds became significantly poorer; where thresholds were once present they were now absent). The Stenger was performed at 500 and 1,000 Hz and was positive, indicating false responses. The type of hearing loss could not be determined due to patient inconsistency during bone conduction threshold testing. The SRT revealed a slight loss in the ability to receive speech and was in poor agreement with the PTA. The WRS revealed very poor recognition ability. Immittance testing was not measured due to the previous otosurgery.

8.4.3 Intervention

The otologist noted a perforation in the left tympanic membrane and otitis media. A CT scan revealed ossicular discontinuity, which the otologist thought was due to a previous cholesteatoma. The patient will return in 2 weeks to have her hearing retested due to inconsistencies and a positive Stenger. She was encouraged to be more consistent with her responses. When she returned she was more consistent and results revealed a bilateral mild to moderate mixed hearing loss. The audiological recommendations included a hearing test annually and post–medical management, a hearing aid evaluation pending medical clearance, HAT, and hearing protection in noise.

8.5 Case 5

8.5.1 Case History

A 14-year-old female was accompanied to the hearing test by her mother, who provided most of the history. The patient was referred for a diagnostic evaluation after not passing a hearing screening at school. Reportedly, a hearing test was completed last month at another center, but was not available for comparison. The patient reported a sudden change in her hearing in the right ear approximately 2 months ago. She reported needing frequent repetition, specifically with her family. She switched using her phone to the left ear because sound is clearer from the left. The patient denied tinnitus, dizziness, or aural fullness or pressure. Intermittent pain was reported for the left ear. No significant history of ear pathology, noise exposure, or familial hearing loss was reported. All developmental milestones were reported to be normal. The patient reported a significant history of migraine headaches.

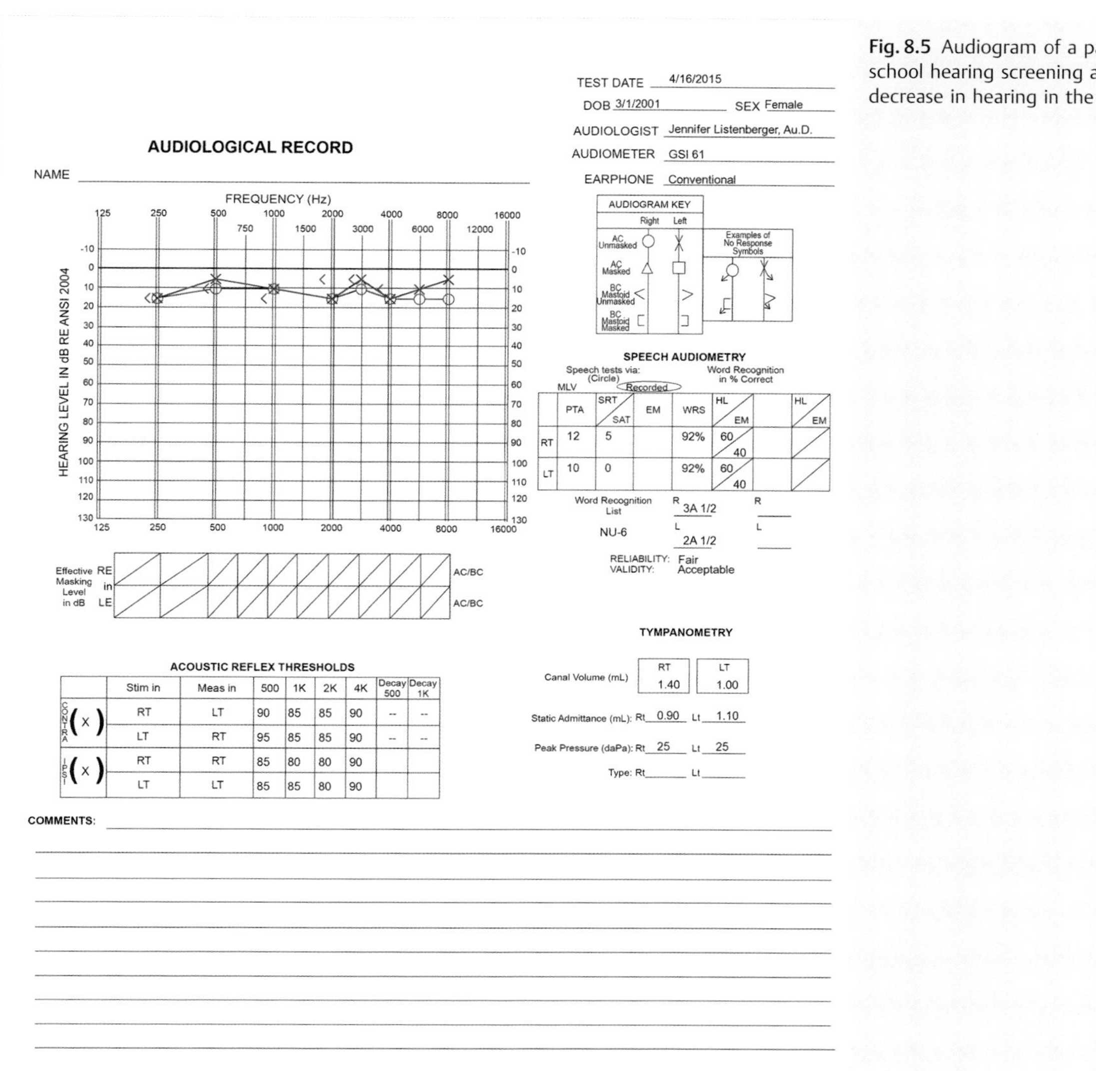

	PTA	SRT / SAT	EM	WRS	HL / EM		HL / EM
RT	12	5		92%	60 / 40		
LT	10	0		92%	60 / 40		

	Stim in	Meas in	500	1K	2K	4K	Decay 500	Decay 1K
CONTRA	RT	LT	90	85	85	90	--	--
	LT	RT	95	85	85	90	--	--
IPSI	RT	RT	85	80	80	90		
	LT	LT	85	85	80	90		

Fig. 8.5 Audiogram of a patient who failed a school hearing screening and reported a sudden decrease in hearing in the right ear.

8.5.2 Interpretation

Right ear—Pure-tone air and bone conduction threshold testing revealed normal hearing sensitivity at 250 through 8,000 Hz. The SRT revealed a normal ability to receive speech and was in agreement with the PTA. The WRS revealed a normal ability to recognize speech. Immittance testing revealed a normal tympanogram. The acoustic reflex thresholds were present and normal for ipsilateral and contralateral stimulation at 500, 1,000, 2,000, and 4,000 Hz. Acoustic reflex decay was negative for contralateral stimulation at 500 and 1,000 Hz.

Initially, the patient was not consistent with responses to pure-tone stimulation in the right ear. Her initial responses were elevated to levels of a mild and a moderate hearing loss, but changed immediately after reinstruction and the use of an ascending presentation method. Improved responses were also obtained after rapidly switching between presenting to the left and right ears and having the patient identify where the sound was.

Left ear—Pure-tone air and bone conduction threshold testing revealed normal hearing sensitivity at 250 through 8,000 Hz. The SRT revealed a normal ability to receive speech and was in agreement with the PTA. The WRS revealed a normal ability to recognize speech. Immittance testing revealed a normal tympanogram. The acoustic reflex thresholds were present and normal for ipsilateral and contralateral stimulation at 500, 1,000, 2,000, and 4,000 Hz. Acoustic reflex decay was negative for contralateral stimulation at 500 and 1,000 Hz.

8.5.3 Intervention

The patient was referred to the otologist. The patient's family was encouraged to obtain the previous hearing test to be used for comparison. A 6-month hearing test was recommended to monitor hearing sensitivity due to family concerns and patient observations.

9 Practice Cases

The following supplemental audiograms are included for further practice for the reader. This section can also be used by teachers and professors as an assignment to examine a student's ability to interpret audiograms and write a report.

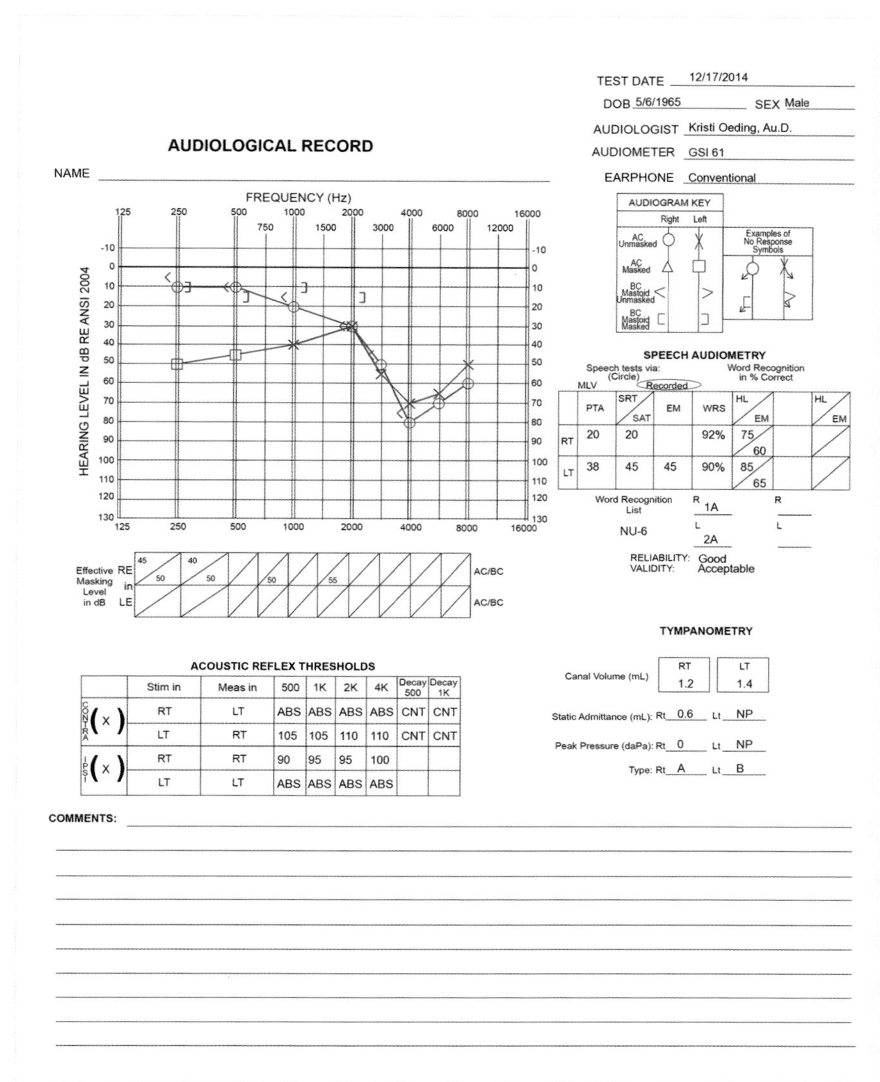

TEST DATE 12/17/2014
DOB 5/6/1965 SEX Male
AUDIOLOGIST Kristi Oeding, Au.D.
AUDIOMETER GSI 61
EARPHONE Conventional

AUDIOLOGICAL RECORD

NAME

Effective Masking Level in dB

	125	250	500	750	1000	1500	2000	3000	4000	6000	8000	
RE in	45 / 50	40 / 50		50		55						AC/BC
LE												AC/BC

SPEECH AUDIOMETRY

Speech tests via: (Circle) MLV Recorded (circled)

Word Recognition in % Correct

	PTA	SRT / SAT	EM	WRS	HL / EM		HL / EM
RT	20	20		92%	75 / 60		
LT	38	45	45	90%	85 / 65		

Word Recognition List NU-6: R 1A, L 2A; R ___, L ___

RELIABILITY: Good
VALIDITY: Acceptable

TYMPANOMETRY

	RT	LT
Canal Volume (mL)	1.2	1.4

Static Admittance (mL): Rt 0.6 Lt NP
Peak Pressure (daPa): Rt 0 Lt NP
Type: Rt A Lt B

ACOUSTIC REFLEX THRESHOLDS

	Stim in	Meas in	500	1K	2K	4K	Decay 500	Decay 1K
CONTRA (X)	RT	LT	ABS	ABS	ABS	ABS	CNT	CNT
	LT	RT	105	105	110	110	CNT	CNT
IPSI (X)	RT	RT	90	95	95	100		
	LT	LT	ABS	ABS	ABS	ABS		

COMMENTS:

Fig. 9.1 Practice audiogram case 1.

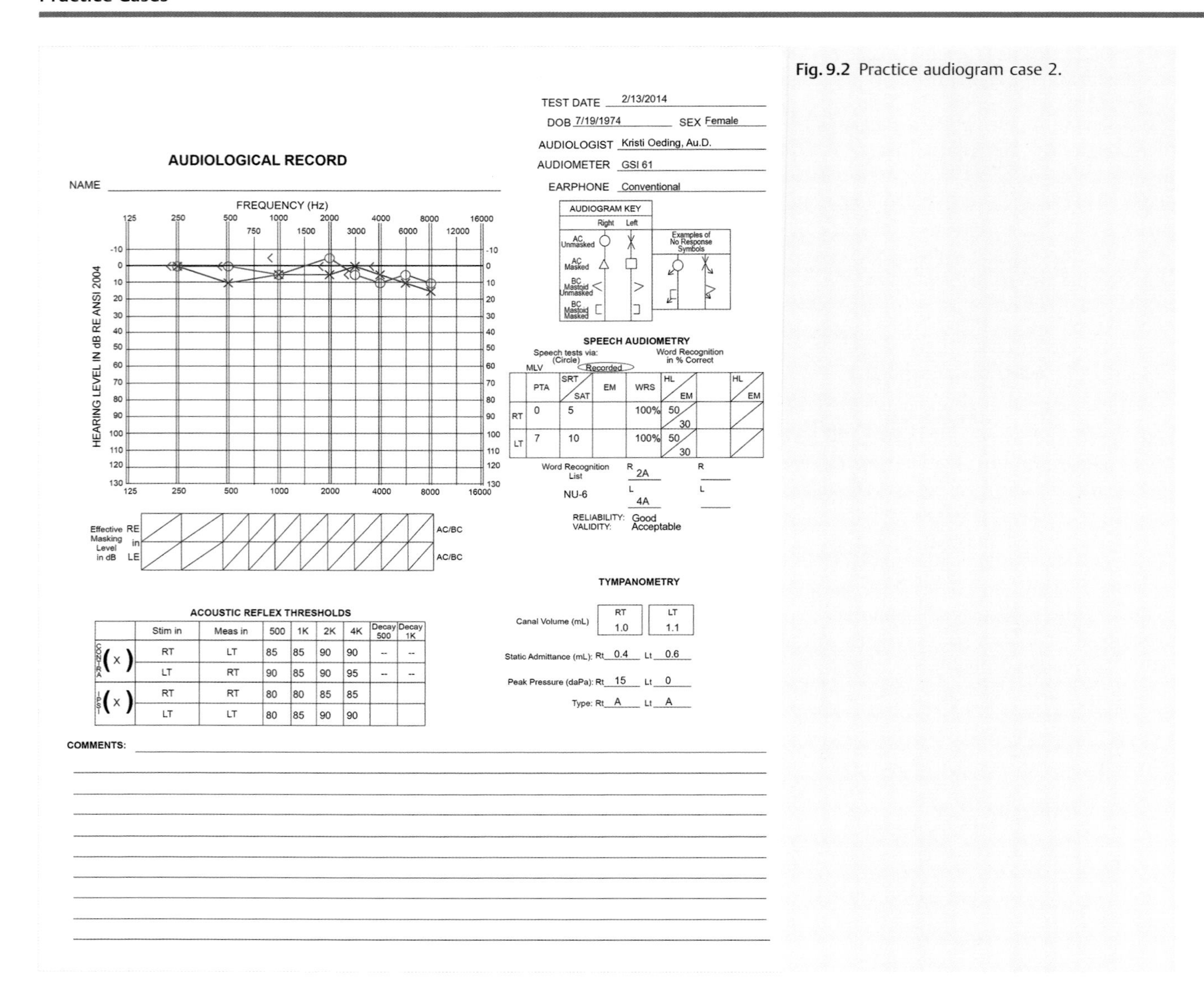

TEST DATE 2/13/2014
DOB 7/19/1974 SEX Female
AUDIOLOGIST Kristi Oeding, Au.D.
AUDIOMETER GSI 61
EARPHONE Conventional

AUDIOLOGICAL RECORD

NAME

SPEECH AUDIOMETRY

Speech tests via: (Circle) MLV Recorded

Word Recognition in % Correct

	PTA	SRT / SAT	EM	WRS	HL / EM		HL / EM
RT	0	5		100%	50 / 30		
LT	7	10		100%	50 / 30		

Word Recognition List: R 2A, L 4A
NU-6

RELIABILITY: Good
VALIDITY: Acceptable

TYMPANOMETRY

	RT	LT
Canal Volume (mL)	1.0	1.1

Static Admittance (mL): Rt 0.4 Lt 0.6
Peak Pressure (daPa): Rt 15 Lt 0
Type: Rt A Lt A

ACOUSTIC REFLEX THRESHOLDS

	Stim in	Meas in	500	1K	2K	4K	Decay 500	Decay 1K
CONTRA (X)	RT	LT	85	85	90	90	--	--
	LT	RT	90	85	90	95	--	--
IPSI (X)	RT	RT	80	80	85	85		
	LT	LT	80	85	90	90		

COMMENTS:

Fig. 9.2 Practice audiogram case 2.

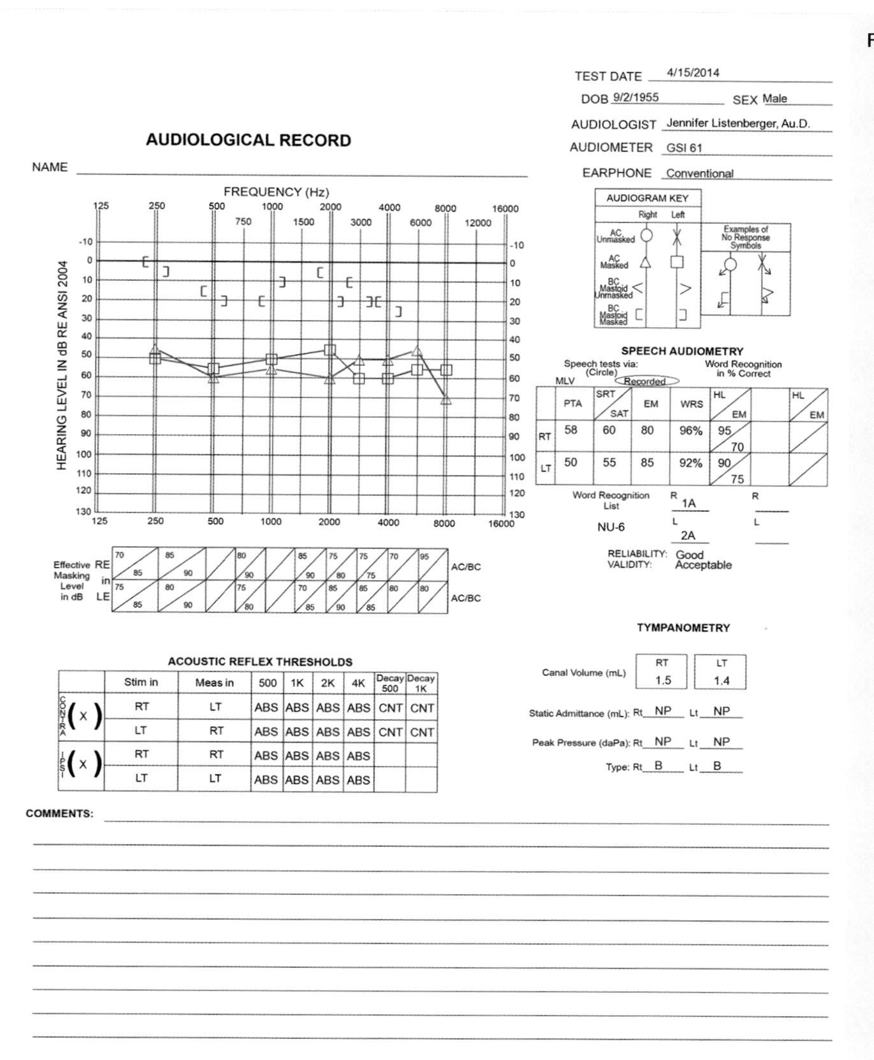

AUDIOLOGICAL RECORD

NAME

TEST DATE 4/15/2014
DOB 9/2/1955 SEX Male
AUDIOLOGIST Jennifer Listenberger, Au.D.
AUDIOMETER GSI 61
EARPHONE Conventional

Effective Masking Level in dB

RE in	70 / 85	85 / 90		80 / 90		85 / 90	75 / 80	75 / 75	70 /	95 /	AC/BC
LE in	75 / 85	80 / 90		75 / 80		70 / 85	85 / 90	85 / 85	80 /	80 /	AC/BC

SPEECH AUDIOMETRY

Speech tests via: (Circle) MLV Recorded (circled: Recorded)

Word Recognition in % Correct

	PTA	SRT / SAT	EM	WRS	HL / EM		HL / EM
RT	58	60	80	96%	95 / 70		
LT	50	55	85	92%	90 / 75		

Word Recognition List: NU-6 — R 1A, L 2A; R ___ L ___

RELIABILITY: Good
VALIDITY: Acceptable

TYMPANOMETRY

Canal Volume (mL): RT 1.5, LT 1.4
Static Admittance (mL): Rt NP Lt NP
Peak Pressure (daPa): Rt NP Lt NP
Type: Rt B Lt B

ACOUSTIC REFLEX THRESHOLDS

	Stim in	Meas in	500	1K	2K	4K	Decay 500	Decay 1K
CONTRA (X)	RT	LT	ABS	ABS	ABS	ABS	CNT	CNT
	LT	RT	ABS	ABS	ABS	ABS	CNT	CNT
IPSI (X)	RT	RT	ABS	ABS	ABS	ABS		
	LT	LT	ABS	ABS	ABS	ABS		

COMMENTS:

Fig. 9.3 Practice audiogram case 3.

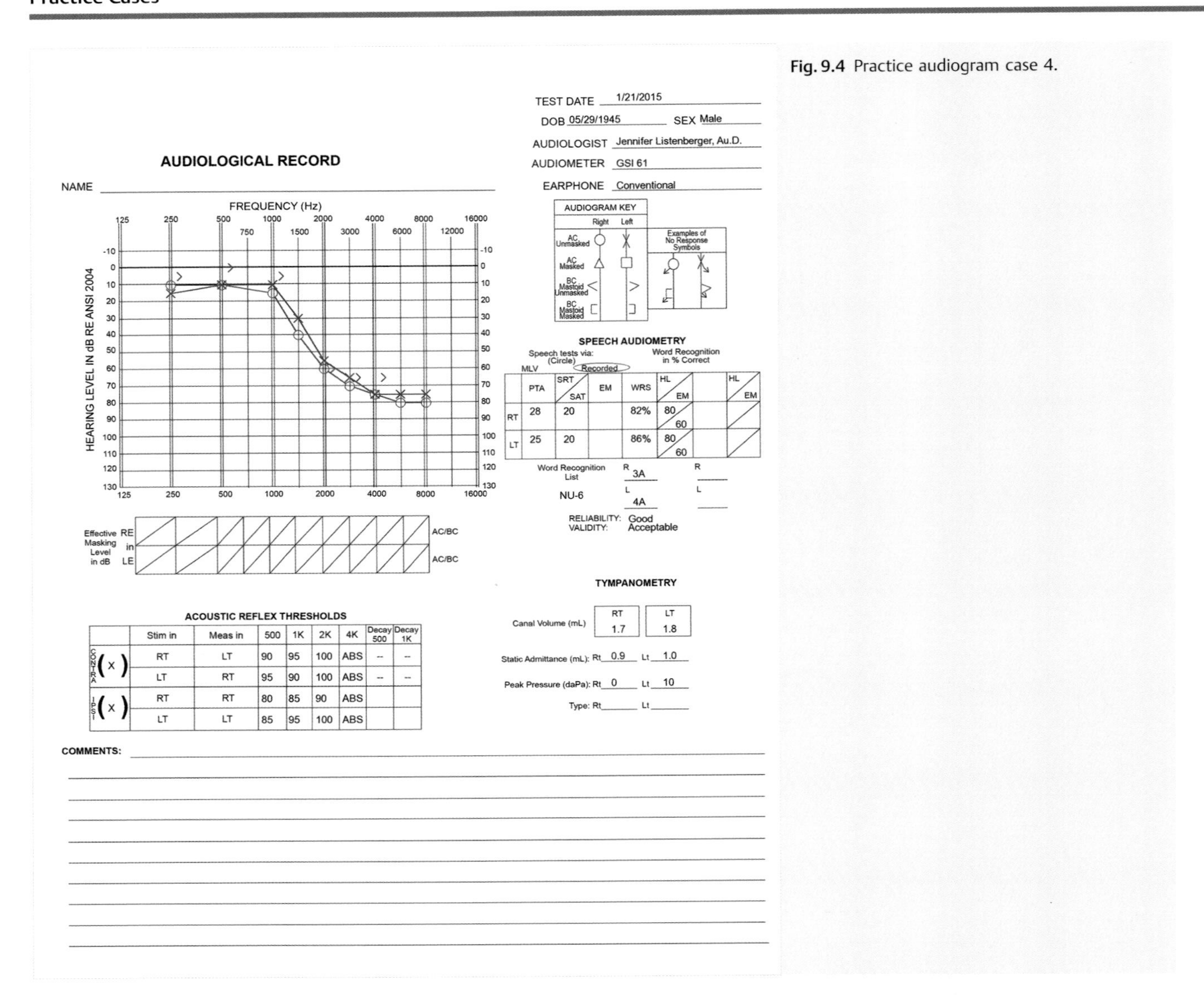

AUDIOLOGICAL RECORD

TEST DATE 1/21/2015
DOB 05/29/1945 SEX Male
AUDIOLOGIST Jennifer Listenberger, Au.D.
AUDIOMETER GSI 61
EARPHONE Conventional

NAME

SPEECH AUDIOMETRY

Speech tests via: (Circle) MLV Recorded

Word Recognition in % Correct

	PTA	SRT / SAT	EM	WRS	HL / EM		HL / EM
RT	28	20		82%	80 / 60		
LT	25	20		86%	80 / 60		

Word Recognition List: R 3A, L 4A; R ___, L ___

NU-6

RELIABILITY: Good
VALIDITY: Acceptable

TYMPANOMETRY

	RT	LT
Canal Volume (mL)	1.7	1.8

Static Admittance (mL): Rt 0.9 Lt 1.0

Peak Pressure (daPa): Rt 0 Lt 10

Type: Rt ___ Lt ___

ACOUSTIC REFLEX THRESHOLDS

	Stim in	Meas in	500	1K	2K	4K	Decay 500	Decay 1K
CONTRA (x)	RT	LT	90	95	100	ABS	--	--
	LT	RT	95	90	100	ABS	--	--
IPSI (x)	RT	RT	80	85	90	ABS		
	LT	LT	85	95	100	ABS		

COMMENTS:

Fig. 9.4 Practice audiogram case 4.

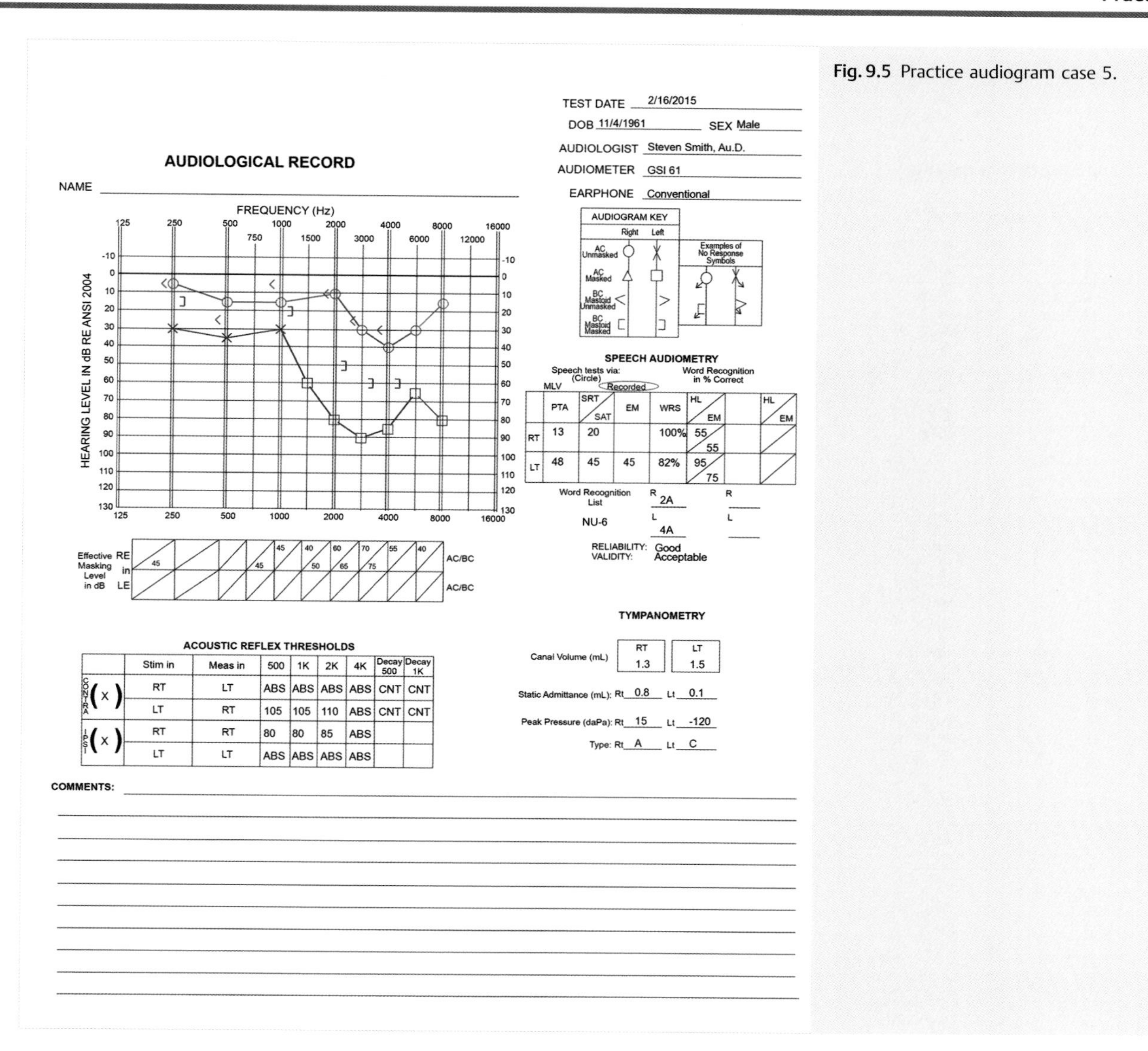

AUDIOLOGICAL RECORD

NAME

TEST DATE 2/16/2015

DOB 11/4/1961 SEX Male

AUDIOLOGIST Steven Smith, Au.D.

AUDIOMETER GSI 61

EARPHONE Conventional

SPEECH AUDIOMETRY

Speech tests via: (Circle) MLV Recorded

Word Recognition in % Correct

	PTA	SRT / SAT	EM	WRS	HL / EM		HL / EM
RT	13	20		100%	55 / 55		
LT	48	45	45	82%	95 / 75		

Word Recognition List NU-6: R 2A, L 4A; R ___, L ___

RELIABILITY: Good

VALIDITY: Acceptable

TYMPANOMETRY

Canal Volume (mL): RT 1.3, LT 1.5

Static Admittance (mL): Rt 0.8 Lt 0.1

Peak Pressure (daPa): Rt 15 Lt -120

Type: Rt A Lt C

ACOUSTIC REFLEX THRESHOLDS

	Stim in	Meas in	500	1K	2K	4K	Decay 500	Decay 1K
CONTRA (x)	RT	LT	ABS	ABS	ABS	ABS	CNT	CNT
	LT	RT	105	105	110	ABS	CNT	CNT
IPSI (x)	RT	RT	80	80	85	ABS		
	LT	LT	ABS	ABS	ABS	ABS		

COMMENTS:

Fig. 9.5 Practice audiogram case 5.

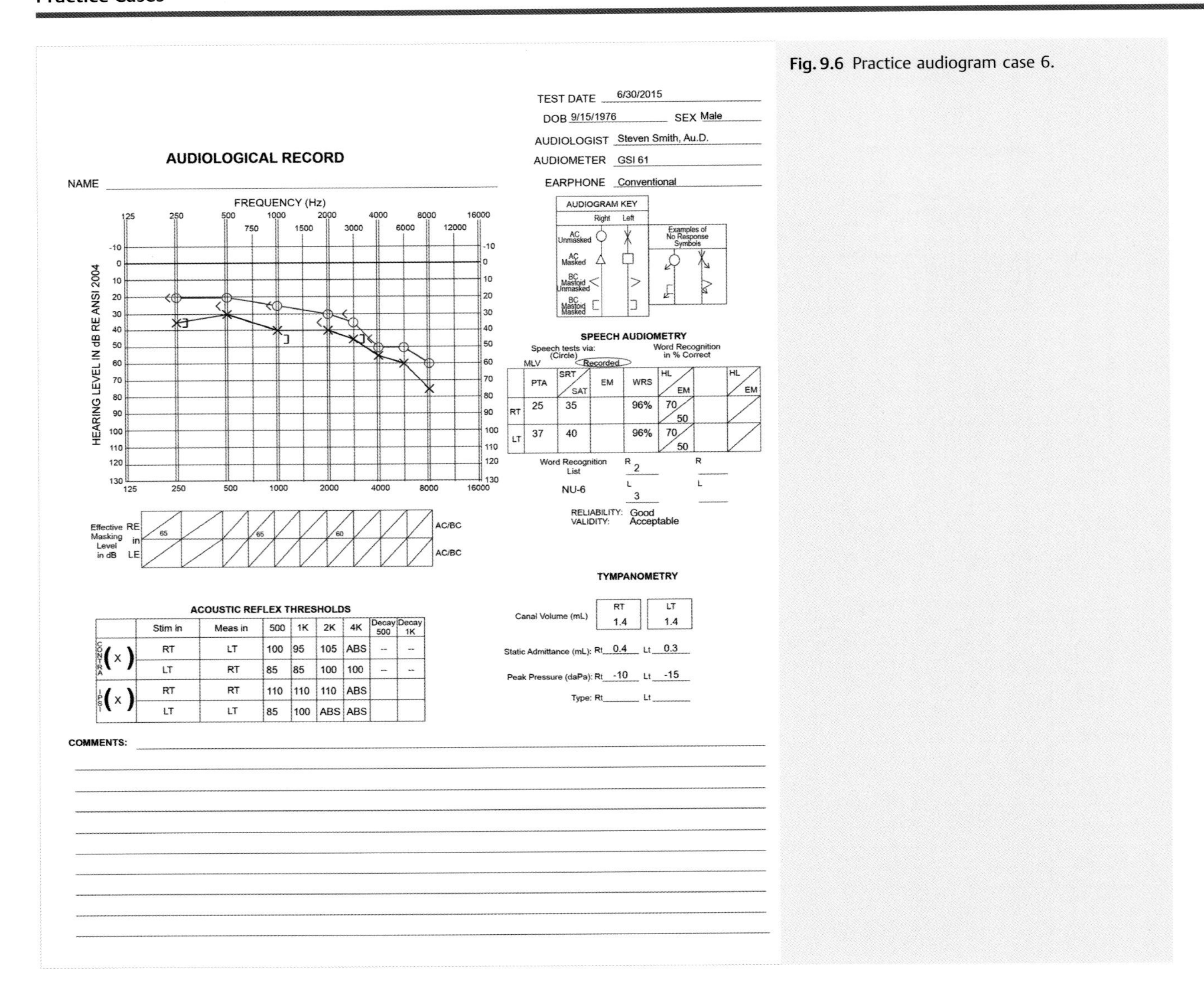

TEST DATE 6/30/2015

DOB 9/15/1976 SEX Male

AUDIOLOGIST Steven Smith, Au.D.

AUDIOMETER GSI 61

EARPHONE Conventional

AUDIOLOGICAL RECORD

NAME

FREQUENCY (Hz)

HEARING LEVEL IN dB RE ANSI 2004

AUDIOGRAM KEY

	Right	Left
AC Unmasked	O	X
AC Masked	△	□
BC Mastoid Unmasked	<	>
BC Mastoid Masked	[	]

Examples of No Response Symbols

Effective Masking Level in dB

RE in	65		65			60					AC/BC
LE											AC/BC

SPEECH AUDIOMETRY

Speech tests via: (Circle) MLV Recorded

Word Recognition in % Correct

	PTA	SRT / SAT	EM	WRS	HL / EM	HL / EM
RT	25	35		96%	70 / 50	
LT	37	40		96%	70 / 50	

Word Recognition List: R 2, L 3; R ___, L ___

NU-6

RELIABILITY: Good

VALIDITY: Acceptable

ACOUSTIC REFLEX THRESHOLDS

	Stim in	Meas in	500	1K	2K	4K	Decay 500	Decay 1K
CONTRA (x)	RT	LT	100	95	105	ABS	--	--
	LT	RT	85	85	100	100	--	--
IPSI (x)	RT	RT	110	110	110	ABS		
	LT	LT	85	100	ABS	ABS		

TYMPANOMETRY

	RT	LT
Canal Volume (mL)	1.4	1.4

Static Admittance (mL): Rt 0.4 Lt 0.3

Peak Pressure (daPa): Rt -10 Lt -15

Type: Rt ___ Lt ___

COMMENTS:

Fig. 9.6 Practice audiogram case 6.

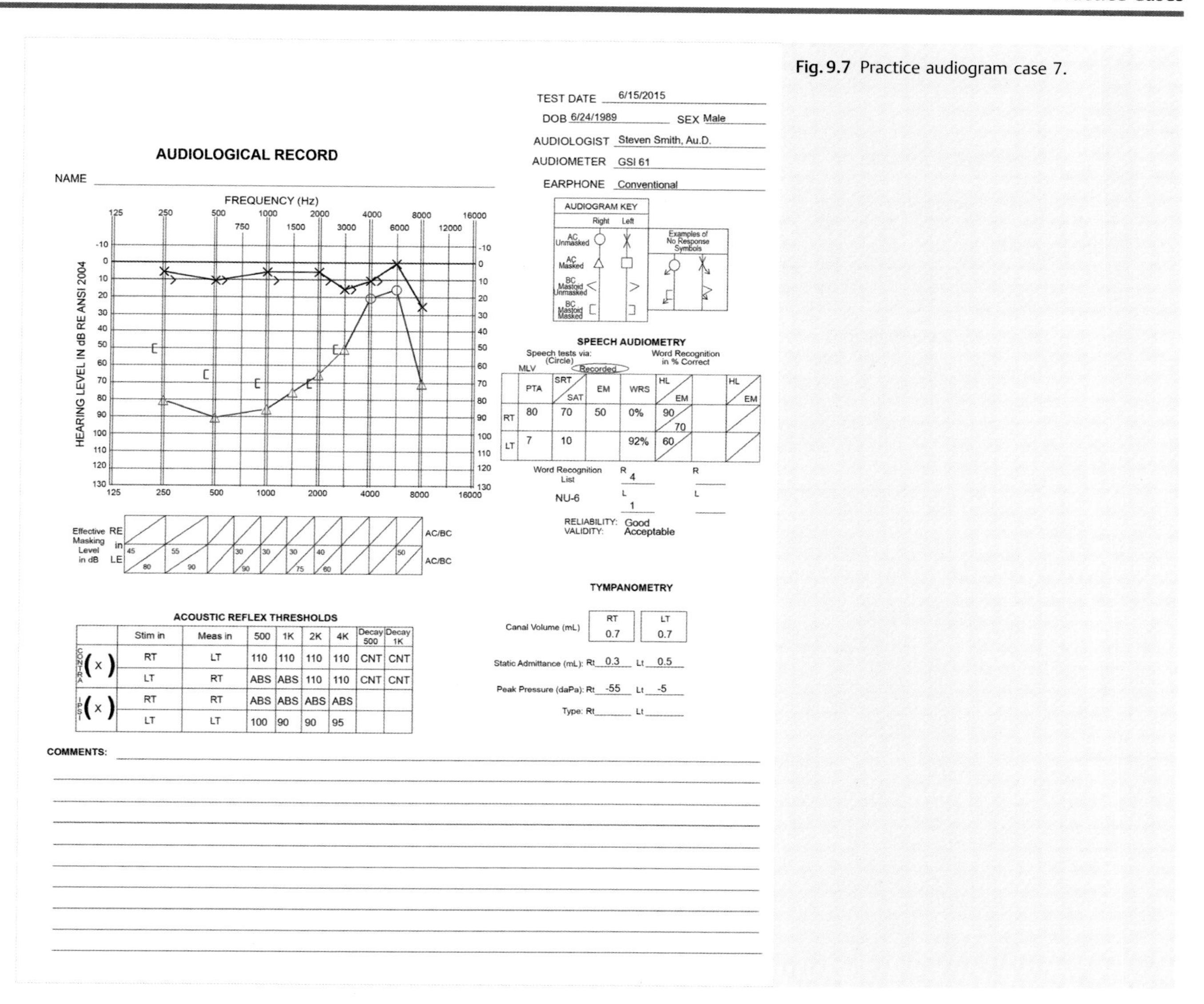

TEST DATE 6/15/2015

DOB 6/24/1989 SEX Male

AUDIOLOGIST Steven Smith, Au.D.

AUDIOMETER GSI 61

EARPHONE Conventional

AUDIOLOGICAL RECORD

NAME

Effective Masking Level in dB												
RE												AC/BC
LE	45 / 80	55 / 90		30 / 90	30	30 / 75	40 / 60				50	AC/BC

SPEECH AUDIOMETRY

Speech tests via: (Circle) MLV Recorded — Word Recognition in % Correct

	PTA	SRT / SAT	EM	WRS	HL / EM	HL / EM
RT	80	70	50	0%	90 / 70	
LT	7	10		92%	60	

Word Recognition List NU-6: R 4, L 1; R ____, L ____

RELIABILITY: Good
VALIDITY: Acceptable

ACOUSTIC REFLEX THRESHOLDS

	Stim in	Meas in	500	1K	2K	4K	Decay 500	Decay 1K
CONTRA (x)	RT	LT	110	110	110	110	CNT	CNT
	LT	RT	ABS	ABS	110	110	CNT	CNT
IPSI (x)	RT	RT	ABS	ABS	ABS	ABS		
	LT	LT	100	90	90	95		

TYMPANOMETRY

	RT	LT
Canal Volume (mL)	0.7	0.7

Static Admittance (mL): Rt 0.3 Lt 0.5

Peak Pressure (daPa): Rt -55 Lt -5

Type: Rt ____ Lt ____

COMMENTS:

Fig. 9.7 Practice audiogram case 7.

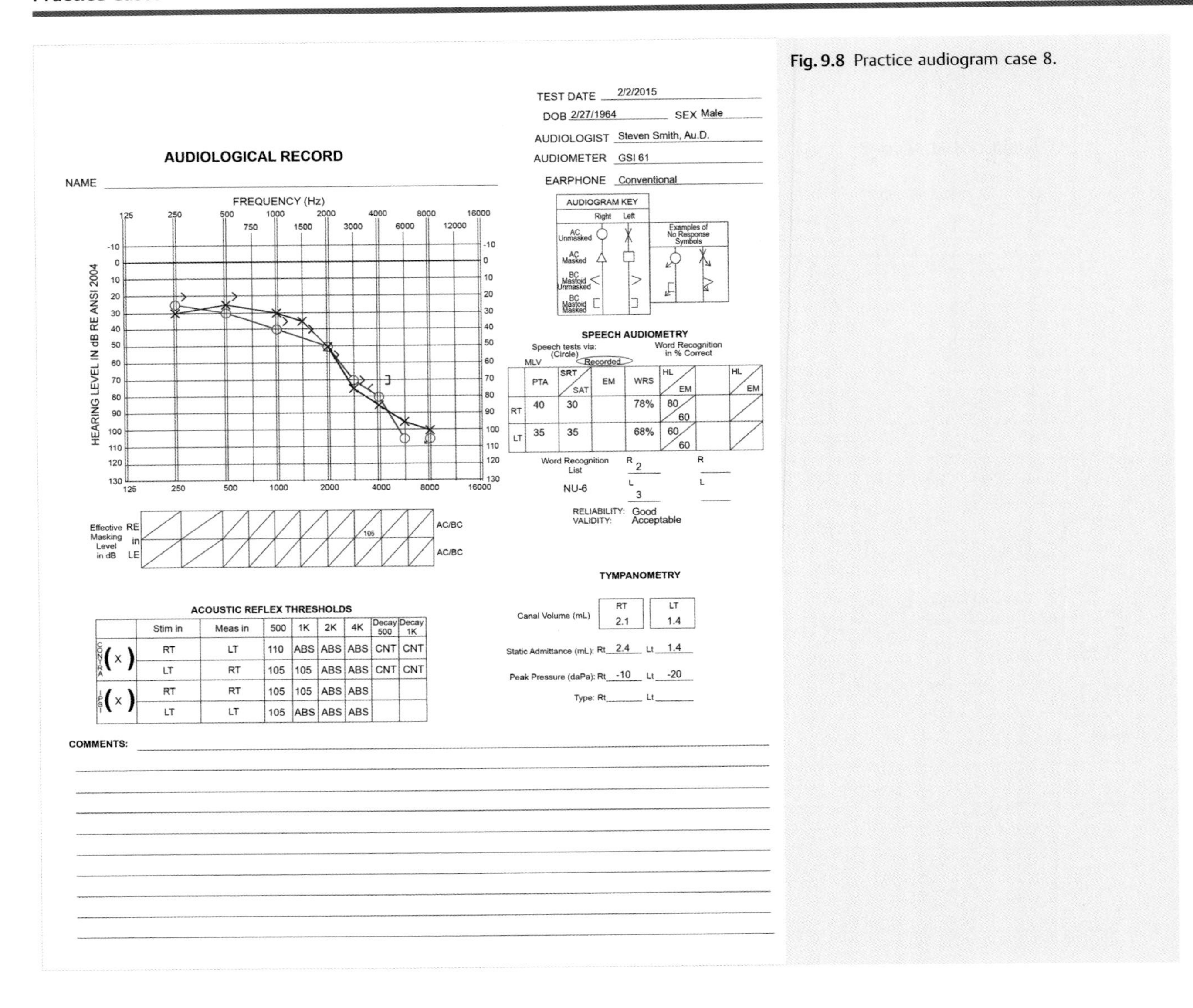

AUDIOLOGICAL RECORD

NAME

TEST DATE 2/2/2015
DOB 2/27/1964 SEX Male
AUDIOLOGIST Steven Smith, Au.D.
AUDIOMETER GSI 61
EARPHONE Conventional

Effective Masking Level in dB — RE in AC/BC; LE in AC/BC: 105

SPEECH AUDIOMETRY

Speech tests via: (Circle) MLV / Recorded (circled)
Word Recognition in % Correct

	PTA	SRT / SAT	EM	WRS	HL / EM		HL / EM
RT	40	30		78%	80 / 60		
LT	35	35		68%	60 / 60		

Word Recognition List NU-6: R 2, L 3; R ___, L ___

RELIABILITY: Good
VALIDITY: Acceptable

ACOUSTIC REFLEX THRESHOLDS

	Stim in	Meas in	500	1K	2K	4K	Decay 500	Decay 1K
CONTRA (x)	RT	LT	110	ABS	ABS	ABS	CNT	CNT
	LT	RT	105	105	ABS	ABS	CNT	CNT
IPSI (x)	RT	RT	105	105	ABS	ABS		
	LT	LT	105	ABS	ABS	ABS		

TYMPANOMETRY

	RT	LT
Canal Volume (mL)	2.1	1.4

Static Admittance (mL): Rt 2.4 Lt 1.4
Peak Pressure (daPa): Rt -10 Lt -20
Type: Rt ___ Lt ___

COMMENTS:

Fig. 9.8 Practice audiogram case 8.

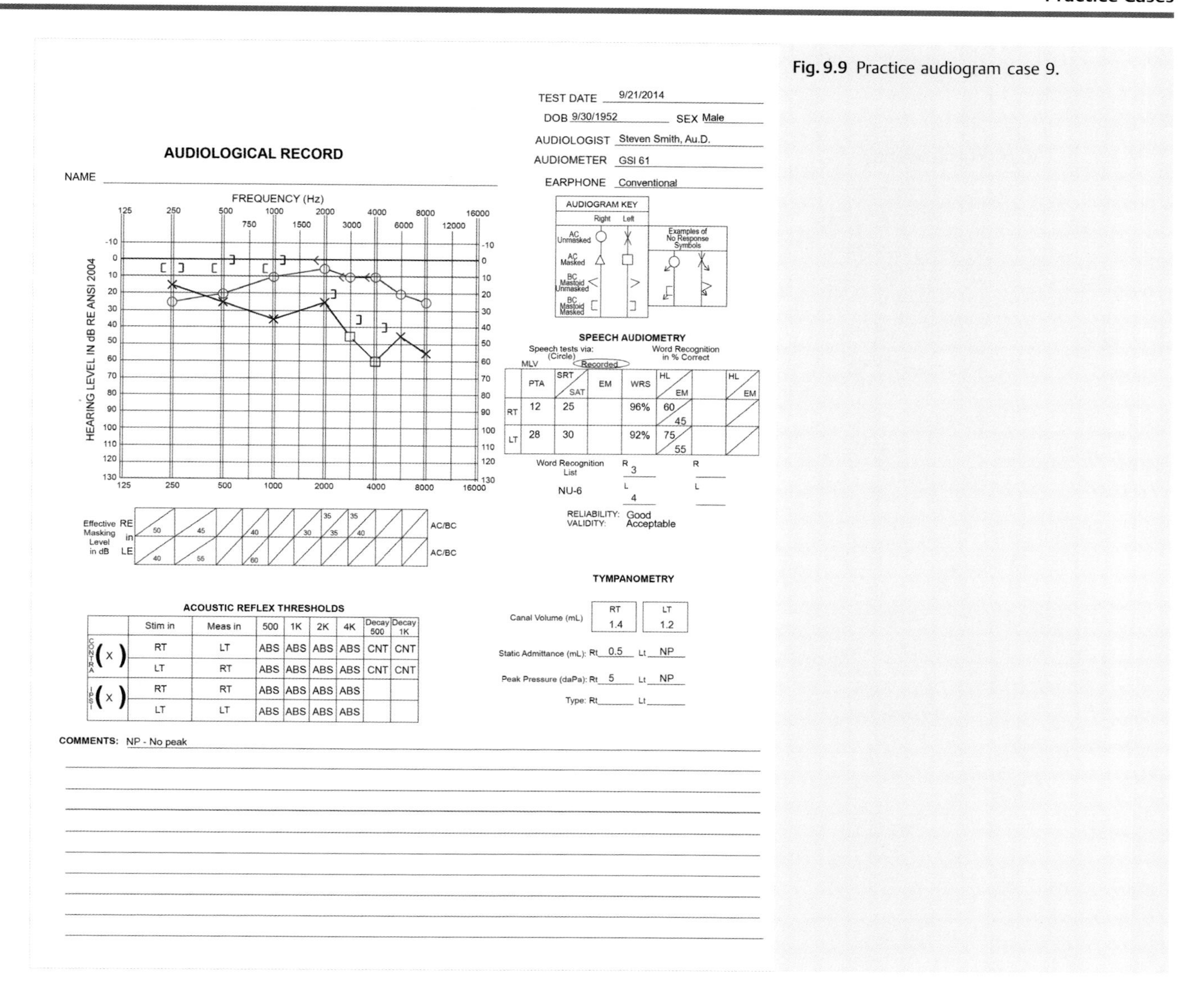

TEST DATE 9/21/2014
DOB 9/30/1952 SEX Male
AUDIOLOGIST Steven Smith, Au.D.
AUDIOMETER GSI 61
EARPHONE Conventional

AUDIOLOGICAL RECORD

NAME

SPEECH AUDIOMETRY

Speech tests via: (Circle) MLV Recorded
Word Recognition in % Correct

	PTA	SRT / SAT	EM	WRS	HL / EM	HL / EM
RT	12	25		96%	60 / 45	
LT	28	30		92%	75 / 55	

Word Recognition List: R 3, L 4
NU-6

RELIABILITY: Good
VALIDITY: Acceptable

TYMPANOMETRY

	RT	LT
Canal Volume (mL)	1.4	1.2

Static Admittance (mL): Rt 0.5 Lt NP
Peak Pressure (daPa): Rt 5 Lt NP
Type: Rt Lt

ACOUSTIC REFLEX THRESHOLDS

	Stim in	Meas in	500	1K	2K	4K	Decay 500	Decay 1K
CONTRA (x)	RT	LT	ABS	ABS	ABS	ABS	CNT	CNT
	LT	RT	ABS	ABS	ABS	ABS	CNT	CNT
IPSI (x)	RT	RT	ABS	ABS	ABS	ABS		
	LT	LT	ABS	ABS	ABS	ABS		

COMMENTS: NP - No peak

Fig. 9.9 Practice audiogram case 9.

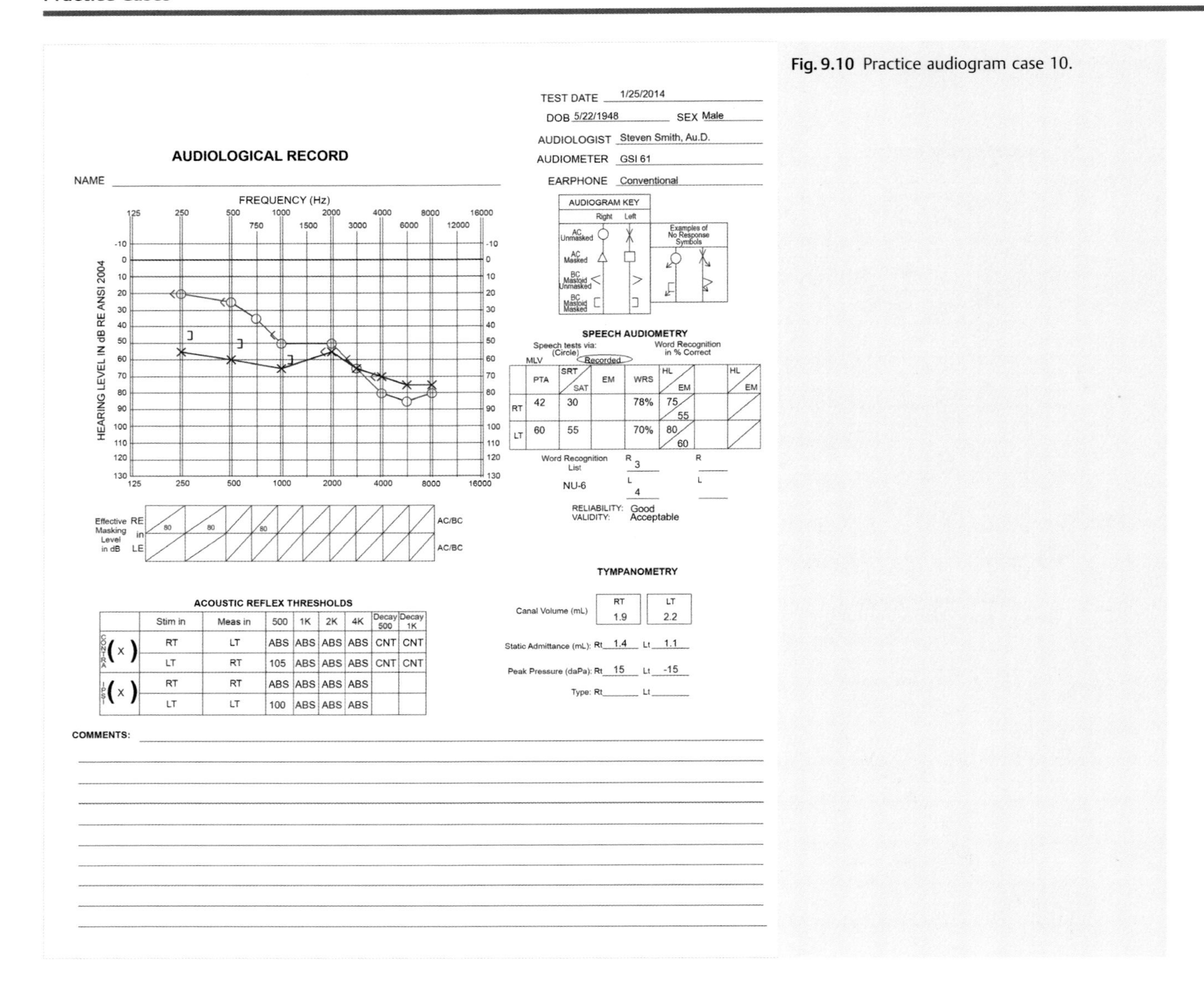

TEST DATE 1/25/2014
DOB 5/22/1948 SEX Male
AUDIOLOGIST Steven Smith, Au.D.
AUDIOMETER GSI 61
EARPHONE Conventional

AUDIOLOGICAL RECORD

NAME

AUDIOGRAM KEY

	Right	Left
AC Unmasked	○	X
AC Masked	△	□
BC Mastoid Unmasked	<	>
BC Mastoid Masked	[	]

Examples of No Response Symbols

Effective Masking Level in dB — RE in: 80, 80, 80 — AC/BC; LE in — AC/BC

SPEECH AUDIOMETRY

Speech tests via: (Circle) MLV Recorded

Word Recognition in % Correct

	PTA	SRT / SAT	EM	WRS	HL / EM		HL / EM
RT	42	30		78%	75 / 55		
LT	60	55		70%	80 / 60		

Word Recognition List NU-6: R 3; L 4

RELIABILITY: Good
VALIDITY: Acceptable

TYMPANOMETRY

	RT	LT
Canal Volume (mL)	1.9	2.2

Static Admittance (mL): Rt 1.4 Lt 1.1
Peak Pressure (daPa): Rt 15 Lt -15
Type: Rt Lt

ACOUSTIC REFLEX THRESHOLDS

	Stim in	Meas in	500	1K	2K	4K	Decay 500	Decay 1K
CONTRA (x)	RT	LT	ABS	ABS	ABS	ABS	CNT	CNT
	LT	RT	105	ABS	ABS	ABS	CNT	CNT
IPSI (x)	RT	RT	ABS	ABS	ABS	ABS		
	LT	LT	100	ABS	ABS	ABS		

COMMENTS:

Fig. 9.10 Practice audiogram case 10.

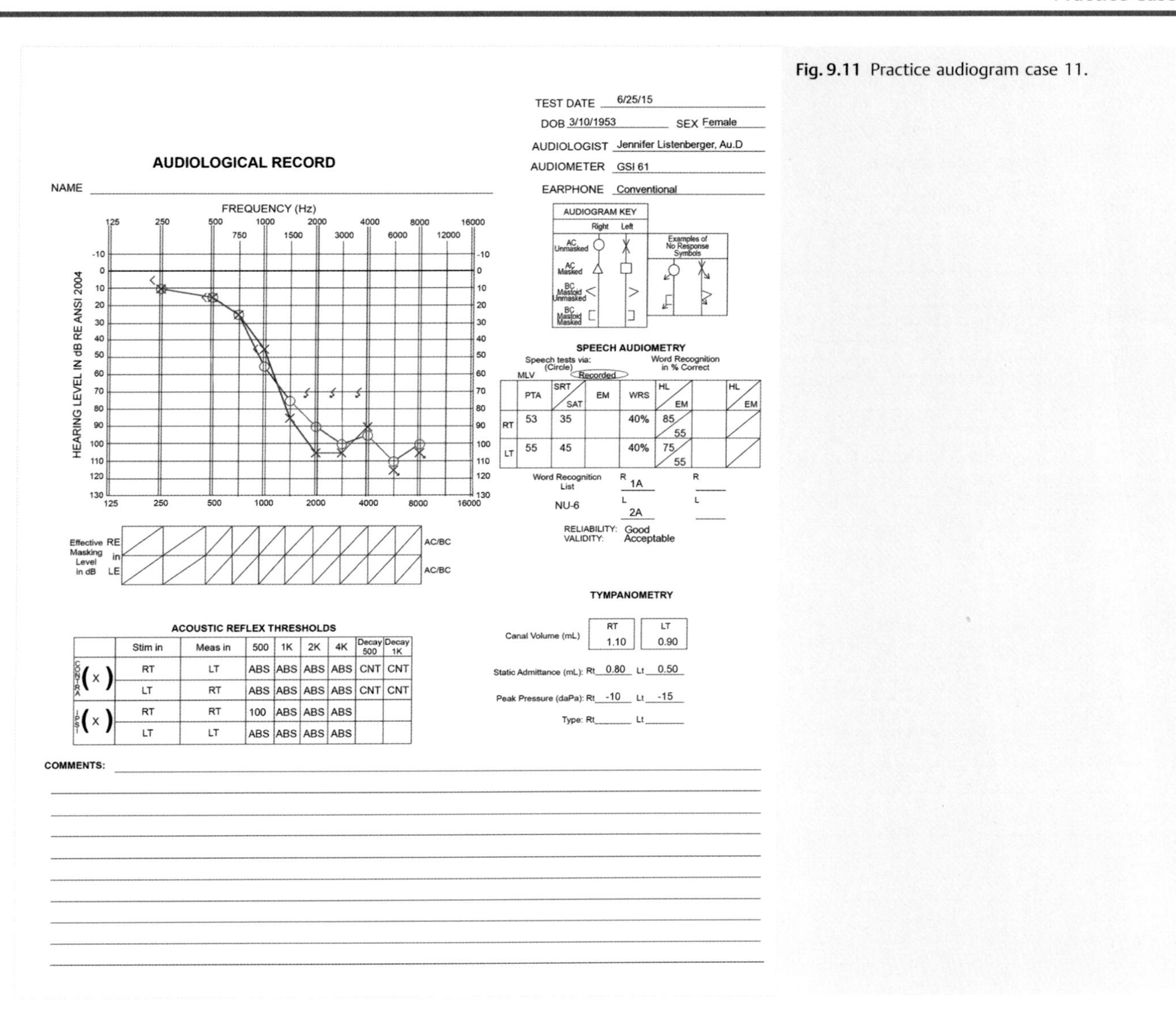

AUDIOLOGICAL RECORD

NAME

TEST DATE 6/25/15
DOB 3/10/1953 SEX Female
AUDIOLOGIST Jennifer Listenberger, Au.D
AUDIOMETER GSI 61
EARPHONE Conventional

SPEECH AUDIOMETRY

Speech tests via: (Circle) MLV Recorded (circled)
Word Recognition in % Correct

	PTA	SRT / SAT	EM	WRS	HL / EM		HL / EM
RT	53	35		40%	85 / 55		
LT	55	45		40%	75 / 55		

Word Recognition List NU-6: R 1A, L 2A; R ___, L ___

RELIABILITY: Good
VALIDITY: Acceptable

ACOUSTIC REFLEX THRESHOLDS

	Stim in	Meas in	500	1K	2K	4K	Decay 500	Decay 1K
CONTRA (X)	RT	LT	ABS	ABS	ABS	ABS	CNT	CNT
	LT	RT	ABS	ABS	ABS	ABS	CNT	CNT
IPSI (X)	RT	RT	100	ABS	ABS	ABS		
	LT	LT	ABS	ABS	ABS	ABS		

TYMPANOMETRY

	RT	LT
Canal Volume (mL)	1.10	0.90

Static Admittance (mL): Rt 0.80 Lt 0.50
Peak Pressure (daPa): Rt -10 Lt -15
Type: Rt ___ Lt ___

COMMENTS:

Fig. 9.11 Practice audiogram case 11.

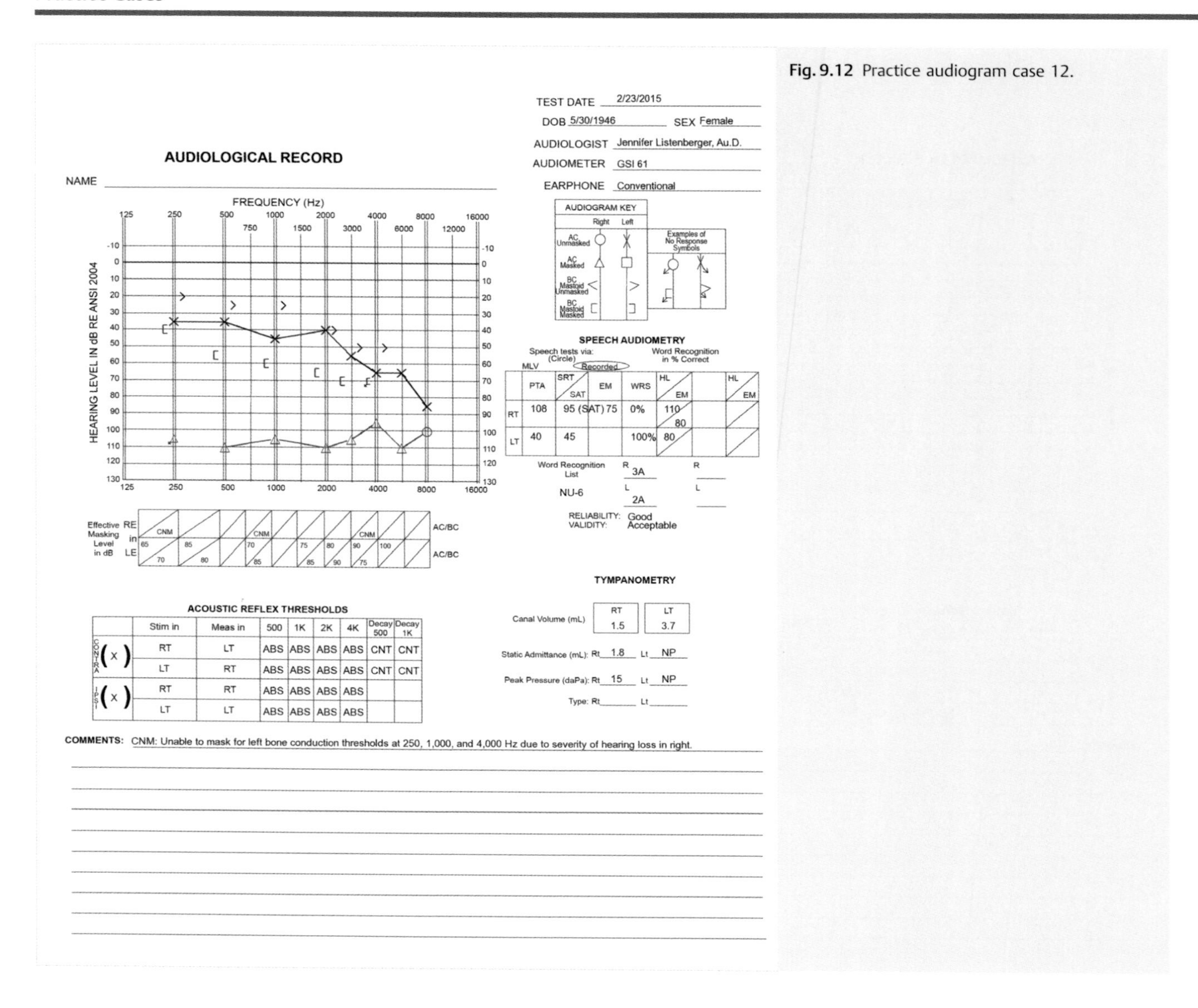

TEST DATE 2/23/2015
DOB 5/30/1946 SEX Female
AUDIOLOGIST Jennifer Listenberger, Au.D.
AUDIOMETER GSI 61
EARPHONE Conventional

AUDIOLOGICAL RECORD

NAME

SPEECH AUDIOMETRY

Speech tests via: (Circle) MLV Recorded

Word Recognition in % Correct

	PTA	SRT / SAT	EM	WRS	HL / EM	HL / EM
RT	108	95 (SAT) 75		0%	110 / 80	
LT	40	45		100%	80	

Word Recognition List: R 3A; L 2A

NU-6

RELIABILITY: Good
VALIDITY: Acceptable

ACOUSTIC REFLEX THRESHOLDS

	Stim in	Meas in	500	1K	2K	4K	Decay 500	Decay 1K
CONTRA (x)	RT	LT	ABS	ABS	ABS	ABS	CNT	CNT
	LT	RT	ABS	ABS	ABS	ABS	CNT	CNT
IPSI (x)	RT	RT	ABS	ABS	ABS	ABS		
	LT	LT	ABS	ABS	ABS	ABS		

TYMPANOMETRY

	RT	LT
Canal Volume (mL)	1.5	3.7

Static Admittance (mL): Rt 1.8 Lt NP

Peak Pressure (daPa): Rt 15 Lt NP

Type: Rt ____ Lt ____

COMMENTS: CNM: Unable to mask for left bone conduction thresholds at 250, 1,000, and 4,000 Hz due to severity of hearing loss in right.

Fig. 9.12 Practice audiogram case 12.

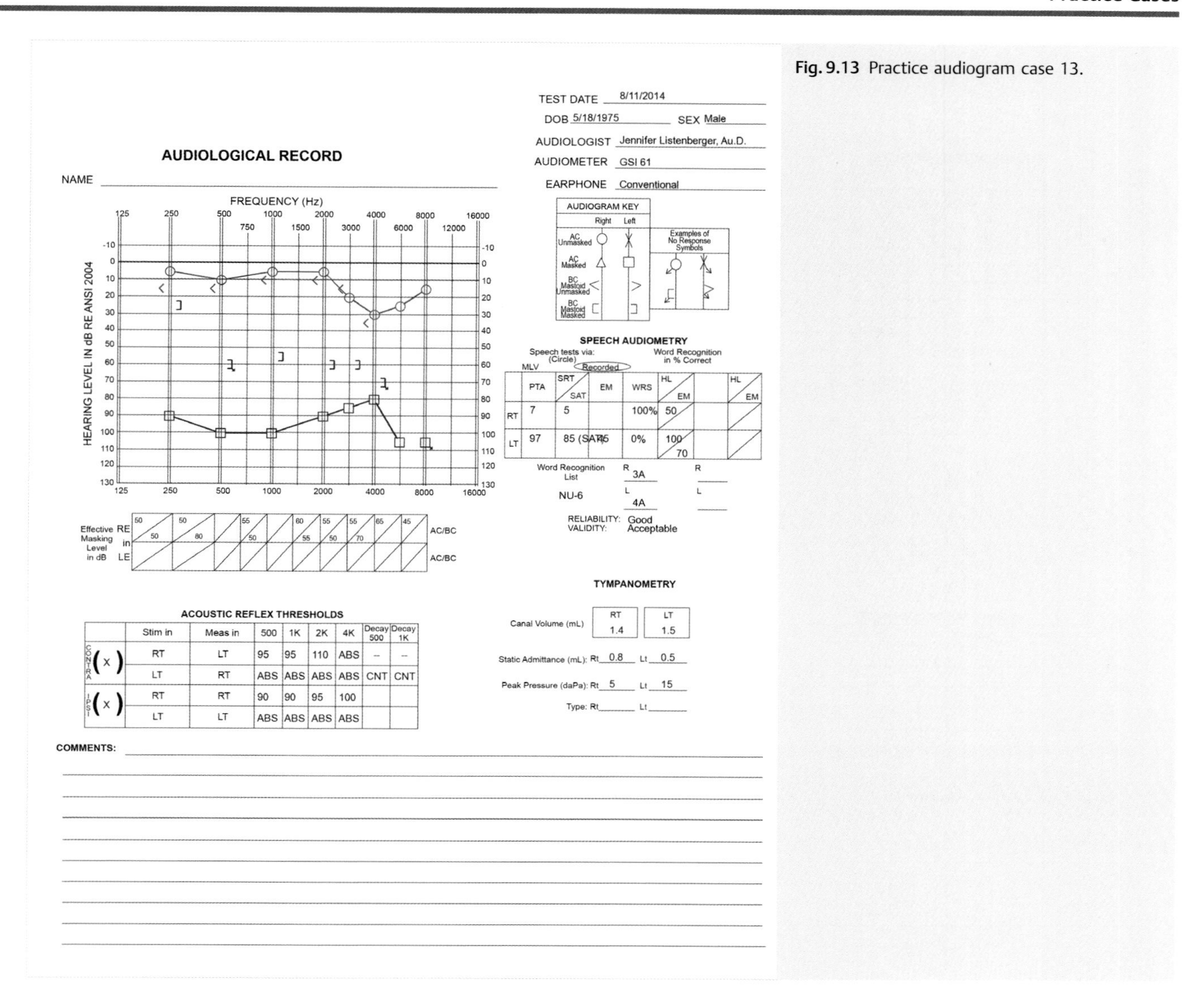

TEST DATE 8/11/2014

DOB 5/18/1975 SEX Male

AUDIOLOGIST Jennifer Listenberger, Au.D.

AUDIOMETER GSI 61

EARPHONE Conventional

AUDIOLOGICAL RECORD

NAME

Effective Masking Level in dB											
RE in	50/50	50/80		55/50		60/55	55/50	55/70	65/	45/	AC/BC
LE in											AC/BC

SPEECH AUDIOMETRY

Speech tests via: (Circle) MLV Recorded

Word Recognition in % Correct

	PTA	SRT/SAT	EM	WRS	HL/EM		HL/EM
RT	7	5		100%	50/		
LT	97	85 (SAT)	45	0%	100/70		

Word Recognition List: R 3A; L 4A — R ____; L ____

NU-6

RELIABILITY: Good
VALIDITY: Acceptable

TYMPANOMETRY

	RT	LT
Canal Volume (mL)	1.4	1.5

Static Admittance (mL): Rt 0.8 Lt 0.5

Peak Pressure (daPa): Rt 5 Lt 15

Type: Rt ____ Lt ____

ACOUSTIC REFLEX THRESHOLDS

	Stim in	Meas in	500	1K	2K	4K	Decay 500	Decay 1K
CONTRA (X)	RT	LT	95	95	110	ABS	--	--
	LT	RT	ABS	ABS	ABS	ABS	CNT	CNT
IPSI (X)	RT	RT	90	90	95	100		
	LT	LT	ABS	ABS	ABS	ABS		

COMMENTS:

Fig. 9.13 Practice audiogram case 13.

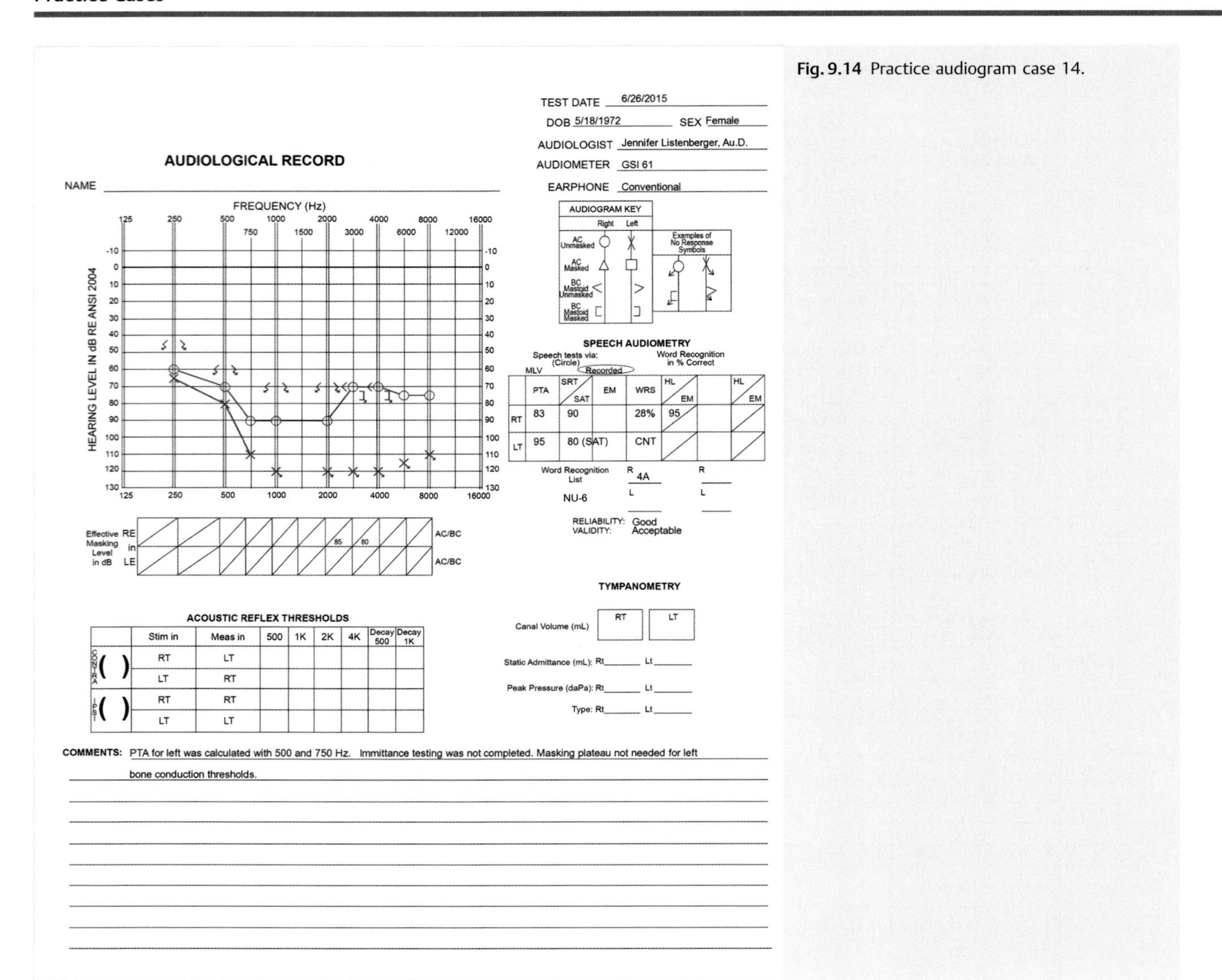

AUDIOLOGICAL RECORD

NAME

TEST DATE 6/26/2015

DOB 5/18/1972 SEX Female

AUDIOLOGIST Jennifer Listenberger, Au.D.

AUDIOMETER GSI 61

EARPHONE Conventional

SPEECH AUDIOMETRY

Speech tests via: (Circle) MLV Recorded

Word Recognition in % Correct

	PTA	SRT / SAT	EM	WRS	HL / EM		HL / EM
RT	83	90		28%	95		
LT	95	80 (SAT)		CNT			

Word Recognition List NU-6: R 4A

RELIABILITY: Good

VALIDITY: Acceptable

TYMPANOMETRY

Canal Volume (mL) RT LT

Static Admittance (mL): Rt____ Lt____

Peak Pressure (daPa): Rt____ Lt____

Type: Rt____ Lt____

ACOUSTIC REFLEX THRESHOLDS

	Stim in	Meas in	500	1K	2K	4K	Decay 500	Decay 1K
CONTRA ( )	RT	LT						
	LT	RT						
IPSI ( )	RT	RT						
	LT	LT						

COMMENTS: PTA for left was calculated with 500 and 750 Hz. Immittance testing was not completed. Masking plateau not needed for left bone conduction thresholds.

Fig. 9.14 Practice audiogram case 14.

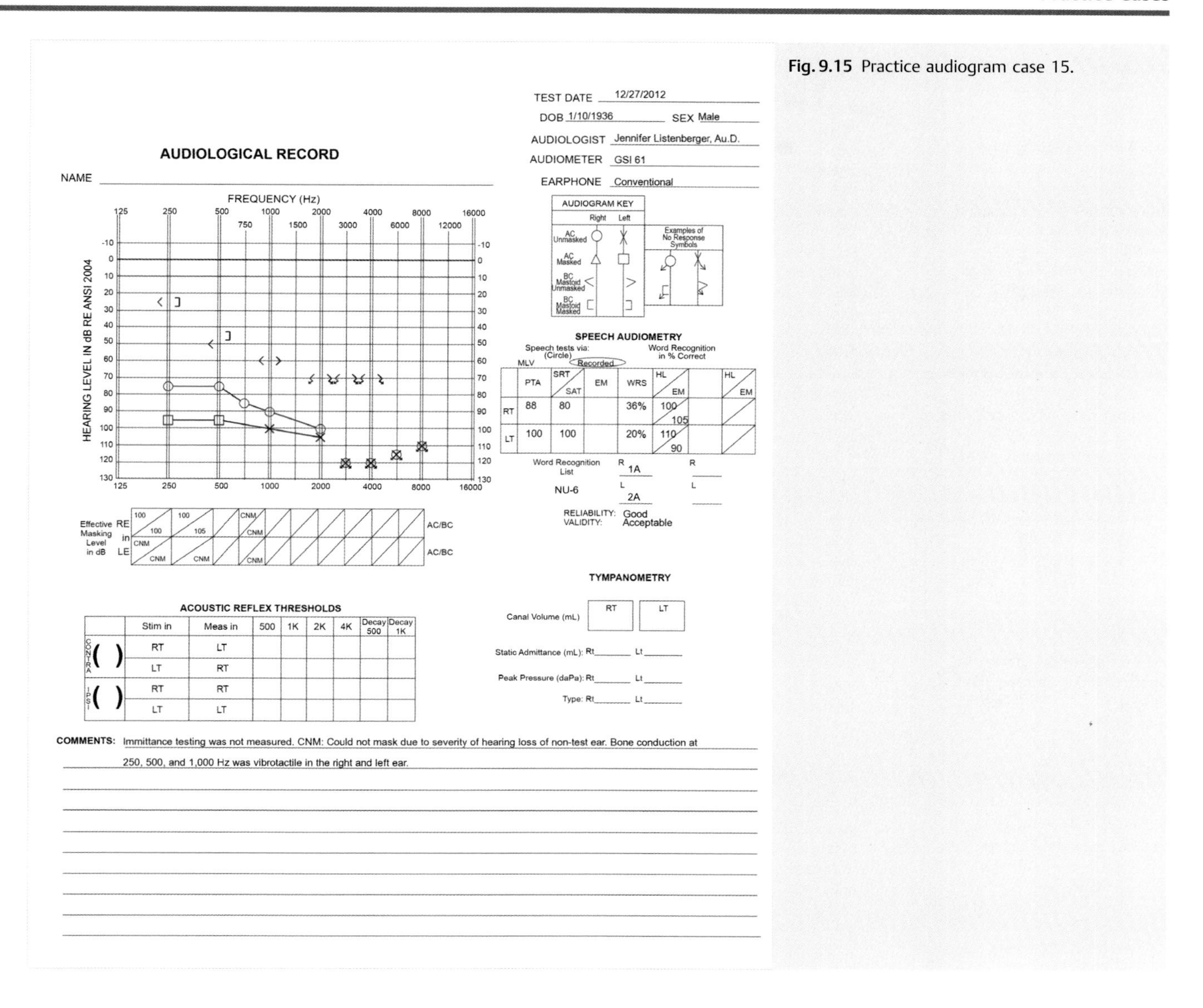

AUDIOLOGICAL RECORD

TEST DATE 12/27/2012
DOB 1/10/1936 SEX Male
AUDIOLOGIST Jennifer Listenberger, Au.D.
AUDIOMETER GSI 61
EARPHONE Conventional

NAME

Effective Masking Level in dB

	250	500	1000								
RE	100 / 100	100 / 105	CNM / CNM								AC/BC
LE	CNM / CNM	CNM	CNM								AC/BC

SPEECH AUDIOMETRY

Speech tests via: (Circle) MLV Recorded
Word Recognition in % Correct

	PTA	SRT/SAT	EM	WRS	HL/EM		HL/EM
RT	88	80		36%	100/105		
LT	100	100		20%	110/90		

Word Recognition List R 1A R
NU-6 L 2A L

RELIABILITY: Good
VALIDITY: Acceptable

ACOUSTIC REFLEX THRESHOLDS

	Stim in	Meas in	500	1K	2K	4K	Decay 500	Decay 1K
CONTRA ( )	RT	LT						
	LT	RT						
IPSI ( )	RT	RT						
	LT	LT						

TYMPANOMETRY

Canal Volume (mL) RT LT
Static Admittance (mL): Rt______ Lt______
Peak Pressure (daPa): Rt______ Lt______
Type: Rt______ Lt______

COMMENTS: Immittance testing was not measured. CNM: Could not mask due to severity of hearing loss of non-test ear. Bone conduction at 250, 500, and 1,000 Hz was vibrotactile in the right and left ear.

Fig. 9.15 Practice audiogram case 15.

Index

M

N

O

P

R

S

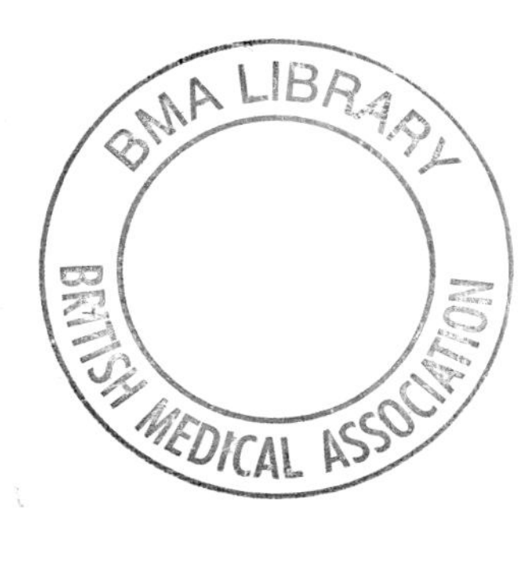